Techniques in the Management of Gallstone Disease

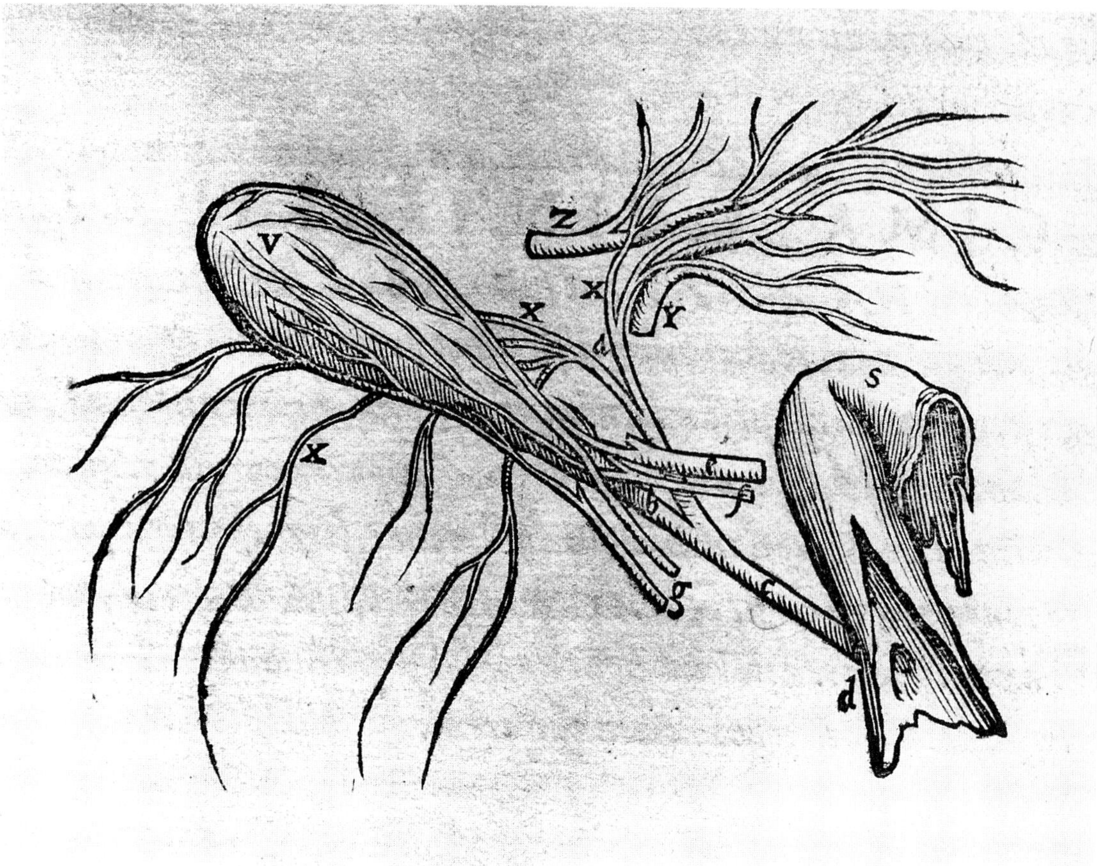

Frontispiece The extrahepatic biliary tree. (Vesalius A. *De Humani Corporis Fabrica, Liber V*. Basle, 1543.)

Techniques in the Management of Gallstone Disease

EDITED BY

Ara Darzi MD, FRCSI
Consultant Surgeon
Department of Surgery
Central Middlesex Hospital
London

Pierce A. Grace
MCh, FRCSI
Consultant Senior Lecturer
Department of Surgery
Royal Postgraduate Medical School
The Hammersmith Hospitals Trust
London

Henry A. Pitt MD
Professor and Vice-Chairman
Department of Surgery
Johns Hopkins Medical Institution
Baltimore

David Bouchier-Hayes
MCh, FRCS, FRCSI, FACS
Professor of Surgery
Royal College of Surgeons in Ireland
Dublin

b
Blackwell
Science

Editorial Offices:
Osney Mead, Oxford OX2 0EL
25 John Street, London WC1N 2BL
23 Ainslie Place, Edinburgh EH3 6AJ
238 Main Street, Cambridge
Massachusetts 02142, USA
54 University Street, Carlton
Victoria 3053, Australia

Other Editorial Offices:
Arnette Blackwell SA
1, rue de Lille, 75007 Paris
France

Blackwell Wissenschafts-Verlag GmbH
Kurfürstendamm 57
10707 Berlin, Germany

Blackwell MZV
Feldgasse 13, A-1238 Wien
Austria

First published 1995

Set by Excel Typesetters Co., Hong Kong
Printed and bound in Great Britain
at the University Press, Cambridge

DISTRIBUTORS

Marston Book Services Ltd
PO Box 87
Oxford OX2 0DT
(*Orders*: Tel: 01865 791155
Fax: 01865 791927
Telex: 837515)

North America
Blackwell Science, Inc.
238 Main Street
Cambridge, MA 02142
(*Orders*: Tel: 800 215-1000
617 876-7000
Fax: 617 492-5263)

Australia
Blackwell Science Pty Ltd
54 University Street
Carlton, Victoria 3053
(*Orders*: Tel: 03 347-5552)

A catalogue record for this title is available from the British Library

ISBN 0-632-03675-3

Library of Congress
Cataloging in Publication Data

Techniques in the management of
gallstone disease/edited by Ara Darzi
... [et al.].
p. cm.
Includes bibliographical references
and index.
ISBN 0-632-03675-3
1. Gallstones. 2. Gallstones–Surgery.
I. Darzi, Ara.
[DNLM: 1. Cholelithiasis–surgery.
2. Cholecystectomy–methods.
WI 755 T255 1995]
RC850.T43 1995
616.3′65–dc20

Contents

List of contributors

M.Z. Abedin PhD, Assistant Professor of Surgery, Medical College of Pennsylvania, 3300 Henry Avenue, Philadelphia, PA 19129, USA

I.S. Benjamin BSc, MD, FRCS, Professor of Surgery, King's College School of Medicine and Dentistry, Denmark Hill, London SE5 9RS, UK

D. Bouchier-Hayes MCh, FRCS, FRCSI, FACS, Professor of Surgery, Royal College of Surgeons in Ireland, 123 St Stephen's Green, Dublin 2, Ireland

T.G. Brennan FRCS, Consultant Surgeon, Department of Surgery, St. James's University Hospital, Beckett Street, Leeds LS9 7TF, UK

P.J. Broe MCh, FRCSI, Consultant Surgeon, Beaumont Hospital, Beaumont Road, Dublin 9

H.J. Burhenne MD, FRCPC, FACR, FRCS, Professor of Radiology, Department of Radiology, Vancouver General Hospital, 10th Avenue and Heather Street, Vancouver, BC V5Z 1M9, Canada

W.C. Chapman MD, Department of Surgery, Vanderbilt University Medical Center, Nashville, TN, USA

S.C. Sydney Chung LRCP, SI, MB, BCh, BAO, FRCS, MRCP(UK) MD Senior Lecturer in Surgery and Chief Combined Endoscopy Unit, Prince of Wales Hospital, The Chinese University Hong Kong, Shatin, New Territories, Hong Kong

A. Darzi MD, FRCSI Consultant Surgeon, Department of Surgery, Central Middlesex Hospital, Acton Lane, Park Royal, London NW10 7NS, UK

T.R. Gadacz Department of Surgery, Medical College of Georgia, 1120 15th Street, Augusta, GA 30912, USA

J.G. Geraghty MCh, FRCSI, Senior Registrar in Surgery, Beaumont Hospital, Beaumont Road, Dublin 9, Ireland

E.J. Gibney FRCSI, Consultant Surgeon, Lloydminster Hospital, Lloydminster, Alberta, Canada

P.A. Grace MCh, FRCSI, Consultant Senior Lecturer, Department of Surgery, Royal Postgraduate Medical School, The Hammersmith Hospitals Trust, London

R.M. Howerton MD, Assistant Professor, General Surgery, Bowman-Gray School of Medicine, Wake Forest University, Winston, Salem, NC, USA

F.B.V. Keane MD, FRCS, FRCSI, Consultant Surgeon, Department of Clinical Surgery, Meath and Adelaide Hospitals, Heytesbury Street, Dublin 8, Ireland

A.L. Leahy MCh, FRCS, FRCSI, Lecturer in Surgery, Department of Surgery, Royal College of Surgeons in Ireland, 123 St Stephen's Green, Dublin 2, Ireland

P.A. Lipsett MD, Assistant Professor of Surgery, Attending Surgeon and Attending Critical Care Medicine, Johns Hopkins University School of Medcine, 600 Wolfe Street, Blalock 688, Baltimore, MD 21287, USA

A.J. McMahon FRCS (Glas), FRCS (Edin), Research Fellow in Surgery, Western Infirmary, Glasgow G11 6NT, UK

K. Mealy MD, FRCSI, Senior Registrar in General Surgery, 13 The Square, Irishtown, Dublin 4, Ireland

S. Mikami MD, The First Department of Medicine, Chiba University School of Medicine, 1-8-1 Inohana, Chiba 260, Japan

P.M. Murchan FRCSI, Surgical Registrar, Department of Surgery, St James's University Hospital, Beckett Street, Leeds LS9 7TF, UK

P.J. O'Dwyer FRCSI, Senior Lecturer in Surgery, Department of Surgery, Western Infirmary, Glasgow G11 6NT, UK

M. Ohto MD, Professor and Chairman, The First Department of Internal Medicine, Chiba University School of Medicine, 1-8-1 Inohana, Chiba 260, Japan

D.H. Osborne MD, FRCSI, Consultant Surgeon, Beaumont Hospital, Beaumont Road, Dublin 9, Ireland

H.A. Pitt MD, Professor and Vice-Chairman, Department of Surgery, Johns Hopkins Medical Institution, 600 North Wolfe Street, Blalock 688, Baltimore, MD 21287, USA

J.J. Roslyn MD, Alma Dea Morani Professor and Chairman, Department of Surgery, The Medical College of Pennsylvania, 3300 Henry Avenue, Philadelphia, PA 19129, USA

R.C.G. Russell MS, FRCS, Consultant Surgeon, The Middlesex Hospital, Mortimer Street, London W1N 8AA, UK

H. Saisho MD, Associate Professor, The First Department of Internal Medicine, Chiba University School of Medicine, 1-8-1 Inohana, Chiba 260, Japan

T. Sauerbruch MD, Medizinschen Universitatsklinik, Sigmund-Freud-Str. 25, 53105, Bonn 1, Germany

R. Sherry MD, Department of Surgery, Medical College of Georgia, 1120 15th Street, Augusta, GA 30912, USA

A.D. Spigelman FRASC, Senior Lecturer and Honorary Consultant Surgeon, Academic Surgical Unit, St. Mary's Hospital Medical School, Imperial College of Science, Technology and Medicine, Norfolk Place London W2 1PQ

J. Stewart MD, FRCS, Consultant Surgeon, Walsall General Hospital, Walsall, West Midlands, UK

W.A. Tanner MD, FRCSI, Consultant Surgeon, Department of Clinical Surgery, Meath and Adelaide Hospitals, Heytesbury Street, Dublin 8, Ireland

J.L. Thistle MD, Gastroenterology and Internal Medicine, Mayo Clinic, Rochester, MN 55905, USA

Y. Tsuchiya MD, Assistant Professor, The First Department of Medicine, Chiba University School of Medicine, 1-8-1 Inohana, Chiba 260, Japan

T. Tsuyuguchi MD, Senior Fellow, The First Department of Internal Medicine, Chiba University School of Medicine, 1-8-1 Inohana, Chiba, Japan

A.F. Watkinson MB, BS, BSc, MSc, FRCS, FRCR, Lecturer in Interventional Radiology, X-Ray Department, Guy's Hospital, St. Thomas Street, London

M.M. Wiley Head, Health Project Research Centre, The Economic and Social Research Institute, 4 Burlington Road, Dublin 4 Ireland.

R.C.N. Williamson MA, MD, MChir, FRCS Hon, Professor and Director of Surgery, Royal Postgraduate Medical School, Hammersmith Hospital, Du Cane Road, London W12 0HS, UK

T. Yamaguchi MD, Assistant Professor, The First Department of Internal Medicine, Chiba University School of Medicine, 1-8-1 Inohana, Chiba 260, Japan

H. Yugi MD, Research Fellow, The First Department of Internal Medicine, Chiba University School of Medicine, 1-8-1 Inohana, Chiba 260, Japan

Preface

Gallstones, and the clinical and pathological conditions which arise from them, have plagued humankind and intrigued and exasperated doctors for centuries. Over the last 130 years, effective treatments for gallstone disease have been developed, and more recently unprecedented attention has been given to elucidating the aetiology and refining the clinical management of these troublesome little stones. While much has been learned, gallstone disease continues to emerge in communities where it was hitherto unknown and remains a major health care problem in Western societies.

In his book *The Structure of Scientific Revolutions*, the philosopher Thomas Kuhn argued that towards the end of a scientific epoch, most energies are directed not towards new discoveries, but to the refinement of the old model and that change, when it occurs, does so in a revolutionary manner resulting in a new model—the paradigm shift. Similarly, the theoretical concept of chaos has recently added a new dimension to the reductionist view of science with much consideration being given to the notion that the whole cannot be explained in terms of the parts. Such perspectives may change received wisdom. As we approach the end of the century, can we detect a paradigm shift or the influence of chaos in our understanding of the natural history and management of cholelithiasis? Unfortunately, only with hindsight will we be able to answer these questions.

This book attempts to provide an overview of the current state of our knowledge about cholelithiasis. It summarizes the recent developments in relation to aetiology, pathology, natural history, clinical manifestations and management of gallstone disease. Each of the chapters has been commissioned from experts in particular areas. The authors have provided a comprehensive view of their subject, based on their own personal experience and perspective. We believe that it is this feature which renders this a most valuable text. The insights gained from experience cast a bright light, and to paraphrase the words of physicist Alvin Weinberg: '. . . that field has the most merit which contributes most heavily to and illuminates most brightly its neighbouring disciplines'. We hope that this book will illuminate the several disciplines involved in the management of gallstones and thereby help physicians care for their patients with this ubiquitous disease.

Ara Darzi
Pierce A. Grace
Henry A. Pitt
David Bouchier-Hayes

Chapter 1
Gallstone pathogenesis

M.Z. Abedin & J.J. Roslyn

Introduction

The presence of gallstones has long been recognized as a cause of significant clinical problems. Archaeological studies have uncovered gallstones in members of the Royal Egyptian family dating back several thousand years. For millenia, inquisitive students of alchemy and medicine have pondered innovative ways to make these 'unpleasant little stones' disappear. Some of these techniques were based on sound scientific principles, some on mechanical factors, and others on myths and misinformation.

In the Middle Ages, patients suffering from biliary colic were told to drink spa water rich in magnesium sulphate, a substance now known to be a potent stimulus of gallbladder contraction. The surgeon barbers and alchemists of the day probably did not appreciate the merit of this treatment regimen given our current understanding of the importance of gallbladder stasis in the pathogenesis of gallstones. Surgical removal of gallstones was introduced in the mid-1800s. Although this was an attractive idea, the hazards of the procedure and the realization that recurrence was quite likely, doomed this operation. The first successful cholecystectomy, performed in 1882 by Carl Langenbuch, heralded the era of surgery as the gold standard of therapy for patients with gallstones. For the last 100 years, open cholecystectomy has been the primary modality of treatment for this problem. In recent years, a number of new and interesting methods of gallstone treatment have been tested and evaluated. The rationale for many of these have been derived from our ever-expanding knowledge of the pathogenesis of gallstones.

The earliest theories regarding the pathogenesis of gallstones focussed on the role of the gallbladder, as evidenced by the recommendations that patients plagued with biliary colic drink waters rich in magnesium sulphate. The predominance of cholesterol gallstones in Western civilization led to investigation of factors responsible for cholesterol gallstone formation. In the early 1900s, it was suggested that the failure of cholesterol to remain in solution was critical to the formation of cholesterol gallstones. This concept remained dormant until 1968, when Admirand and Small [1] in a classic report, suggested that the hepatic secretion of cholesterol-saturated bile was the critical factor in the formation of cholesterol gallstones. For the next 15 years, this notion dominated the thinking of investigators in this area. Data from the last 10 years suggests that neither the liver nor the gallbladder alone has an exclusive aetiological role in the formation of cholesterol gallstones. Current theory postulates a dynamic interaction between these two organs which alters normal hepatic and gallbladder function and promotes the nucleation and agglomeration of cholesterol crystals into stones. Identification of the factors responsible for cholesterol solubilization and transport is critical to our understanding of the pathogenesis of gallstones. The recognition that cholesterol, which is virtually insoluble in water (the major component of bile), is normally transported by cholesterol-phospholipid vesicles and by micelles, has provided new insights into the physicochemical phenomena associated with cholesterol gallstone formation.

The predominance of cholesterol calculous disease in Western countries has been largely responsible for the disproportionate research efforts which have focussed on cholesterol versus pigment gallstones. World-wide, pigment gallstones are much more common than cholesterol stones. Recent efforts have been directed toward elucidating the aetiological factors critical to the formation of pigment gallstones.

Biliary physiology

Composition of normal bile

Bile is a complex solution produced by the hepatocytes. It is composed primarily of water, inorganic electrolytes, and organic solutes. Under normal circumstances, bile is isotonic and resembles extracellular fluid in terms of electrolyte composition. The principal electrolytes in bile are (mEq/L): Na^+ 146–165, K^+ 2.7–4.9, Cl^- 88–115, Ca^{2+} 2.5–4.8, and HCO_3^- 27–55. The three main organic solutes: bile salts; cholesterol; and phospholipids account for approximately 90% of the dry weight of bile (Fig. 1.1).

Enterohepatic circulation of bile acids

Metabolism of bile acids is a key component of digestive function by virtue of their ability to facilitate fat absorption through the intestinal tract. Moreover, bile acids can be viewed as the 'water soluble form of cholesterol', and as a major determinant of cholesterol solubility. The regulation of bile acid synthesis and concentration, therefore, is of critical importance to homoeostasis and normal function.

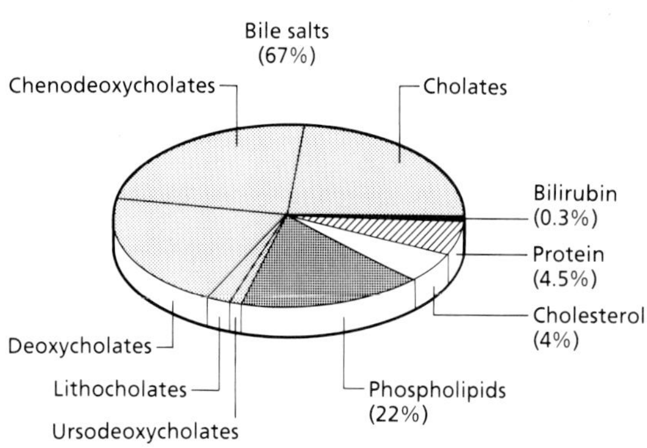

Fig. 1.1 Typical solute composition (expressed as weight percentage) of hepatic and gallbladder biles in healthy humans. (From Carey *et al.* [167].)

Bile salts (interchangeably used with bile acids) are classified as either primary or secondary. The primary bile acids, cholic and chenodeoxycholic acid, are synthesized in the liver from cholesterol and then conjugated with either glycine or taurine having a pK_a well below the physiological range of biliary pH, and are, therefore, present as anions (referred to as bile salts) rather than as undissociated bile acids. Ultimately, less than 5% of the circulating bile salt pool enters the colon, where it undergoes bacteria-mediated deconjugation and dehydroxylation, resulting in the formation of the secondary bile acids, deoxycholic, and lithocholic acids.

The enterohepatic circulation (EHC) provides an efficient means of reabsorption and recirculation of primary bile acids. The hepatic synthesis of bile acids is, to some extent, controlled by a feedback mechanism. The conjugated primary bile acids are excreted in bile. During interdigestive periods, most of the bile acids are stored in the gallbladder where reabsorption of water and solutes results in concentration of bile. After consumption of a meal, cholecystokinin (CCK) is released by the duodenum, and gallbladder contraction is stimulated. Bile is evacuated from the gallbladder and enters the duodenum. Although some passive absorption of bile acids occurs during passage through the small intestine, most of the bile acids reach the terminal ileum. Here, an active transport process is initiated which results in the reabsorption of approximately 90% of the bile acids. This relatively large amount of bile acids is then transported by the portal venous system back to the liver, where the process begins all over again. As stated above, less than 5% of the circulating bile acid pool reaches the colon, where secondary bile acids are formed by bacterial enzymes. Ultimately, this small amount is excreted in the faeces and is obviously lost from the EHC. Derangements in the EHC due to functional or anatomic alterations can result in a reduced circulating bile acid pool and may predispose to gallstone formation.

Cholesterol solubilization

Most cholesterol present in bile is synthesized *de novo* in the liver. The dietary contribution to this pool is minimal. Cholesterol is virtually insoluble in water, and bile is an aqueous solution. The mechanism of cholesterol solubilization in bile is accordingly very complex. For many years, investigators believed that the formation of mixed micelles was exclusively responsible for the maintenance of cholesterol solution in bile. The term micelle refers to small polymolecular aggregates which, in the case of bile results from the molecular dissymmetry of one of the bile acid molecules being hydrophobic and the other being hydrophilic. The polar ends of bile acid molecules are oriented outwardly and the non-polar ends point inwardly. This configuration occurs when bile acid concentration exceeds a certain level, the critical micellar concentration (CMC). Bile acid micelles have a relatively small capacity for solubilization of cholesterol, but they are capable of solubilizing and incorporating lecithin in the micelle. As lecithin, which is itself comparatively insoluble in water, enters this cylindrical aggregate, the micelle swells, facilitating the incorporation of cholesterol. Cholesterol molecules are ultimately transported within the matrix of this structure. In essence, bile acid and lecithin act as a solvent for cholesterol. This relationship between the relative concentrations of bile acids, phospholipids, and cholesterol has been thought to be critical to the understanding of cholesterol gallstone formation. This concept has been expressed schematically by Admirand and Small [1] and others [2, 3], as well as by a number of mathematical formulae.

The concept of mixed micelle formation and its central role in the formation of cholesterol gallstones has recently been challenged by the demonstration that much of the biliary cholesterol exists in a vesicular form [4–9]. These vesicles were first reported in human bile by Sömjen and Gilat in 1983 [4]. Structurally, these vesicles are made up of lipid bilayers, similar to those found in cell membranes. The amphipathic molecules of lecithin and bile acids form this lipid bilayer. Cholesterol is solubilized within the non-polar portion of the bilayer. Greater quantities of cholesterol are solubilized in these vesicles than in micelles. The exact amount of biliary cholesterol that is carried in these respective vehicles is unclear, although estimates have suggested that up to 70% is transported in vesicles [5, 7–9]. As hepatic bile becomes more dilute, the amount that is carried in the vesicular phase actually increases. Figure 1.2 represents cholesterol carried in vesicle fractions of control and cholestertol gallstone patients. Quasielastic light-scattering studies have confirmed the presence and composition of these vesicles [4, 6, 9]. The diameter of these structures is reported to be between 600 and 700 Å [4, 9].

A dynamic equilibrium exists between the micelles and vesicles in normal hepatic bile. Cholesterol is predominantly in the vesicular form when it is secreted from the hepatocyte into the canaliculus. These vesicles mature in the

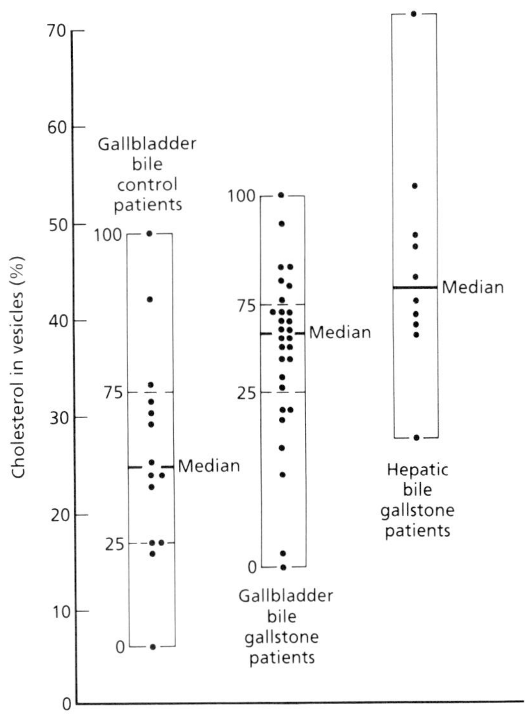

Fig. 1.2 Percentage of total cholesterol carried in vesicle fractions of control and cholesterol gallstone patients. The difference between gallbladder bile in stone patients and control was significant. (From Harvey *et al.* [168].)

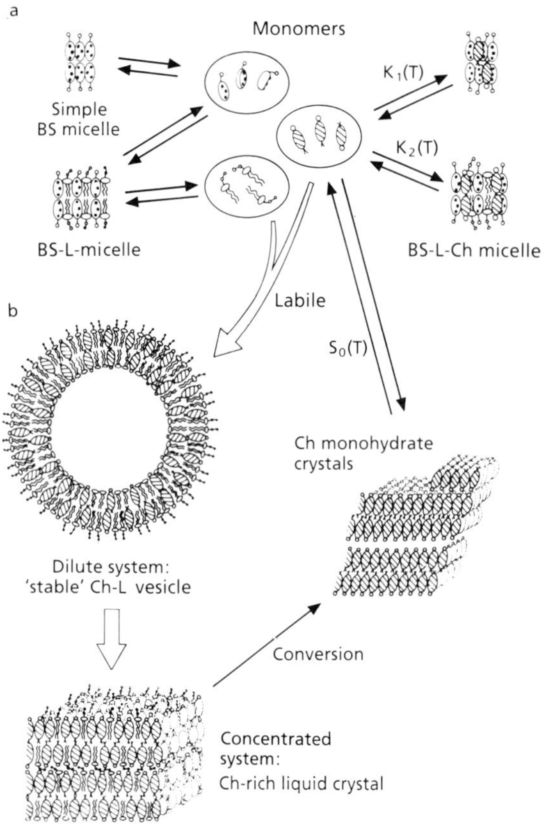

Fig. 1.3 Schematic diagram of the aggregative behaviour of aqueous taurocholate (BS = bile salt, L = lecithin, Ch = cholesterol) systems with physiological L/BS ratios as determined by quasielastic light scattering (QLS). (a), in unsaturated systems, Ch is solubulized in simple BS and mixed BS-L micelles. Ch is present within the hydrophobic, non-polar core of the micelle. (b), in supersaturated systems, the micellar phase is saturated at equilibrium, and excess Ch monohydrate crystals exist. Rapid temperature change experiments demonstrate that labile precipitation into Ch-rich vesicles (dilute systems) or Ch-rich liquid crystals (concentrated systems) eventually occurs. With time, Ch-rich liquid crystals convert to solid Ch monohydrate crystals. (From Mazer [169].)

presence of bile salts to form micelles during passage into the gallbladder. As micelles form, the remaining vesicles become enriched with cholesterol. If the capacity of micelles to solubilize cholesterol is exceeded, as in supersaturated bile, cholesterol is contained in the less stable vesicular phase. Figure 1.3 depicts this equilibrium of micelles and vesicles both with respect to micellar cholesterol saturation and to bile salt concentration. In the presence of supersaturated bile, vesicular cholesterol is transformed into cholesterol liquid crystals, from which cholesterol monohydrate crystals form in a process known as nucleation. It is this process which is believed to be critical to the formation of cholesterol gallstones.

Extrahepatic biliary tract motility

The postprandial delivery of bile to the small intestine requires the coordination and integration of a series of complex motor activities of the gallbladder and sphincter of Oddi which are regulated in part by gut peptides and neural influences. These factors work in concert to facilitate storage of bile in the gallbladder during interdigestive periods and evacuation of bile after meal stimulation. Gallbladder motility is controlled in part by parasympathetic, sympathetic, and peptidergic fibres. The effect of CCK on gallbladder and sphincter motor activity was first described by Ivy over 50 years ago [10]. In recent years, a number of other gut peptides have also been implicated in this intricate process. These include vasoactive intestinal peptide (VIP) [11], motilin [12], and pancreatic polypeptide [13]. Alteration in gallbladder motor activity has been proposed by a number of authors as an important aetiological factor in the pathogenesis of cholesterol gallstone formation [14, 15].

Gallbladder absorption

It has been more than 300 years since Diemerbroek [16] first recognized that bile enters the gallbladder, '. . . to acquire greater strength and digestive power.' In 1902, Brand [17] suggested that the differences between gallbladder and hepatic bile could be explained by gallbladder reabsorption of isotonic NaCl and $NaHCO_3$. Rous and McMaster [18] provided further evidence for this hypothesis by comparing concentration of bile pigments in gallbladder and hepatic bile. Subsequent studies by Ravdin and coworkers [19] demonstrated that the normal canine

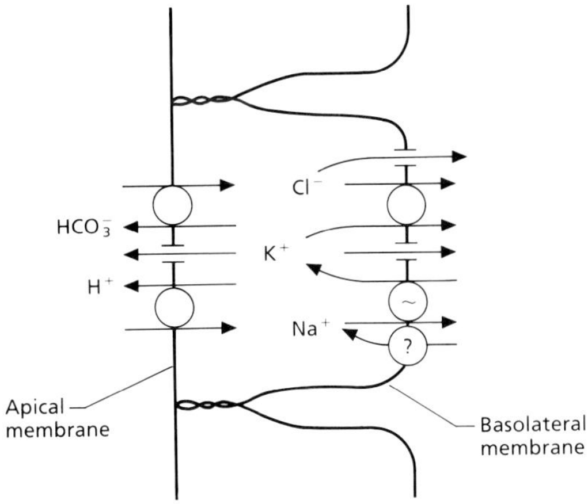

Fig. 1.4 Transepithelial ion transport model for *Necturus* gallbladder. Directions of fluxes observed in steady state are depicted. Apical membrane NaCl entry is via parallel Na^+/H^+ and Cl^-/HCO_3^- exchangers. Basolateral Na^+ extrusion is via Na^+–K^+–ATPase pump; Cl^- exit is by KCl cotransport and a Cl^- conduction pathway. There are K^+ selective channels in both membranes, but K^+ recycles mostly at the basolateral border, which has much higher K^+ conductance. There is also some basolateral Na^+ recycling. (From Reuss [170].)

gallbladder reabsorbs approximately 60% of its volume per hour without any significant alteration in the absolute amounts of bile acids, bile pigment, or cholesterol which are initially present. They concluded that these constituents of bile were neither absorbed nor secreted by the gallbladder, but increased in concentration as a result of an absolute decrease in gallbladder bile volume. The gallbladder is capable of concentrating the solutes contained in hepatic bile by a factor of 5–10 times and reducing its volume by 80–90%. Gallbladders transport large volumes of isotonic fluid, such that despite a dramatic increase in sodium concentration, gallbladder bile is isomotic to plasma.

Reabsorption of gallbladder fluid is largely determined by transport of sodium. This cation traverses the apical membrane down an electrochemical gradient which is maintained by its active extrusion across the basolateral membrane by an energy-dependent Na^+–K^+ ATPase [20]. The application of electrophysiological principles and techniques has facilitated a broader understanding of the mechanism and site of ion transport. It has been demonstrated that independent (although simultaneous) carriers exist at the apical membrane which determine entry of $Na^+(Na^+/H^+)$ and $Cl^-(Cl^-/HCO_3^-)$ into the cell [21]. The result is a 'silent' or electrically neutral coupled entry mechanism. Removal of sodium or chloride [22] from the bathing solution abolishes fluid transport. The identification of carrier-specific transport inhibitors (amiloride, 4,4′-diisothiocyanostilbene-2,2′-disulphonic acid (DIDS) and bumetanide) have greatly facilitated studies of ion transport [23, 24]. A working hypothesis of ion transport mechanism in gallbladder epithelium is described in Fig. 1.4.

Absorption of water by the gallbladder is a passive process and is linked to active solute transport. Substitution of K^+ for Na^+ in luminal solution, or addition of ouabain to serosal solution prevents water absorption. Furthermore, there is a direct correlation between water and electrolyte absorption with time. Evidence suggests that water transport occurs as a result of local osmotic forces and is intimately related to the ultrastructure of the cell [25]. The precise mechanism and site of water absorption, however, remain unclear.

Gallstone classification

Gallstones are typically classified based on their site of origin, location or composition. In the USA and most Western countries, biliary calculi are formed and are present in the gallbladder. When stones are located in the bile duct, they are almost certainly stones that have migrated into the choledochus from their site of origin within the gallbladder. In other parts of the world, particularly in Asia, primary bile duct and intrahepatic pigment stone disease (in the absence of gallbladder stones) is quite frequent. Based on composition, stones are generally classified as either cholesterol, mixed, or pigment gallstones. This latter group can be further classified as either 'brown' or 'black' stones. While classification of stones based on composition may not be critical for therapeutic decision-making, the recent introduction of agents or modalities which are capable of dissolving [26–29] or fragmenting stones

[30, 31], has provided an important rationale for being able to talk about the different stone types.

There is some debate as to how much cholesterol a stone should contain by dry weight in order to be considered a 'cholesterol gallstone.' Most authorities will classify stones as being primarily cholesterol if they contain more than 70% cholesterol by dry weight. Most stones in the USA are in fact mixed stones, containing significant amounts of substances other than cholesterol.

Pigment gallstones usually contain a relatively high concentration of bilirubin (usually in excess of 40%) and a minimal amount of cholesterol. The distinction between brown and black stones is important from the perspective of associated disorders and in the understanding of the aetiologies. Brown stones occur with greater frequency than do other types of pigment stones. They tend to be earthy, soft, easily crushable, have a composition similar to primary common bile duct stones, and can be found both in the gallbladder and throughout the hepatobiliary tract. Black stones have a different appearance as they are typically black or tarry in appearance, multiple in number, small, and tend to originate exclusively in the gallbladder. Similar to cholesterol gallstones, black pigment gallstones noted in the bile duct are generally gallbladder stones that have passed out of the gallbladder down through the cystic duct and have come to lie in the common bile duct. These stones typically occur in patients with cirrhosis or haemolytic disorders.

Intrahepatic stone disease appears to be a separate entity from gallbladder stones and is particularly common in parts of Asia and the Orient. Studies of the chemical composition of intrahepatic stones reveal that most are composed largely of calcium bilirubinate [32]. As with brown pigment stones found elsewhere in the biliary tract, biliary infection and stasis play a significant role in the formation of intrahepatic stones.

Pathogenesis of cholesterol gallstones

Perspective

Gallstone disease continues to be a major national health problem with estimates indicating that the incidence of gallstones in the USA is 10%, with the majority of these being cholesterol in nature [33]. Despite considerable investigations, the pathogenesis of cholesterol gallstones is still not completely understood. For years, the formation of cholesterol gallstones has been conveniently separated into three stages:

1 cholesterol saturation;
2 nucleation;
3 stone growth.

Since the documentation of the physicochemical basis of cholesterol gallstone formation by Admirand and Small [1], the hepatic secretion of cholesterol-saturated bile has generally been accepted as a prerequisite for gallstone formation. It is becoming increasingly apparent that the pathogenesis of cholesterol gallstones is multifactorial and there is an essential inter-relationship between altered hepatic metabolism and gallbladder function [34].

Understanding the mechanisms by which cholesterol is solubilized in bile would appear to be critical to the elucidation of the pathogenesis of cholesterol gallstones. Several independent investigators have recently demonstrated that while some cholesterol is solubilized in mixed bile acid lecithin micelles, much of the biliary cholesterol normally present actually exists in a vesicular form [4–9]. Moreover, fusion and aggregation of unilamellar vesicles in cholesterol saturated bile leads to the formation of larger multilamellar vesicles and represents the critical first step in the precipitation of cholesterol monohydrate crystals and gallstone formation [35]. The factors responsible for initiating and promoting these processes remain unclear.

Although our understanding of vesicles and their formation is rapidly expanding, the precise relationship between vesicle formation and nucleation continues to be an area of intense investigation. The elucidation of factors governing vesicle formation is the immediate challenge to investigators interested in gallstone research. Understanding the cause and effect relationships between the hepatic secretion of cholesterol saturated bile, alterations in gallbladder motor secretory, and absorptive function, and the specific factors present in cholesterol saturated bile which

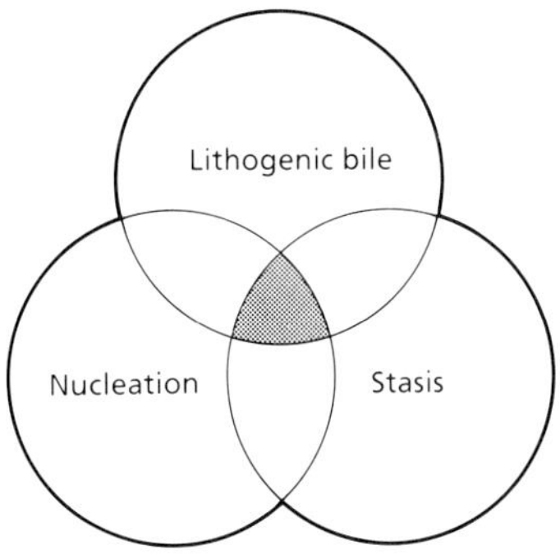

Fig. 1.5 Three main elements in the pathogenesis of gallstones.

affect these activities continues to be elusive. Although somewhat simplistic, it is helpful to conceptualize cholesterol gallstone formation as requiring three essential elements:

1 cholesterol saturation of bile;
2 a nucleation defect;
3 gallbladder stasis or hypomotility (Fig. 1.5).

Cholesterol saturation of bile is indeed a prerequisite for stone formation, but will not occur unless a nucleation defect exists concurrently. Precipitation and agglomeration of monohydrate crystals is facilitated by mucin hypersecretion and stasis of bile within the gallbladder.

Cholesterol saturation

Many years ago, early investigators recognized that the amount of cholesterol present in bile was somehow related to the propensity to develop cholesterol gallstones. Although Findlay suggested in 1924 that the total amount of biliary cholesterol was the most important factor in determining gallstone formation, this concept was not fully appreciated until 25 years ago. In 1968, Admirand and Small [1] utilized model bile solutions to demonstrate that it was the relative molar concentrations of cholesterol, phospholipids, and bile salts which defined cholesterol solubility and precipitation. The results of these studies described the essential relationship between cholesterol, phospholipids, and bile salts in health and disease, and helped chart the course of gallstone research for many years. Their data have

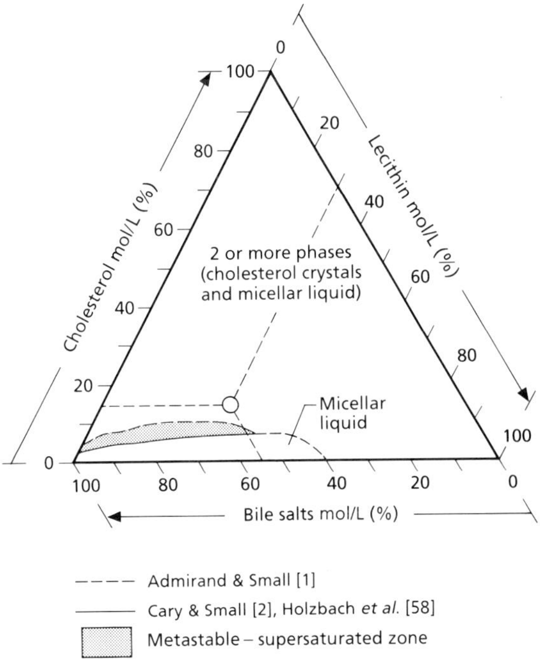

Fig. 1.6 Tricoordinate phase diagram for determination of cholesterol saturation index (CSI). A given single point represents the relative molar ratios of bile salts, lecithin, and cholesterol. The range of concentrations consistent with a clear micellar solution (where cholesterol is fully solubilized) is limited to a small region in the lower left. The shaded area directly above this region corresponds to a 'metastable' zone, in which bile initially appears clear but develops cholesterol crystals with time. All other regions (including the designated point) represent bile solutions in which the cholesterol solubilization capacity is exceeded and cholesterol crystals form rapidly. (After Holzbach [171].)

been displayed using triangular coordinates (Fig. 1.6). Using this schema, the relative molar ratios of these biliary lipids can be expressed by a single point. More recently, a number of authors have modified this schema to reflect our current understanding of the dynamic equilibrium which exists between the various phases of crystal formation [36]. In addition, a number of mathematical formulae have been developed which describe these relationships and provide for quantitative analyses [37, 38].

Cholesterol supersaturation of bile resulting in its inability to completely solubilize cholesterol is a critical step in the pathogenesis of cholesterol gallstones. Saturation of bile with cholesterol occurs when the amount of cholesterol present in bile exceeds its solubilizing capacity. Theoretically, this situation can occur as a result of altered secretion of any of the three biliary lipids: for example, a relative decrease in phospholipid or in bile salt secretion; or a relative increase in cholesterol secretion. Interruption in the enterohepatic circulation of bile salts, either by surgical resection of the terminal ileum or by diseases such as Crohn's disease, has been associated with reduced biliary secretion of bile salts and predisposition to gallstone formation [39]. Loss of bile salts, as a result of physiological sequestration within the gallbladder during periods of fasting [40], or as a consequence of medications such as cholestyramine [41], leads to cholesterol saturation of bile. Dietary-induced alterations in phospholipid metabolism have been proposed as an explanation for the increased risk of cholesterol gallstone formation noted in the Chilean population [42]. Although these abnormalities in phospholipid and bile salt metabolism may be causally linked with cholesterol gallstone formation in these specific clinical settings, the majority of evidence suggests that cholesterol hypersecretion is the most common abnormality noted in patients with cholesterol gallstones [43]. Considerable evidence has documented the relationship between increased biliary secretion of cholesterol and a very high incidence of cholesterol gallstones in obese patients [44], and in certain specific populations such as the Pima Indians. Furthermore, similar findings have been reported in non-obese patients with gallstones [43], and these seem to be correlated with age [45].

The specific cellular factors responsible for increased biliary secretion of cholesterol in patients with cholesterol gallstones remain obscure. Clinical [46] and experimental studies [47] have suggested that oestrogens influence the lithogenicity of bile. Recent data suggests that this may occur by subtle alterations in the relative concentrations of bile salts (cholate and deoxycholate) and their ability to carry and solubilize cholesterol [48]. Understanding the regulation of biliary cholesterol synthesis and secretion will help unravel the metabolic factors which predispose to cholesterol saturation, a prerequisite for cholesterol gallstone formation. Although supersaturation of bile is a necessary state for crystal formation to occur, its presence does not ensure that nucleation and ultimately stone formation will follow.

Nucleation

Nucleation refers to the complex process by which cholesterol monohydrate crystals form and agglomerate. The early observation that patients without gallstones secrete cholesterol saturated bile in a physiological manner at various times during the day [49], suggested that factors other than the hepatic secretion of cholesterol-saturated bile might be important in the formation of cholesterol gallstones. In 1979, Holan and colleagues [50] provided evidence that nucleation of cholsterol crystals was the earliest event in the evolution of cholesterol gallstones that '... reliably distinguishes patients who form gallstones from normal patients' [51]. At that time, they described a technique for determining the rate of cholesterol crystal nucleation in bile. Using the *in vitro* incubation of bile, they defined nucleation time as the time interval required for the initial appearance of cholesterol monohydrate crystals. These

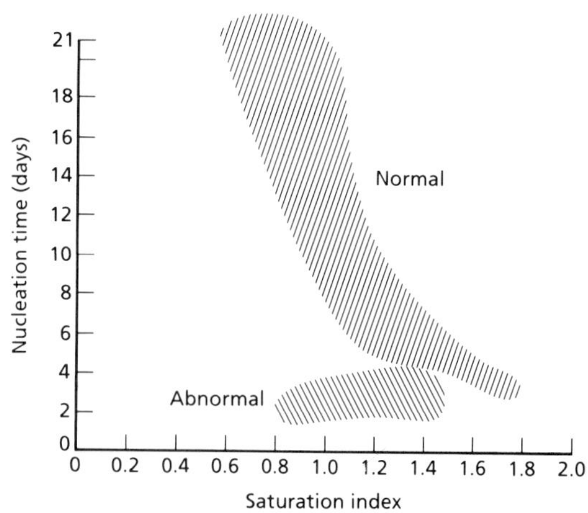

Fig. 1.7 Nucleation time as a function of cholesterol saturation index (CSI) for bile in patients with cholesterol gallstones (abnormal) and in control subjects (normal). (From Busch and Holzbach [172].)

data and subsequent studies have clearly demonstrated that bile from patients with cholesterol gallstones nucleates more rapidly than from individuals with cholesterol-saturated bile but without gallstones [52] (Fig. 1.7). The time required for nucleation appears to correlate with a number of important factors which have been implicated in the formation of cholesterol gallstones. While the process of nucleation is still not completely understood, its importance to the cascade of events resulting in gallstone formation is now a well accepted principle. Compelling evidence suggests that a 'nucleation defect' exists in patients with cholesterol gallstones although the exact nature of this abnormality has yet to be defined. The prevailing hypothesis to explain nucleation presupposes the presence of different biliary proteins and kinetic factors which have opposing functions: promoting and inhibiting nucleation. In a simplistic manner, one can view the normal, non-gallstone state as being characterized by a balance between these factors, whereas gallstone formation occurs when there is an imbalance in this system.

In 1983, Burnstein and co-workers [53] demonstrated that cholesterol crystal nucleation was accelerated by the presence of specific biliary proteins whose molecular weight was less than 300 kD. Subsequent studies have further characterized these as heat-labile, non-mucin glycoproteins [54]. In a series of elegant studies, Groen and colleagues [55, 56] have demonstrated the presence of a Concanavalin-binding protein which has pronucleating properties. This same non-mucin protein has been shown to induce a shift of cholesterol and phospholipids from the micellar to the vesicular fraction and appears to interact directly with the vesicles to facilitate their aggregation and nucleation [57].

As stated above nucleation can also be explained by a loss or relative diminution of nucleation inhibitors. Holzbach *et al.* [58] have reported the presence of low molecular weight proteins in normal bile capable of inhibiting nucleation. Further studies have suggested that apolipoproteins, which stabilize lipid structures in serum, [59] also prolong nucleation time of cholesterol supersaturated bile [60]. The genesis of these purported pro- and anti-nucleating factors, and their relative importance to this process continues to be the subject of considerable controversy and debate. One of the more intriguing substances which may hold the key to understanding the process of crystal agglomeration and nucleation is mucin, the principal organic constituent of mucus.

Mucus hypersecretion

Mucin, normally present in bile prior to gallstone formation, is a high molecular weight glycoprotein which is the main factor responsible for the viscoelastic properties of mucus gel [61]. Considerable evidence has been compiled over the last several years which links mucus hypersecretion to nucleation and gallstone formation. As stated, mucin is the main component of the mucus gel which lines the gallbladder epithelium; it is in this gel layer that nucleation occurs [62]. Indirect evidence based on electron microscopy studies of gallstone structure suggest that mucin may be the nidus in which cholesterol crystals nucleate and agglomerate [63]. Retention of microscopic crystals within the viscus mucus gel layer may facilitate the growth of these crystals to a sufficient size which would promote their stability and precludes their dissolution or spontaneous passage out of the gallbladder. A number of studies have indicated that hypersecretion of mucus precedes cholesterol gallstone formation in diet induced animal models of cholelithiasis [64]. In addition, evidence has been provided that gallbladder mucus hypersecretion is stimulated by cholesterol-saturated bile [65]. The importance of mucus in the formation of gallstones is underscored by the finding that aspirin prevents mucus hypersecretion and reduces the incidence of gallstones without affecting the lithogenicity of bile [66].

More recent studies have focussed on mucus hypersecretion and its relationship to nucleation *per se* and vesicle formation. Using organ cultures, Lee and co-workers [67] have demonstrated that gallbladder mucus hypersecretion precedes cholesterol nucleation in a diet-induced animal model. Although preliminary data indicated that this process was prostaglandin mediated [68], more recent

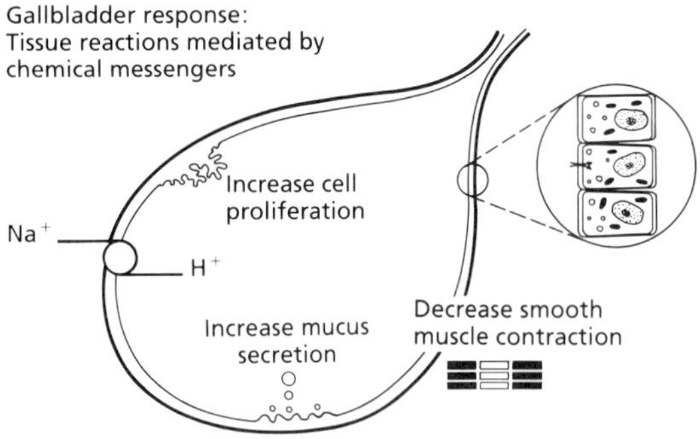

Fig. 1.8 Schematic representation of the contributory role of the gallbladder in biliary sludge formation. The hypothesis is based on the ability of the epithelial cells (insert) to respond to a 'noxious' stimulus, either in the form of a change in the chemical composition of bile or, as a result of obstruction. This triggers the release of chemical messengers (cyclic AMP, inositol triphosphate) resulting in a spectrum of tissue reactions that are known to be present in the process of gallbladder sludge/stone formation. (From Lee [173].)

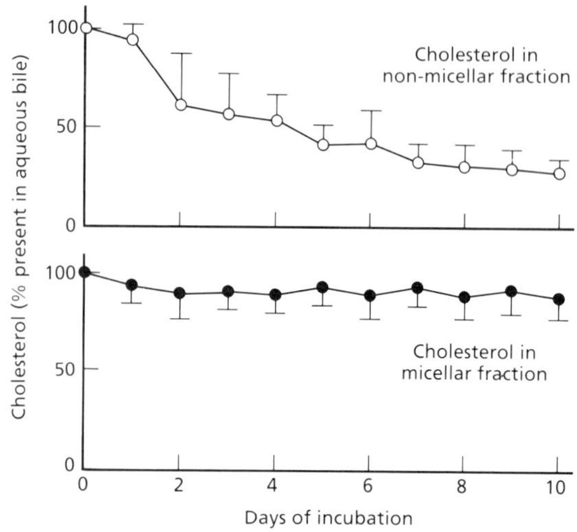

Fig. 1.9 Nucleation time of micellar and nonmicellar (vesicular) cholesterol. Results represent means ± SD of six gallbladder bile specimens. Nucleated (crystalline) cholesterol originates almost exclusively from the non-micellar (vesicular) fraction. (From Lee *et al.* [174].)

findings suggest that inhibition of prostaglandin synthesis does not prevent gallbladder mucin hypersecretion in cholesterol-fed prairie dogs, suggesting that this issue is far from resolved [69].

Studies by Lee and Smith [70] indicate that nucleation of vesicular cholesterol and micellar cholesterol is significantly accelerated in the presence of bovine gallbladder mucin. In a subsequent study, the physical properties of bovine gallbladder mucin were examined to determine whether noncovalent interactions between gallbladder mucins contribute to polymerization [71]. The results of this study suggest that the physicochemical behaviour of gallbladder mucin is influenced by the concentration of mucin and electrolytes at the epithelial surface of the gallbladder. Figure 1.8 represents a schematic diagram of the contributory role of gallbladder in biliary sludge formation.

Vesicles and nucleation

Biliary cholesterol is in a dynamic equilibrium between the micellar and vesicular phases. Upon secretion from the hepatocyte into the canaliculus, cholesterol is predominantly in the vesicular form. These vesicles mature in the presence of bile salts to form micelles during their passage into the gallbladder. As micelles form, the remaining vesicles become enriched with cholesterol. If the capacity of micelles to solubilize cholesterol is exceeded, as in supersaturated bile, cholesterol is contained in the less stable vesicular phase. In the presence of supersaturated bile, vesicular cholesterol is transformed into cholesterol liquid crystals and ultimately cholesterol monohydrate crystals. Evidence is rapidly emerging which suggests that aggregation of these cholesterol-phospholipid vesicles is critical to the nucleation process. Analysis of human bile from patients undergoing cholecystectomy reveals that there is a significant correlation between the cholesterol saturation index, the vesicular cholesterol fraction, and the presence of cholesterol crystals [72]. In addition, the nucleation time of gallbladder and hepatic bile correlates with the nucleation time of vesicles as opposed to that of micelles [73] (Fig. 1.9). Video-enhanced microscopic studies have demonstrated that the formation of cholesterol-phospholipid vesicles precedes the nucleation of cholesterol crystals [74]. Based on studies performed using both human and model bile solutions, Peled and colleagues [75] have suggested that the nucleation of micellar cholesterol occurs through the formation of cholesterol-phospholipid vesicles and that these vesicles appear to be the final common pathway for cholesterol nucleation in bile.

It is currently believed that vesicular aggregation into large multilamellar liquid crystals is promoted by specific proteins which are present in cholesterol saturated bile. Concanavalin A binding protein has been shown to induce a shift of cholesterol and phospholipids from the thermonuclear-stable micellar to the more unstable cholesterol-rich vesicular fraction and appears to interact directly with the vesicles to facilitate their aggregation and nucleation [76]. Harvey *et al.* [77] have recently presented information suggesting that IgM and possibly IgA are pronucleating agents particularly important in the aggregation of vesicles. Although it is clear that vesicles play an important role in the pathogenesis of cholesterol gallstones, our difficulty in identifying the factors responsible for promoting their aggregation has limited our ability to understand the 'nucleation defect' that characterizes patients with this disorder.

Gallbladder stasis

In 1856, Meckel von Helmsbach first suggested that stasis of bile within the gallbladder might be a critical factor in the formation of cholesterol gallstones [78]. Despite the fact that gallstones form almost exclusively in the gallbladder, little attention was directed towards this concept until relatively recently. Over the last 20 years numerous clinical and experimental studies have documented stasis of bile within the gallbladder and detected a number of specific defects in gallbladder motility in patients with gallstones. It has been suggested that stasis is the critical link between the hepatic secretion of cholesterol-saturated bile and gallstone formation [79]. In 1978, Meyer *et al.* [80] demonstrated the presence of gallbladder bile stasis in cholesterol-fed animals at a time when bile was saturated with cholesterol, but prior to stone formation. Development of the prairie dog and ground squirrel models of cholelithiasis have been of enormous benefit in understanding the factors which account for these observations. Early manometric studies in the prairie dog suggested that gallstone formation was associated with increased resistance to outflow through the cystic duct [81] and decreased gallbladder emptying [82]. Subsequent *in vitro* studies in the cholesterol-fed ground squirrel indicate a reduction in isometric tensions generated by gallbladder muscle strips in response to a variety of stimuli consistent with a reduction in gallbladder contractility as compared to controls [83]. Decreased gallbladder contractility in response to CCK has also been observed in cholesterol-fed prairie dogs utilizing quantitative cholescintigraphy [84]. Li and co-workers [85] have extended this finding and have reported that cholesterol feeding induces a shift in gallbladder smooth muscle actin isoforms at the same time that there is an observable decrease in gallbladder contractility.

Impaired gallbladder emptying has been viewed as a causative factor in the increased incidence of gallstones reported in patients maintained on long-term total parenteral nutrition [86, 87], following truncal vagotomy [88, 89], and in women during the latter stages of pregnancy [90, 91]. A series of cholescintigraphic studies in humans have suggested that there are subsets of gallstone patients who have reduced gallbladder emptying and contractility [92, 93, 94], perhaps as a consequence of reduced endogenous cholecystokinin production [95] (Fig. 1.10).

Other evidence which suggests the presence of gallbladder hypomotility in gallstone patients includes: persistence of a motility defect in patients undergoing lithotripsy despite the clearance of all stones [96]; decrease in gallbladder emptying as bile lithogenicity increases [97]; demonstration of motor defect in diabetics without gallstones [98]; and the recent report that populations of patients with a low incidence of gallstones have more complete gallbladder emptying than other groups with a higher incidence of cholelithiasis [99].

The mechanism(s) by which stasis of bile within the gallbladder promotes cholesterol gallstone formation remains unclear. One possible consequence is the sequestration of bile acids within the gallbladder and the associated reduction in

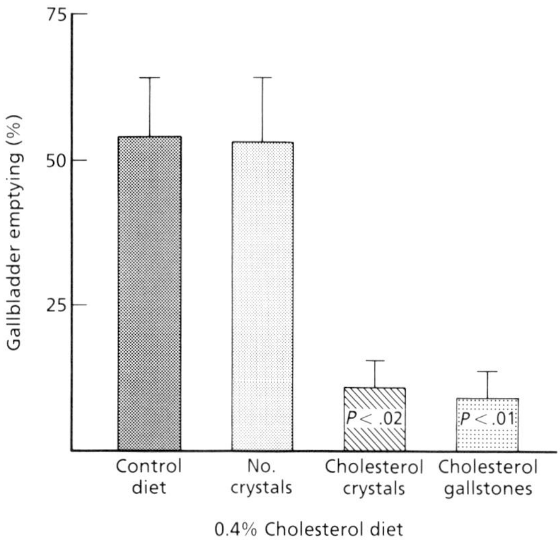

Fig. 1.10 Effect of cholesterol feeding on percent of gallbladder emptying in prairie dogs. Gallbladder emptying was significantly diminished when either cholesterol crystals or gallstones were present. Vertical bars represent mean ± SEM. (From Doty *et al.* [175].)

the pool of bile acids available for cholesterol solubilization. Intuitively, it would appar that a stagnant pool of bile provides an ideal milieu for the precipitation and agglomeration of cholesterol crystals into gallstones. Stasis of bile will increase the exposure time of the gallbladder mucosa to luminal factors present within cholesterol-saturated bile which may alter normal gallbladder physiology. The relationship between biliary stasis and the concentration of nucleating or antinucleating factors is an area of current investigation.

Biliary calcium

The importance of biliary calcium as an aetiological factor in the formation of calcium bilirubinate gallstones has long been recognized. For many years, clinical dogma suggested that calcium was present in less than 30% of all patients with cholesterol gallstones. This concept has been questioned by the recent observation that calcium salts exist in the central matrix of many, if not all, cholesterol gallstones [100]. *In vitro* studies have shown that the crystal structures of calcium carbonate and cholesterol monohydrate are similar enough to support the growth of one crystal on the framework of another [101]. Recent preliminary studies suggest that gallbladder bile from patients with gallstones is supersaturated with calcium [102]. Moreover, animal studies indicate that gallbladder bile (and not hepatic bile) from gallstone animals contains significantly more total and ionized calcium as compared with controls [103].

In addition to potentially serving as a nidus for nucleation and crystal growth, Moore [104] and Been et al. [100] have advanced the hypothesis that Ca^{++} ions promote aggregation and fusion of cholesterol-phospholipid vesicles. These thoughts are based on the observations that free Ca^{++} ions:
1 promote fusion of vesicles in bile [105] and acidic phospholipid vesicles *in vitro* [106];
2 promote cholesterol phase transitions [107]; promote cholesterol crystal growth [108];
3 decrease solubility of mucin [109] and bile salts [110];
4 appear to lower the critical micellar concentration of bile salts [111].

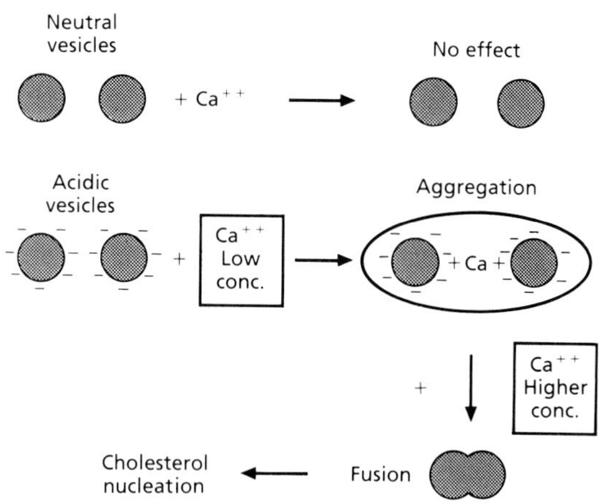

Fig. 1.11 Schematic illustration of potential interactions between Ca^{++} ions and PL (phospholipid) vesicles. It is predicted that neutral vesicles (as with pure phosphatidylcholine) would have low Ca^{++}-binding affinity, so that Ca^{++} ion would have little tendency to promote vesicle aggregation. In contrast, Ca^{++} in very low concentrations may induce aggregation of acidic vesicles, with fusion at higher Ca^{++} concentrations. (From Moore [176].)

Understanding the precise role of calcium in gallstone formation may facilitate the development of strategies designed to reduce calcium precipitation and thereby prevent gallstones. Figure 1.11 illustrates the potential interactions between Ca^{++} ions and phospholipid vesicles.

Altered gallbladder absorption

Although the primary function of the gallbladder is to concentrate bile during interdigestive periods by absorption of sodium and water, the manner in which this activity is altered during gallstone formation has only recently become the focus of investigation. Conflicting data have been reported regarding absorption of bile salts, water, and sodium in experimental and human studies. Using electrophysiological parameters as indices of ion transport and absorptive function, a decrease in potential difference has been observed in humans with chronic cholelithiasis [112]. *In vitro* studies with diet-induced models of gallstone disease indicate that gallbladder fluid transport actually increases during the formation of experimentally induced non-cholesterol [113] and cholesterol gallstones [114]. Subsequent studies have suggested that this observed early alteration in transport function is due to luminal factors present within cholesterol saturated bile and not to an irreversible change in mucosal function [115, 116]. Although some alteration in gallbladder ion transport and absorption appears to occur during early gallstone formation, the specific defects in unidirectional flux associated with this phenomenon remain obscure. The realization that altered gallbladder absorptive function may occur during the early stages of gallstone formation is particularly intriguing given our current understanding of the factors and relationships which govern the stability of vesicles.

Gallstone formation and prostaglandins

Recent studies indicate that gallbladder synthesis of prostaglandins is altered prior to the formation of experimentally-induced cholesterol gallstones [117, 118, 119]. While the mechanism of the observed alterations is unclear, a role for elevated biliary cholesterol has been suggested by studies which have examined the effect of cholesterol on prostaglandin production by platelets. Cholesterol enrichment of platelet membranes resulted in increased arachidonic acid release and increased production of thromboxane [120, 121]. Interestingly, the various prostanoids appear to mediate several different aspects of cholesterol gallstone pathogenesis, including mucin secretion, gallbladder stasis, and absorptive function.

Specifically, increased gallbladder synthesis of $PGF_{2\alpha}$, PGE_2, prostacyclin PGI_2 and thromboxane have been shown to precede, and likely to be causally related to, increased gallbladder mucin production in prairie dogs [122, 123]. Treatment of cholesterol-fed animals with aspirin, a known cyclooxygenase inhibitor, reduces mucin hypersecretion and cholesterol gallstone formation without affecting bile lithogenicity [66]. More recent studies utilizing indomethacin failed to confirm this earlier finding as cholesterol-fed animals went on to demonstrate mucin hypersecretion and gallstone formation [69]. The role of altered prostaglandin metabolism and gallbladder mucin hypersecretion is far from resolved.

In vivo and *in vitro* studies both suggest that prostaglandins affect gallbladder motility [124, 125]. Ion and fluid transport is mediated by prostanoids, as demonstrated in frog skin, toad bladder, mammalian collecting duct, and human intestine [126]. In the rabbit gallbladder, studies using a gravimetric technique for measuring fluid absorption have demonstrated inhibition of normal gallbladder absorptive function with exogenous PGE_2, $PGF_{2\alpha}$, PGA_2 and PGI_2 [127]. Recently completed studies in the prairie dog model suggest that indomethacin has a significant proabsorptive effect on gallbladder epithelium, converting the gallbladder to a Cl^- absorptive organ and stimulating Na^+ absorption [128]. Exposure to PGE_2 reversed the effects of indomethacin and exerted a significant secretory stimulus on gallbladder Cl^- and water transport. These studies when taken together, suggest that endogenous concentrations of prostanoids mediate gallbladder ion transport and that changes in tissue levels may mediate changes in ion transport and mucus secretion during gallstone formation. The importance of prostaglandins as potential mediators of gallbladder absorptive function is underscored by reports linking prostaglandins in gallbladder distension and abdominal pain in patients with acute cholecystitis [129].

Bacteria and cholesterol gallstones

In 1966, Maki [130] elucidated the essential aetiologic role of bacteria in the pathogenesis of calcium bilirubinate gallstones. The recent observation that bacteria are present in a finite percentage of cholesterol gallstones [131], suggests that bacteria may play a similar role in the formation of cholesterol gallstones. This attractive hypothesis remains to be confirmed.

Unified hypothesis for cholesterol gallstone formation

It is becoming increasingly evident that the pathogenesis of cholesterol gallstones is a multifactorial process. Almost certainly, there is a dynamic interaction between the liver and the gallbladder such that hepatic secretion of cholesterol-saturated bile induces alterations in gallbladder motility, secretion and absorption which may promote cholesterol precipitation, crystal agglomeration and stone growth. Figure 1.12 is a schematic representation of the major pathogenetic abnormalities that occur during gallstone formation. First, supersaturation of bile with cholesterol (lithogenic bile) is a thermodynamic requirement for cholesterol stone formation, but stones do not form unless a defect in nucleation induces precipitation of cholesterol monohydrate crystals. This process is affected by the levels of biliary proteins and calcium, which may be elevated owing to increased gallbladder absorption. Prostaglandins play an important role in the regulation of gallbladder ion transport and water absorption. Finally, the cholesterol crystals must remain in the gallbladder long enough to grow and agglomerate into gallstones. This event is facilitated by gallbladder hypomotility (stasis) and mucus hypersecretion, which may be mediated by prostaglandins. Alterations in prostaglandins may be due to changes in chemical species of biliary lecithins secreted by the liver. Although tremendous progress in the understanding of the pathogenesis of cholesterol gallstones has been made in the last decade, the molecular basis of all the pathogenetic abnormalities and the interactions among them continue to be elusive.

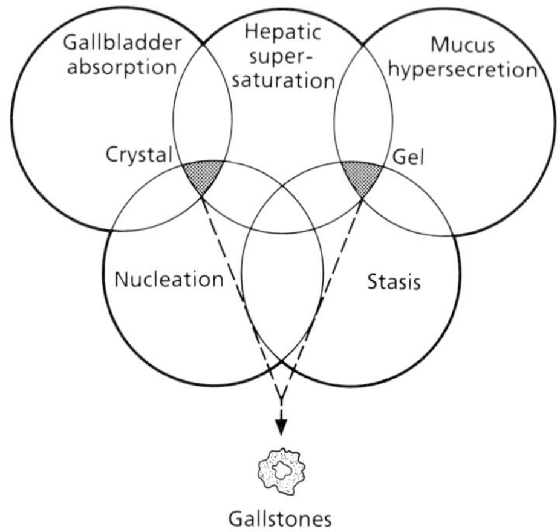

Fig. 1.12 Cascade of events that may occur in the liver and the gallbladder during cholesterol gallstone formation. Cholesterol-saturated bile secreted by the liver induces a series of alterations in gallbladder motility, secretion and absorption which play critical roles in cholesterol precipitation, crystal growth and agglomeration, and stone formation. See text for details. (After Carey *et al.* [177].)

Pathogenesis of pigment gallstones

Overview

Worldwide, pigment gallstones are the most common type of calculi found in the gallbladder. The epidemiology of pigment gallstone disease is evolving. While pigment stones were generally considered to account for less than 10% of all stones found in the USA [33, 132], more recent studies suggest this figure to be closer to 25–30% [133]. In contrast, the incidence of this stone type is actually decreasing in Japan—coincident with an increase in cholesterol gallstones [134, 135]. Autopsy studies suggest that pigment gallstones are being found with increasing frequency in the elderly [136]. Despite the magnitude of pigment gallstone disease from a global perspective and our expansion of knowledge in this area, there are still many unanswered questions regarding the factors responsible for their formation.

Classification

Traditionally, pigment gallstones were viewed as a single entity with a common pathogenesis. As recently as 1977, a classic text devoted 18 pages to the formation of cholesterol gallstones and less than a single page to pigment gallstones [137]. Current schema classify pigment stones as either brown or black. These stones are morphologically and chemically distinct, and occur in different clinical settings.

Brown stones occur with great frequency in Asia and are much more common than black stones [138]. Brown stones are similar in appearance and composition to primary common bile duct stones, can be located throughout the intrahepatic or extrahepatic biliary tract, and are typically associated with infection. Morphologically, these stones tend to be laminated with alternating regions of brown and tan material with a central core. Brown stones contain more cholesterol than black stones, but it still only accounts for less than 15% of dry weight. In addition, brown stones consist of calcium salts of bilirubin (calcium bilirubinate makes up more than 60% of dry weight) and fatty acid in a glycoprotein matrix. Brown pigment stones have been associated with diet [139], long-term administration of total parenteral nutrition (TPN) [140], and are almost always found in patients with biliary infection [141]. The difference in composition of brown and black pigment stones is described in Table 1.1.

Black pigment stones tend to be radio-opaque due to the presence of calcium carbonate or phosphate. In contrast to brown stones, the black variety contains appreciable amounts of calcium carbonate (15%) and phosphate (10% of dry weight) and only 40% calcium bilirubinate. The net effect is that black stones contain more inorganic calcium salts and less cholesterol than brown stones. Black pigment gallstone disease has been reported with increased frequency in patients with haemolytic anaemias [142], alcoholic cirrhosis [143], malaria [144], and in patients on long-term TPN [145]. These stones are usually limited to the gallbladder and bacterial infection of bile is thought not to be an important factor.

Table 1.1 Average composition of pigment gallstones

Component (% dry wt)	Gallstone type: Black	Brown
Calcium bilirubinate	40	60
Calcium palmitate	Rarely present	25
Calcium phosphate	9	Not detected
Calcium carbonate	15	Rarely present
Cholesterol	2	11
Bile salts	2	2
Unmeasured	30	10

From Trotman [166].

Pathogenesis

Since 1966, when Maki [130] first described the enzymatic deconjugation of bilirubin glucuronide by beta glucuronidase of bacterial origin, infection has been recognized as an important factor in the formation of pigment gallstones. The realization that pigment gallstones occur in a variety of different clinical settings as indicated above, and that there are at least two distinct subtypes of pigment calculi, suggests that the pathogenesis of this disorder is multifactorial and cannot be explained by a simple, single hypothesis.

Brown pigment gallstones are indeed associated with biliary infection as manifested by the presence of bacteria in the interstices of brown stones [146, 147], and by the ability to culture bacteria from the bile of these patients [148]. The combination of bacterobilia and stasis leads to the enzymatic deconjugation of bilirubin and alteration in phospholipid and bile salt moieties, ultimately resulting in increased concentrations of unconjugated bilirubin, free fatty acids and lysolecithin, and unconjugated bile salts [149, 150]. These alterations promote cholesterol saturation, and the precipitation of cholesterol with calcium bilirubinate.

Although bacterial infection of bile is not believed to be an essential component of black pigment gallstone disease, specific alterations in hepatic bile composition as a consequence of non-bacterial-mediated hydrolysis of bilirubin have been shown to occur in patients with these stones [151]. The production of relatively large amounts of unconjugated bilirubin may be facilitated as well by the presence of biliary stasis [153]. It has been suggested that black pigment gallstones can occur as a result of too much bilirubin, as in the case of patients with haemolytic anaemias [142, 153], or due to decreased secretion of bile salts which leads to reduced solubilization of unconjugated bilirubin, as has been reported in patients with cirrhosis [154].

Pathogenesis of common bile duct stones

Classification

The nomenclature of common bile duct (CBD) stones which has evolved through the years is somewhat confusing. One system classifies stones as being either retained or recurrent. The former refers to stones which arise in the gallbladder, pass through the cystic duct into the CBD, and are left in the duct after cholecystectomy. Recurrent stones are considered to be those which develop primarily in the CBD and become manifest at some time after removal of the gallbladder. A more popular and widely used system utilizes the terms 'primary' and 'secondary' to designate the site of origin of the stones. Primary stones are those that form exclusively in the CBD, whereas secondary stones arise in the gallbladder and pass through the cystic duct into the CBD. Although some authors have suggested that primary stones account for the majority of CBD calculi [155], epidemiological data indicates most stones found within the common duct are of gallbladder origin and, therefore, would be classified as secondary or retained stones [156].

The aetiology of secondary stones is quite different than for primary ones. Most patients with cholesterol CBD stones also have cholesterol gallbladder stones of identical biochemical composition, underscoring the origin of the common duct stones from within the gallbladder. In contrast, most primary stones are composed of calcium bilirubinate. Considerable evidence suggests that stasis and bacteria are two critical factors for the formation of primary or recurrent biliary stones.

Primary common bile duct stones

Experimental and clinical studies indicate that stasis of bile within the biliary tract as a consequence of either strictures [157], severe ductal dilatation [158], or motor abnormalities of the sphincter mechanism [159], is associated with the presence of primary ductal stones. While much of this evidence is anecdotal, recent manometric studies reporting elevated common duct pressures at operation in patients with choledocholithiasis [160] provides further support for the hypothesis that abnormal sphincter of Oddi motor activity is a causal factor in the formation of primary common duct stones. This issue remains controversial, insofar as endoscopically performed manometric studies have failed to confirm these findings [161, 162].

The role of bacteria and enzymatic hydrolysis of bilirubin diglucuronide in the formation of pigment stones has been detailed above (see page 15). Studies have clearly defined the presence of bacteria (both Gram-negative aerobes and Gram-positive anaerobes) in the matrices of primary common ductal stones [156]. In addition, all of the bacteria isolated possessed β-glucuronidase activity at physiologic pH, consistent with the above stated hypothesis. Further studies are needed to clarify the relationship between biliary stasis, bacteria, and primary common duct stone disease.

Pathogenesis of intrahepatic stones

A better definition of the factors responsible for formation of primary ductal stones will facilitate our understanding of the pathogenesis of intrahepatic stone disease. This entity, although relatively uncommon in Western countries, is endemic in East Asia [163, 164]. Analyses of the composition of these stones demonstrates that the majority of them are calcium bilirubinate [32]. As with other stones containing calcium bilirubinate, biliary infection and stasis would appear to be critical aetiologic factors.

Considerable clinical experience indicates that ductal dilatation and strictures are found with great frequency in patients with intrahepatic stone disease [164]. What remains unclear, however, is the cause and effect relationship between this finding and stone formation. The incidence of bacterial infection with intrahepatic stones is virtually 100% [32]. Recent studies suggest that the observed increase in prevalence of hepatolithiasis in East Asia might be secondary to a decrease in biliary inhibition of bacterial β-glucuronidase activity as a consequence of a diet-induced factor (glucaro-1,4-lactone) which is present in low-fat, low protein diets [165]. The huge number of patients world-wide who suffer with this malady underscores the importance of elucidating the factors responsible for the formation of intrahepatic stones.

References

1 Admirand WH, Small DM. The physicochemical basis of cholesterol gallstone formation in man. *J Clin Invest* 1968;**47**:1043–52.

2 Carey MC, Small DM. The physical chemistry of cholesterol solubility in bile: relationship to gallstone formation and dissolution in man. *J Clin Invest* 1978;**61**:998–1026.

3 Holzbach RT, Pak CY. Metastable supersaturation physicochemical studies provide new insights into formation of renal and biliary tract stones. *Am J Med* 1974;**283**(25):1358–64.

4 Sömjen GJ, Gilat T. A non-micellar mode of cholesterol transport in human bile. *FEBS Lett* 1983; **156**(2):265–8.

5 Sömjen GJ, Gilat T. Contribution of vesicular and micellar carriers to cholesterol transport in human bile. *J Lipid Res* 1985;**26**:699–704.

6 Mazer NA, Schurtenberger P, Carey MC *et al.* Quasi-elastic light scattering of native hepatic bile from the dog: comparison with the aggregative behavior of model biliary lipid systems. *Biochemistry* 1984;**23**: 1994–2005.

7 Pattinson NR. Solubilisation of cholesterol in human bile. *FEBS Lett* 1985;**181**:339–42.

8 Ulloa N, Garrido J, Nervi F. Ultracentifugal isolation of vesicular carriers of biliary cholesterol in native human and rat bile. *Hepatology* 1987;**7**:235–44.

9 Lee SP, Park HZ, Madani H *et al.* Partial characterization of a nonmicellar system of cholesterol solubilization in bile. *Am J Physiol* 1987;**252**:G374–83.

10 Ivy AC, Oldberg E. A hormone mechanism for gallbladder contraction and evacuation. *Am J Physiol* 1928;**86**:599–613.

11 Nyberg B, Sonnenfeld T, Einarsson K. Vasoactive intestinal peptide and secretin: effects of combined and separate intravenous infusions on bile secretion in man. *Scand J Gastroenterol* 1991;**26**:109–18.

12 Bloom SR, Adrian TE, Mitchenere P *et al.* Motilin-induced gallbladder contraction—a new mechanism. *Gastroenterology* 1981;80(2):1113. (Abstract).

13 Adrian TE, Mitchenere P, Sagor G, *et al.* Effect of pancreatic polypeptide on gallbladder pressure and hepatic bile secretion. *Am J Physiol* 1982;**243**:G207–12.

14 Pomeranz IS, Shaffer EA. Abnormal gallbladder emptying in a subgroup of patients with gallstones. *Gastroenterology* 1985;**88**:787–91.

15 Thompson JC, Fried GM, Ogden WD, *et al.* Correlation between release of cholecystokinin and contraction of the gallbladder in patients with gallstones. *Ann Surg* 1982;**195**:670–5.

16 Diemerbroek I. *Anatome corpois humani.* Utrecht, 1672.

17 Brand J. Beitrag Zur Kenntris der menschlichen Gall. *Arch Ges Physiol* 1902;**90**:491–22.

18 Rous P, McMaster PD. The concentrating ability of the gallbladder. *J Exp Med* 1921;**34**:347–423.

19 Ravdin IS, Johnson CG, Austin JH *et al.* Studies of gallbladder function IV. The absorption of chloride from bile free gallbladder. *Am J Physiol* 1932;**99**:638–47.

20 Van Os CH, Slegers JFG. Correlation between (Na^+–K^+)-activated ATPase activities and the rate of isotonic fluid transport of gallbladder epithelium. *Biochim Biophys Acta* 1971;**241**:89–96.

21 Reuss L. Independence of apical membrane Na^+ and Cl^- entry in Necterus gallbladder epithelium. *J Gen Physiol* 1984;**84**:423–45.

22 Ericson AC, Spring KR. Volume regulation by Necterus gallbladder: Apical Na^+–H^+ and Cl^-–HCO_3^- exchange. *Am J Physiol* 1982;**243**:C146–50.

23 Adragna NC, Perkins CM, Lauf PK. Furosemide-sensitive Na^+–K^+ cotransport and cellular metabolism in human erythrocytes. *Biochim Biophys Acta* 1985;**812**:293–6.

24 Smith PL, Sullivan SK, McCabe RD. Concentration-dependent effects of disulfonic stilbenes on colonic chloride transport. *Am J Physiol* 1986;**250**:G44–9.

25 Diamond JM, Tormey JM. Role of long extra-cellular channels in fluid transport across epithelia. *Nature* 1966;**210**:817–20.

26 Schoenfield LJ, Lachin JM *et al.* Chenodiol (chenodeoxycholic acid) for dissolution of gallstones: the National Cooperative Gallstone Study. *Ann Int Med* 1981;**95**:257–82.

27 Roda E, Bazzoli F, Labate AMM *et al.* Ursodeoxycholic acid vs. chenodeoxycholic acid as cholesterol gallstone dissolving agents: a comparative randomized study. *Hepatology* 1982;**2**:804–10.

28 Hofmann AF. Rationale of bile acid therapy after biliary lithotripsy. In: Ferruci JT, Deius M, Burhenne

HJ, eds. *Biliary Lithotripsy*. Chicago: Year Book Medical, 1989:151–7.

29 Saunders KD, Cates JA, Abedin MZ, Roslyn JJ. Lovastatin and gallstone dissolution: A preliminary study. *Surgery* 1993;**113**(1):28–35.

30 Schachler R, Sauerbruch T, Wosiewitz V *et al.* Fragmentation of gallstones during extracorporeal shock waves: An *in vitro* study. *Hepatology* 1988; **8**:925–9.

31 Sachmann M, Delius M, Suerbruch T *et al.* Shock-wave lithotripsy of gallbladder stones–the first 175 patients. *N Engl J Med* 1988;**318**:393–7.

32 Suzuki N, Takahashi W, Sato T. Types and chemical composition of intrahepatic stones. In: Okuda K, Nakayama F, Wong J, eds. *Intrahepatic Calculi*. New York: Alan R Liss, 1984:71–80.

33 Friedman GD, Kann WB, Dawber TR. Epidemiology of gallbladder disease: observation in the Framingham study. *J Chronic Dis* 1966;**19**:273–92.

34 La Morte WW, Schoetz DJ Jr, Birkett DH *et al.* The role of the gallbladder in the pathogenesis of cholesterol gallstones. *Gastroenterology* 1979;**77**:580–92.

35 Halpern Z, Dudley MA, Kibe A *et al.* Rapid vesicle formation and aggregation in abnormal human bile. *Gastroenterology* 1986;**90**:875–85.

36 Holzbach RT. Pathogenesis and medical treatment of gallstones. In: Sleisenger NH, Fordtran JS, eds. *Gastrointestinal Disease*. Philadelphia: Saunders, 1989:1356–72.

37 Carey MC: Critical tables for calculating the cholesterol saturation of native bile. *J Lipid Res* 1978; **19**:945–55.

38 Mazer NA, Carey MC. Mathematical model of biliary lipid secretion: a quantitative analysis of physiological and biochemical data from man and other species. *J Lipid Res* 1984;**25**:932–53.

39 Heaton KW, Read AE. Gallstones in patients with disorders of the terminal ileum and disturbed bile salt metabolism. *Br Med J* 1969;**3**:495–6.

40 Metzger AL, Adler R, Heymsfield S. Diurnal variation in biliary lipid composition. *N Engl J Med* 1973;**288**:333–6.

41 Chiang JYL, Miller MF, Lin GM. Regulation of cholesterol 7α-hydroxylase in the liver. Purification of cholesterol 7α-hydroxylase and the immunochemical evidence for the induction of cholesterol 7α-hydroxylase by cholestyramine and circadian rhythm. *J Biol Chem* 1990;**265**:3889–97.

42 Nervi F, Covarrubias C, Bravo P *et al.* Influence of legume intake on biliary lipids and cholesterol saturation in young Chilean men. *Gastroenterology* 1989;**96**:825–830.

43 Nilsell K, Angelin B, Liljeqvist L *et al.* Biliary lipid output and bile acid kinetics in cholesterol gallstone disease. Evidence for an increased hepatic secretion of cholesterol in Swedish patients. *Gastroenterology* 1985;**89**:287–93.

44 Madura JA, Loomis RC, Harris RA *et al.* Relationship of obesity to bile lithogenicity in man. *Ann Surg* 1979;**189**(1):106–11.

45 Einarsson K, Nilsell K, Leijd B *et al.* Influence of age on secretion and synthesis of bile acids by the liver. *New Engl J Med* 1985;**313**:277–82.

46 Bennion LJ, Mott DM, Howard BV. Oral contraceptives raise the cholesterol saturation of bile by increasing biliary cholesterol secretion. *Metabolism* 1980;**29**:18–22.

47 Henriksson P, Einarsson K, Eriksson A *et al.* Estrogen-induced gallstone formation in males. *J Clin Invest* 1989;**84**:811–16.

48 Heuman DM, Valhcevic ZR, Bailey ML. Regulation of bile acid synthesis. II. Effect of bile acid feeding on enzyme regulating hepatic cholesterol and bile acid synthesis in the rat. *Hepatology* 1988;**8**:892–7.

49 Northfield TC, Hofmann AF. Biliary lipid output during three meals and an overnight fast: relationship to bile acid pool size and cholesterol saturation of bile in gallstone and control subjects. *Gut* 1975; **16**(1):1–11.

50 Holan KR, Holzbach RT, Hermann RE *et al.* Nucleation time: a key factor in the pathogenesis of cholesterol gallstone disease. *Gastroenterology* 1979;**77**:611–17.

51 Holzbach RT, Marsh M, Olszwski M, Holan KR. Cholesterol solubility in bile: evidence that supersaturated bile is frequent in healthy man. *J Clin Invest* 1973;**52**:1467–79.

52 Sedaghat A, Grundy SM. Cholesterol crystals and the formation of cholesterol gallstones. *N Engl J Med* 1980;**302**:1274–7.

53 Burnstein MJ, Ilson RG, Petrunka CN *et al.* Evidence for a potent nucleating factor in the gallbladder bile of patients with cholesterol gallstones. *Gastroenterology* 1983;**85**:801–7.

54 Gallinger S, Taylor RD, Harvey PRC *et al.* Effect of mucous glycoprotein on nucleation time of human bile. *Gastroenterology* 1985;**89**:648–58.

55 Groen AK, Stout JPJ, Drapers JAG *et al.* Cholesterol-nucleation influencing activity in T-tube bile. *Hepatology* 1988;8(2):347–52.

56 Groen AK, Ottenhoff R, Jansen PLM *et al.* Effect of cholesterol nucleation-promoting activity on cholesterol solubilization in model bile. *J Lipid Res* 1989;**30**:51–8.

57 Busch N, Aoyama N, Tokumo H *et al.* Isolation of a potent inhibitory glycoprotein in normal human gallbladder bile that affects both cholesterol nucleation and crystal growth. *Gastroenterology* 1989;**96**: A581. (Abstract).

58 Holzbach RT, Kibe A, Thiel E *et al.* Biliary proteins: Unique inhibitors of cholesterol crystal nucleation in human gallbladder bile. *J Clin Invest* 1984;**73**:35–45.

59 Sewell RB, Mao ST, Kwamoto T, LaRusso NF. Appolipoproteins of high, low and very low density in human bile. *J Lipid Res* 1983;**42**:391–404.

60 Kibe A, Holzbach RT, LaRusso NF *et al.* Inhibition of

cholesterol crystal formation by apolipoproteins in supersaturated model bile. *Science* 1984;**225**: 514–16.
61 Smith BF, Petermanns JA, Tanaka T *et al.* Subunit interactions and physical properties of bovine gallbladder mucin. *Gastroenterology* 1989;**97**:179–87.
62 Hulten O. Formation of gallstones. II. *Acta Chir Scand* 1968;**134**:557–60.
63 Smith BF, LaMont JT. Identification of gallbladder mucin–bilirubin complex in human cholesterol gallstone matrix. *J Clin Invest* 1985;**76**:439–45.
64 Freston JW, Bouchier IAD, Newman J. Biliary mucous substances in dihydrocholesterol-induced cholelithiasis. *Gastroenterology* 1969;**57**:670–8.
65 Doty JE, Pitt HA, Kuchenbecker SL *et al.* The role of gallbladder mucus in the pathogenesis of cholesterol gallstones. *Am J Surg* 1983;**145**:54–6.
66 Lee SP, Carey MC, LaMont JT. Aspirin prevention of cholesterol gallstone formation in prairie dogs. *Science* 1981;**211**:1429–31.
67 Lee SP, LaMont JT, Carey MC. Role of gallbladder mucus hypersecretion in the evolution of cholesterol gallstones: studies in the prairie dog. *J Clin Invest* 1981;**67**:1712–72.
68 LaMorte WW, LaMont JT, Hale W *et al.* Gallbladder prostaglandins and lysophospholipids as mediators of mucin secretion during cholelithiasis. *Am J Physiol* 1986;**251**:G701–9.
69 O'Leary DP, LaMorte WW, Scott TE *et al.* Inhibition of prostaglandin synthesis fails to prevent gallbladder mucin hypersecretion in the cholesterol-fed prairie dog. *Gastroenterology* 1991;**101**:812–20.
70 Lee TJ, Smith BF. Bovine gallbladder mucin promotes cholesterol crystal nucleation from cholesterol-transporting vesicles in supersaturated model bile. *J Lipid Res* 1989;**30**:491–8.
71 Smith BF. Human gallbladder mucin binds biliary lipids and promotes cholesterol crystal nucleation in model bile. *J Lipid Res* 1987;**28**:1088–97.
72 Peled Y, Halpern Z, Baruch R *et al.* Cholesterol nucleation from its carriers in human bile. *Hepatology* 1988;**8**(4):914–18.
73 Harvey RP, Sömjen GJ, Gilat T *et al.* Vesicular cholesterol in bile. Relationship to protein concentration and nucleation time. *Biochim Biophys Acta* 1988; **958**:10–18.
74 Halpern Z, Dudley MA, Kibe A *et al.* Rapid vesicle formation and aggregation in abnormal human biles. *Gastroenterology* 1986;**90**:875–85.
75 Peled Y, Halpern Z, Eitan B *et al.* Biliary micellar cholesterol nucleates via the vesicular pathway. *Biochim Biophys Acta* 1989;**1003**:246–9.
76 Harvey PRC, Upadhya GA, Toth JL *et al.* A Concanavalin A binding glycoprotein accelerates the nucleation of cholesterol from model bile. *Hepatology* 1987;**7**:1112. (Abstract).
77 Harvey PRC, Upadhya GA, Strasberg SM. Immunoglobulins and nucleating proteins in the gallbladder bile of patients with cholesterol gallstones. *J Biol Chem* 1991;**266**(21):13996–14003.
78 Meckel von Helmsbach JH. Mikrogeologie *Über die Concremente in Tierischen Organismus*. Billroth T, ed. Berlin: Reimer, 1856.
79 Roslyn JJ, DenBesten L, Pitt HA *et al.* Effects of cholecystokinin on gallbladder stasis and cholesterol gallstone formation. *J Surg Res* 1981;**30**:200–6.
80 Meyer PD, DenBesten L, Gurll NJ. Effects of cholesterol gallstone induction on gallbladder function and bile salt pool size in the prairie dog model. *Surgery* 1978;**63**:599–604.
81 Pitt HA, Roslyn JJ, Kuchenbecker S, DenBesten L. The role of increased cystic duct resistance in the pathogenesis of cholesterol cholelithiasis. *J Surg Res* 1981;**30**:508–13.
82 Roslyn JJ, Pitt HA, Kuchenbecker S *et al.* Alterations in biliary tract motility during cholesterol gallstone formation. *Surg Forum* 1980;**31**:205–6.
83 Fridhandler TM, Davison JS, Shaffer EA. Defective gallbladder contractility in the ground squirrel and prairie dogs during early stages of cholesterol gallstone formation. *Gastroenterology* 1983;**85**:830–6.
84 Roslyn JJ, DenBesten L, Pitt HA *et al.* Effects of cholecystokinin on gallbladder stasis and cholesterol gallstone formation. *J Surg Res* 1981;**30**:200–4.
85 Li YF, Bowers RL, Haley-Russell D *et al.* Actin and myosin isoforms in gallbladder smooth muscle following cholesterol feeding in prairie dogs. *Gastroenterology* 1990;**99**:1460–6.
86 Messing B, Borris C, Kunstlinger F *et al.* Does total parenteral nutrition induce gallbladder sludge formation and lithiasis? *Gastroenterology* 1983;**84**: 1012–19.
87 Barth RA, Brasch RC, Filly RA. Abdominal pseudotumor in childhood: distended gallbladder with parenteral hyperalimentation. *Am J Roentgenol* 1981; **136**:341–3.
88 Clave RA, Gaspar MR. Incidence of gallbladder disease after vagotomy. *Am J Surg* 1969;**118**:169–76.
89 Pitt HA, Doty JE, DenBesten L. The role of altered extrahepatic biliary motility in the pathogenesis of gallstones following vagotomy. *Surgery* 1981; **90**:418–25.
90 Braverman DZ, Johnson ML, Kern F Jr. Effects of pregnancy and contraceptive steroids on gallbladder function. *N Engl J Med* 1980;**302**:362–4.
91 Glenn F, McSherry CK. Pregnancy, cholesterol metabolism and gallstones. *Ann Surg* 1969;**169**:712–23.
92 Fisher RS, Stelzer F, Rock E *et al.* Abnormal gallbladder emptying in patients with gallstones. *Dig Dis Sci* 1982;**27**:1019–24.
93 Sylwestrowicz TA, Shaffer EA. Gallbladder function during gallstone dissolution. Effect of bile acid therapy in patients with gallstones. *Gastroenterology* 1988; **95**(3):740–8.
94 Forgacs IC, Maisey MN, Murphy GM *et al.* Influence of gallstones and ursodeoxycholic acid therapy on

gallbladder emptying. *Gastroenterology* 1984;**87**: 299–307.
95 Masclee AAM, Jansen JBMJ, Driessen WMM *et al.* Plasma cholecystokinin and gallbladder responses to intraduodenal fat in gallstone patients. *Dig Dis Sci* 1989;**34**:353–9.
96 Spengler U, Sackmann M, Sauerbruch T *et al.* Gallbladder motility before and after extracorporeal lithotripsy. *Gastroenterology* 1989;**96**:860–3.
97 van der Werf SDJ, van Berge Henegouwen GP, Plasma DMH, Ruben AT. Motor function of the gallbladder and cholesterol saturation of the duodenal bile. *Neth J Med* 1987;30:160–71.
98 Stone BG, Gavaler JS, Belle SH *et al.* Impairment of gallbladder emptying in diabetes melitus. *Gastroenterology* 1988;**95**:170–6.
99 Davion T, Tossou H, Delamarre J *et al.* Racial differences in gallbladder motor function. *Lancet* 1989;1:724–5.
100 Been JM, Bills PM, Lewis D. Microstructure of gallstones. *Gastroenterology* 1979;**76**:548–55.
101 Lonsdale K. Epitaxy as a growth factor in urinary calculi and gallstones. *Nature* 1968;**217**:56–8.
102 Shiffman ML, Sugarman HJ, Kellum JM, *et al.* Free calcium ion [Ca^{++}] is increased in gallbladder bile of patients with all types of gallstones. *Hepatology* 1989;**10**:601. (Abstract).
103 Strichartz SD, Abedin MZ, Abdou MS, Roslyn JJ. Increased biliary calcium in cholesterol gallstone formation. *Am J Surg* 1988;**155**:131–7.
104 Moore EW. Biliary calcium and gallstone formation. *Hepatology* 1990;**12**(3):206S–218S.
105 Kibe A, Dudley MA, Halpern Z *et al.* Factors affecting cholesterol monohydrate nucleation time in model solutions of supersaturated bile. *J Lipid Res* 1985; **26**:1102–11.
106 Papahadijopoulos D, Vail WJ, Pangborn WA, *et al.* Studies on membrane fusion. II. Induction of fusion in pure phospholipid membranes by calcium ions and other divalent metals. *Biochim Biophys Acta* 1976;**448**:265–83.
107 Berenson MM, Cardinal JR. Calcium accelerates cholesterol phase transitions in analog bile. *Experientia* 1985:**41**:1328–30.
108 Toor EW, Evans DF, Cussler EL. The nucleation of cholesterol monohydrate crystals in model bile solution. In: Fisher MM, Goresky CA, Shaffer EA, Strasberg SM, eds. *Gallstones.* New York: Plenum Press, 1979:169–81.
109 Forstner JF. Intestinal mucins in health and disease. *Digestion* 1978;**17**:234–63.
110 Jones CA, Hofmann AF, Mysels KJ, Roda A. The effect of calcium and sodium ion concentration on the properties of dilute aqeuous solution of glycine conjugated bile salts: phase behavior and solubility products of the calcium salts of the common glycine bile acids. *J Colloid Inter Sci* 1986;**114**:452–70.
111 Almong S, Lichtenberg D. Effect of calcium on kinetic and structural aspects of dilution-induced micellar to lamellar phase transformation in phosphatidylcholine–cholate mixures. *Blood* 1988;**27**:873–80.
112 Nahrwold DL, Rose RC, Ward SP. Abnormalities in gallbladder morphology and function in patients with cholelithiasis. *Ann Surg* 1976;**184**:415–21.
113 Lee SP. Enhanced fluid transport across gallbladder mucosa in experimental cholelithiasis. *Am J Physiol* 1978;3:E575–8.
114 Conter RL, Roslyn JJ, Porter-Fink V *et al.* Gallbladder absorption increases during early cholesterol gallstone formation. *Am J Surg* 1986;**151**:184–91.
115 Abdou MS, Strichartz SD, Abedin MZ *et al.* Biliary lipids alter ion transport during cholesterol gallstone formation. *J Surg Res* 1988;**44**:672–8.
116 Roslyn JJ, Abedin MZ, Strichartz SD *et al.* Regulation of gallbladder ion transport: role of biliary lipids. *Surgery* 1989;**155**:207–12.
117 LaMorte WW, Booker ML, Scott TE *et al.* Increases in gallbladder prostaglandin synthesis before the formation of cholesterol gallstones. *Surgery* 1985;**98**: 445–51.
118 Strichartz SD, Abedin MZ, Song MK *et al.* Altered biliary prostaglandins and cholesterol gallstones: an *in vivo* study. *J Surg Res* 1989;**46**:620–4.
119 England DW, Jaffe BM, Webb H, Hoover EL. The prostaglandin response to cholesterol feeding by the rabbit gallbladder *in vitro*. *Surgery* 1988;**103**(1):69–73.
120 Stuart MJ, Gerrard JM, White JG. Effect of cholesterol on production of thromboxane B_2 by platelets *in vitro*. *N Engl J Med* 1980;**302**:6–10.
121 Kramer RM, Jakubowski JA, Vaillancourt R *et al.* Effect of membrane cholesterol on phospholipid metabolism in thrombin-stimulated platelets. *J Biol Chem* 1982;**257**:6844–9.
122 LaMont JT, Turner BS, DiBenedetto D *et al.* Arachidonic acid stimulates mucin secretion in prairie dog gallbladder. *Am J Physiol* 1983;**245**:G92–8.
123 Myers SI, Haley-Russell D, Bartula L *et al.* Long-term cholesterol feeding stimulates increased bile phospholipids and gallbladder prostanoid synthesis. *Surgery* 1991;**109**:656–62.
124 Kotwall CA, Clanachan AS, Baer HP *et al.* Effects of prostaglandins on motility in gallbladders removed from patients with gallstones. *Arch Surg* 1984; **119**:709–12.
125 Andersson KE, Hedner P, Persson CGA. Differentiation of the contractile effects of prostaglandin E_2 and C-terminal octapeptide of cholecystokinin in isolated guinea pig gallbladder. *Acta Physiol Scand* 1974;**90**:657–63.
126 Ramwell PW, Shaw JE. Biological significance of prostaglandins. In: Astwood EB, ed. *Recent Progress in Hormone Research.* New York: Academic Press, 1970: Vol 26, 139.
127 Leyssac P, Bukhave K, Frederikesen O. Inhibitory effect of prostaglandins on isomotic fluid transport

by rabbit gallbladder *in vitro*, and its modification by blockade of endogenous PGE-biosynthesis with indomethacin. *Acta Physiol Scand* 1974;**92**:496–507.
128 Moser AJ, Abedin MZ, Roslyn JJ. Eicosanoids mediate gallbladder (GB) secretory function. 26th Annual Meeting of the Association for Academic Surgeons, Montreal, Canada, Nov 18–21, 1992. (Abstract).
129 Myers SI, Cheung LY. Prostacyclin (PGI) biosynthesis and its effect on luminal fluid absorption in gallbladder. *Surg Forum* 1984;**35**:229–30.
130 Maki T. Pathogenesis of calcium bilirubinate gallstone. *Ann Surg* 1966;**164**:90–100.
131 Vitetta L, Sali A, Moritz V *et al.* Bacteria and gallstone nucleation. *Aust NZ J Surg* 1989;**59**(7):571–7.
132 Miyke H, Johnson CG. Gallstones: Ethnological studies. *Digestion* 1968;**1**:219–28.
133 Trotman BW, Soloway RD. Pigment vs. cholesterol cholelithiasis: clinical and epidemiological aspects. *Am J Dig Dis* 1975;**20**:735–40.
134 Nagase M, Hikasa Y, Soloway RD *et al.* Gallstones in Western Japan. Features affecting the prevalence of intrahepatic gallstones. *Gastroenterology* 1980;**78**: 684–90.
135 van der Linden W, Nakayama F. Gallstone disease in Sweden versus Japan: clinical and etiological aspects. *Am J Surg* 1973;**125**:267–72.
136 Vitteta L, Sali A, Chou ST *et al.* Gallstones at autopsy and cholecystectomy: A comparative study. *Aust NZ J Surg* 1988;**58**:561–8.
137 Schoenfield LJ. Pathogenesis of cholelithiasis. In: Schoenfield LJ, ed. *Disease of the Gallbladder and Biliary System.* New York: Wiley, 1977:81–107.
138 Trotman BW, Soloway RD. Pigment gallstone disease. Summary of the National Institutes of Health International Workshop. *Hepatology* 1982;**2**:879–84.
139 Soloway RD, Trotman BW. Bile pigment gallstones. In Osrow JD, ed. *Bile Pigments and Jaundice*. New York: Marcel Dekker, 1986:581–600.
140 Dotey JE, Pitt HA, Porter-Fink V *et al.* The effect of intravenous fat and total parenteral nutrition on biliary physiology. *J Parenter Enteral Nutr* 1984;**8**: 263–8.
141 Cetta FM. Bile infection documented as initial event in the pathogenesis of brown pigment biliary stones. *Hepatology* 1986;**6**:482–9.
142 Bates GL, Brown GH. Incidence of gallbladder disease in chronic hemolytic anemia (spherocytosis). *Gastroenterology* 1952;**21**:104–9.
143 Bouchier IAD. Postmortem study of the frequency of gallstones in patients with cirrhosis of the liver. *Gut* 1969;**10**:705–10.
144 Tamalet E. La lithiase biliarire d'origine paludeenne. *Journal Medical Français* 1932;**21**:159–64.
145 Roslyn JJ, Pitt HA, Mann LL *et al.* Gallbladder disease in patients on long-term parenteral nutrition. *Gastroenterology* 1983;**84**:148–54.
146 Stewart L, Smith AL, Pellegrini CA *et al.* Pigment gallstones form as a composite of bacterial microcolonies and pigment solids. *Ann Surg* 1987;**206**:242–50.
147 Kaufman HS, Magnuson TH, Lillemoe KD *et al.* The role of bacteria in gallbladder and common duct stone formation. *Ann Surg* 1989;**209**:584–91.
148 Delikaris PG, Michail PO, Klonis GD *et al.* Biliary bacteriology based on intraoperative bile cultures. *Am J Gastroenterol* 1977;**68**:51–5.
149 Cetta F. The role of bacteria in pigment gallstone disease. *Ann Surg* 1991;**213**(4):315–26.
150 Trotman BW. Insight into pigment stone disease. *J Lab Clin Med* 1979;**93**:349–56.
151 Wosiewitz U, Althoff J, Langhans P. Beta-glucuronidase activity in human cholesterol and pigment stone bile. *Z Gastroenterol* 1979;**17**(5):301–9.
152 Everson GT, Nemeth A, Kourourian S *et al.* Gallbladder function is altered in sickle hemoglobinopathy. *Gastroenterology* 1989;**96**:1307–16.
153 Jordan RA. Cholelithiasis in sickle cell disease. *Gastroenterology* 1957;**33**:952–8.
154 Angelin B, Einarsson K, Ewerth S *et al.* Biliary lipid composition in patients with portal cirrhosis of the liver. *Scand J Gastroenterol* 1980;**15**:849–52.
155 Madden JL. Primary common duct stones. *World J Surg* 1978;**2**:465–9.
156 Bartlett MK: Retained and recurrent common duct stones. *Am Surg* 1972;**38**:63–8.
157 Way LW, Bernhoft RA, Thomas MJ: Biliary stricture. *Surg Clin North Am* 1981;**61**:963–72.
158 Lygidikas NJ. Incidence and significance of primary stones of the common bile duct in choledocholithiasis. *Surg Gynecol Obstet* 1983;**157**:434–9.
159 Toouli J, Bushell M, Innanos J *et al.* Preoperative sphincter of Oddi manometry: motility disorder in patients with cholelithiasis. *Aust NZ J Surg* 1986; **56**:625–9.
160 Wong HN, Frey CF, Gagic NM. Intraoperative common duct pressure and flow measurements. *Am J Surg* 1980;**139**:691–5.
161 Toouli J, Jeenen JE, Hogan WJ *et al.* Sphincter of Oddi motor activity: A comparison between patients with common bile duct stones and controls. *Gastroenterology* 1982;**82**:111–17.
162 De Masi E, Coraziarri E, Habib FI *et al.* Manometric study of the sphincter of Oddi in patients with and without common bile duct stones. *Gut* 1984;**25**: 275–8.
163 Nakayama F, Soloway Rd Nakama T *et al.* Hepatolithiasis in East Asia: retrospective study. *Dig Dis Sci* 1986;**31**:21–6.
164 Nakyama F, Koga A. Hepatolithiasis: Present status. *World J Surg* 1984;**8**:9–14.
165 Matshubrio T, Susuki N, Sato T *et al.* Effects of diet on glauaric acid concentration in bile and the formation of calcium bilirubinate gallstones. *Gastroenterology* 1977;**72**:630–8.
166 Trotman BW. Pigment gallstone disease. *Gastroenterol Clin N Am* 1991;**20**:111–26.

167 Carey MC, Cahalane MJ. Enterohepatic circulation. In: Arias IM, Jakoby WB, Popper H, Schachter D, Shafritz DA, eds. *The liver: Biology and Pathobiology.* New York: Raven Press, 1988:573–616.
168 Harvey PRC, Somjen GJ, Gilat T, Gallinger S, Strasberg SM. Vesicular cholesterol in bile: relationship to protein concentration and nucleation time. *Biochem Biophys Acta* 1988;**958**:10–18.
169 Mazer NA. Quasielastic light scattering studies of aqeous biliary lipid systems and native bile. *Hepatology* 1990;**12**:395–445.
170 Reuss L, Segal Y, Altenberg G. Regulation of ion transport across gallbladder epithelium. *Annu Rev Physiol* 1991;53;361–73.
171 Holzbach RT. Pathogenesis and medical treatment of gallstones. In: Sleisinger MH, Fordtran JS, eds. *Gastrointestinal Diseases.* Philadelphia: Saunders, 1989:1356–1372.
172 Busch N, Holzbach RT. Crystal growth-inhibiting proteins in bile. *Hepatology* 1990;**12**(3):195S–9S.
173 Lee SP. Pathogenesis of biliary sludge. *Hepatology* 1990;**12**(3):200S–205S.
174 Lee SP, Park HZ, Mandani H, Kaler EW. Partial characterization of a nonmicellar system of cholesterol solubilization in bile. *Am J Physiol* 1987;**225**:G374–83.
175 Doty JE, Pitt HA, Kuchenbecker SL *el al.* Impaired gallbladder emptying before gallstone formation. *Gastroenterology* 1983;**85**:168–74.
176 Moore EW. Biliary calcium and gallstone formation. *Hepatology* 1990;**12**(3):206S–18S.
177 Carey MC. Formation of cholesterol gallstones; the new paradigms. In: Paumgartner G, Stiehl A, Gerok W, eds. *Trends in Bile Acid Research.* Dordrecht: Kluwer, 1989:259–81.

Chapter 2
Natural history of gallstone disease

E.J. Gibney

Introduction

Despite the high prevalence of gallstones in the adult population of developed countries, there remain many gaps in our knowledge of the natural history of gallstones and of the factors which dictate whether or not they will become symptomatic in a particular patient [1]. Nevertheless, knowledge of the natural history of gallstones is of paramount importance in advising patients with asymptomatic gallstones, as to whether or not treatment is indicated. Such stones are usually confined within the gallbladder. However, it is increasingly recognized that many patients with common bile duct stones may not develop symptoms [2, 3] and often pass such stones asymptomatically through the ampulla of Vater [4, 5]. The advent of laparoscopic cholecystectomy has made the decision-making process in such patients even more relevant today than it formerly has been.

What determines whether or not a gallstone becomes symptomatic is largely unclear [6]. The natural history of gallstones may be influenced by local factors in the gallbladder and biliary tree, and also by systemic factors. It is recognized that gallstones may behave differently in different patient groups. For example, patients with diabetes mellitus form one such group [1]. Stone size and duct anatomy may also be important in determining the course of events and conditions promoting gallbladder stasis are also of relevance in this context. It is clear, therefore, that once the gallbladder contains stones, there are many factors which may possibly influence subsequent events. Therefore, predicting the course of events in an individual patient cannot often be done with great accuracy [7]. Nevertheless, much is known about the natural history and the risks of symptom development in the population in general and in certain subgroups of patients [1]. The relationship between gallstones and the development of gallbladder carcinoma must also be examined when considering the natural history of gallstones, as must the role of gallstones in the aetiology of pancreatitis.

Gallstones: formation and prevalence

Although traditionally gallstones have been classified as cholesterol, pigment, and mixed types, there is often no clear division between these three classifications [8]. Pure cholesterol stones are rare and most stones which are predominantly cholesterol have a significant amount of pigment in them. Cholesterol stones are believed to form primarily because the bile becomes supersaturated with cholesterol and this occurs when an imbalance between the concentrations of cholesterol, lecithin and bile acids takes place [9, 10]. This has been expressed mathematically as a lithogenic index.

The prevalence of pigment stones shows considerable geographical variation and these stones occur typically in conditions which cause haemolysis and in hepatic cirrhosis. In addition, pigment stones may also be formed in association with biliary infections. They are believed to form due to an excess of unconjugated bilirubin in bile leading eventually to the formation of insoluble calcium bilirubinate and subsequent stone formation. Stasis, sludge formation, and the presence of ova or foreign bodies may also play an important role as a nidus for stone formation. The importance of biliary sludge has received increasing attention because of a recognized association with intrinsic gallbladder pathology [11], with pancreatitis [12, 13], and because of the high incidence of subsequent gallstone formation in patients with sludge [14].

Many now believe that gallstones arise because of a combination of supersaturated bile, increased crystal formation, and reduced gallbladder contractility [15]. Once stones have formed, however, there appears to be no evidence to suggest that the likelihood or otherwise of symptom development is related to the type of stone which has formed, unless the primary pathogenic factor is associated with symptoms in its own right (e.g., biliary infection or infestation).

Studies have shown that approximately 10–20% of adults in developed countries have gallstones [16–21], and the prevalence of gallstones has been clearly documented to be higher in women [16, 20–22], in obese patients [23, 24], and to increase with age [16, 20, 21]. Some particular groups are especially prone to the development of gallstones including certain American Indian tribes, where the incidence may reach up to 75% in young adults [25]. Gallstones are common in the Far East and biliary tract infection and infestation play a more important role in the aetiology of gallstones in this part of the world than elsewhere.

The prevalence of common duct stones (as detected by routine operative cholangiography in patients undergoing surgery for cholelithiasis) varies but usually is of the order of 10–15% [26]. The prevalence of symptomatic common duct stones is considerably lower than this [2, 27]. Most common bile duct stones are believed to form in the gallbladder (where concentration of bile and stasis make better conditions for stone formation), and subsequently pass into the common bile duct, but primary common bile duct stones may also occur.

Initial symptoms

Symptomatic gallstone disease generally implies the occurrence of biliary pain, acute cholecystitis, biliary obstruction or pancreatitis in the presence of gallstones. Rarer presentations include bowel obstruction secondary to gallstone ileus. Painless dyspepsia is no longer considerecd to be more frequent in those with gallstones as opposed to those without [20, 21, 28]. There is usually a latent period of several years between stone formation and symptom development in those patients who do develop symptoms. One study, which used carbon dating techniques on retrieved stones, found a mean latent period of 8 years [29].

In patients who become symptomatic, there is considerable dispute as to what the commonest initial symptoms are. Some studies have suggested that uncomplicated biliary pain is the commonest initial manifestation [30, 31], while others have concluded that acute cholecystitis is the most frequent mode of presentation. This occurred as the initial symptom of gallbladder disease in 77% of patients in one study [32]. These differences may to a large degree depend on the criteria used to differentiate cholecystitis from biliary colic. Indeed, there is often a relatively poor correlation between the clinical features, ultrasonic findings, operative appearances, and pathological findings. Since the pathogenic mechanism of both acute cholecystitis and biliary colic (i.e., obstruction of the cystic duct by a stone) is believed to be the same, it is probably not of great importance epidemiologically whether patients' initial symptoms are classified as pure colic or inflammatory and infective.

Although gallstones are a significant cause of pancreatitis, this appears to be the least common initial presenting feature of gallstones. A number of recent studies have suggested, however, that many of what were formerly considered to be cases of idiopathic pancreatitis may in fact be due to gallstones or biliary sludge [12, 13] (Table 2.1).

Table 2.1 Manifestations of gallstones

None–asymptomatic
Biliary pain
Cholecystitis
Pancreatitis
Obstructive jaundice
Cholangitis
Gallstone ileus
Gallbladder carcinoma

Natural history of gallstones

Symptomatic gallbladder stones

Patients with symptomatic gallbladder stones are almost universally advised to undergo cholecystectomy if they are considered medically fit for surgery [33]. Because of this there are few studies which examine the risks of subsequent symptoms or complications in symptomatic patients. Truesdell noted, however, that it was not unusual for a patient to experience a single typical attack of biliary pain followed by a long period of freedom from symptoms—so called quiescent gallstones [34]. In Lund's series there were almost 500 non-operated symptomatic patients followed for 5–20 years after gallstone diagnosis. Between one-third and one-half were shown to develop severe symptoms and/or complications [35]. In a 2-year follow-up of 305 patients assigned to non-operative placebo management of diagnosed gallstone disease, 69% of those who had had one or more episodes of biliary pain in the 12 months before the study reported recurrent pain, compared to only 31% of patients who had been pain-free in the year before the study [36]. McSherry and colleagues studied the natural history of gallstone disease for a mean of 78 months in 691 non-operated patients [37]. Of these, 556 were considered symptomatic, and in the follow-up period about half of those with mild symptoms (40% of the entire symptomatic group) did not experience any increase in symptom severity. These studies suggest that many patients with symptomatic gallstones may not develop severe symptoms or complications over prolonged periods of time. Observations such as these have led to suggestions that a 'delayed surgical strategy' may be advantageous in the management of cholelithiasis [38], and it has also been suggested that higher surgical rates may be associated with increased mortality [38, 39]. Nevertheless, given that it is currently not possible to predict with any great accuracy those patients whose symptoms are likely to remain mild or who will not develop complications, and in the light of the current low morbidity and mortality rates for cholecystectomy, surgeons are likely to continue to recommend cholecystectomy to patients with symptomatic gallbladder stones [37].

Asymptomatic gallbladder stones

Over the years there have been numerous studies which have attempted to define the risks of symptom development in patients with gallstones who are initially asymptomatic at the time of gallstone detection. Most of the earlier reports which addressed this issue recommended cholecystectomy, as the authors concluded that symptom development was common, with an incidence of between about 30 and 45% [34, 40, 41]. These studies, however, were based entirely on groups of patients in whom the detection of gallstones was made initially at laparotomy for other conditions. Such patients, however, may constitute a select group at greater risk of developing symptoms than patients with asymptomatic gallstones detected non-invasively [1]. This matter is further discussed below when considering the effects of gallbladder stasis on symptom development.

Studies on patients in whom asymptomatic gallbladder stones have been detected radiologically, or by ultrasonography, have reached varying conclusions. Lund found that of 34 patients with asymptomatic stones, about one-third went on to develop significant symptoms and he recommended cholecystectomy in patients considered to be good surgical risks [35]. Wenckert and Robertson recommended cholecystectomy for patients with asymptomatic stones. This was based on their study, which found that more than one-third of patients subsequently developed symptoms on follow-up [42]. However, this conclusion is open to criticism because the group of patients studied were not uniformally asymptomatic at the beginning of the observation period.

Two more recent reports, however, have contradicted these earlier findings and concluded with substantially different figures for the risks of symptom development. Gracie and Ransohoff studied 123 patients with asymptomatic stones (detected by cholecystographic screening of a healthy group of university faculty members) and found that only 18% of these became symptomatic during a follow-up period of 15 years [43]. This particular study was by no means ideal in that the majority of the study group were men (110 of the 123 patients), and also because 35 of the group underwent prophylactic cholecystectomy on medical advice soon after gallstone detection. Despite these objections, however, the basic findings of the study are probably valid and suggest that the long-term risk of symptom development in patients with gallstones is somewhere in the order of 20%. Whether the risk would substantially increase after more than 15 years is a matter for conjecture. This tendency for asymptomatic gallbladder stones to remain silent in the medium- to long-term has been confirmed in a study by McSherry *et al.* who followed 135 patients for a mean of 5 years and found that only 10.4% developed symptoms [37].

It is interesting to note that in a small percentage of cases gallbladder stones have been documented to disappear spontaneously [36]. This may occur in one of two ways. Gallstones may fragment (or already be small enough) and pass asymptomatically via the cystic and common bile duct into the gastrointestinal tract. Alternatively, changes in the composition of bile might result in gallstone dissolution. Either way spontaneous disappearance of documented gallbladder stones is an unusual event.

Factors influencing the natural history of gallstones

Diabetes mellitus

There have been many studies over the years which have shown that the presence of gallstones in diabetics constitutes a greater threat to health than in non-diabetics. Traditionally, diabetics with gallstones have been considered to be at greater risk of complication development and indeed of mortality when complications do develop [44, 45]. Thus, most authors have recommended cholecystectomy in diabetics with gallstones regardless of whether or not they have symptoms.

While many believe that gallstones are more common in diabetics, there is little solid evidence to support this belief [24]. However, the results of a number of studies suggest that acute cholecystitis is more common in patients with diabetes mellitus, with combined data from a number of studies suggesting that about 15% of patients with acute cholecystitis have diabetes mellitus [32, 46, 47]. However, this conclusion has been reached largely by indirect evidence showing an over-representation of diabetics among a series of patients who presented with acute cholecystitis. Given the uncertainties with regard to the prevalence of gallstones in diabetics and thus the real risk of symptom development, it is not known with certainty whether diabetics are more prone than non-diabetics to symptom development if they have stones. It may be concluded, however, from the studies that are available, that if symptoms do develop they are more likely to be severe, and more likely to lead to the need for emergency surgery [46], with an attendant higher morbidity and mortality rate [44–47].

It is clear, therefore, that further studies are required to define more precisely the relationship between gallstones and diabetes mellitus. But until the results of such studies are available current knowledge does suggest that the natural history of gallstones is different in the diabetic when compared to the non-diabetic.

Unrelated surgery and gallbladder stasis

The role of stasis in precipitating symptom development in patients with gallbladder disease is well recognized. Even in the absence of gallstones, conditions which promote stasis are among the main predisposing factors for the development of acalculous cholecystitis. The stress of surgery itself is one such stasis-promoting factor and many studies have addressed the issue of the likelihood of symptom development in patients in whom gallstones were first detected at laparotomy. If such patients are compared to those in whom asymptomatic gallstones are initially discovered by ultrasound or other non-invasive techniques, then it appears that patients whose stones are detected initially at laparotomy are at greater risk of subsequent symptom development both in the short-term and in the long-term future.

Table 2.2 Factors which may influence the natural history of gallstones

Intervention (medical, surgical)
Diabetes mellitus
Bile stasis
Unrelated abdominal surgery
Hormonal factors (female sex)

Peterson found that 37.2% of 51 patients developed symptoms, although all of the patients were not strictly asymptomatic at the time of their original surgery [40]. Truesdell followed a similar group of patients (all women) whose stones were detected at laparotomy for pelvic disease and found a high incidence of subsequent symptom development [34]. The group studied by Comfort and colleagues [41] provided less useful information since painless dyspepsia was included as a symptom indicative of gallbladder disease.

More recent studies have also confirmed the tendency for patients with asymptomatic gallstones to become symptomatic following unrelated surgery. Thompson *et al.* studied 23 patients previously asymptomatic, 16 of whom developed biliary symptoms within 6 months of a primary operation [48]. In a study of 11 patients by Ouriel *et al.* [49], eight developed biliary symptoms over a mean follow-up period of 2.9 years, and 13 of 25 patients in a group studied by Saade *et al.* [50] became symptomatic within 2 years, as did 11 of the 17 patients studied by String [51]. From these reports it is apparent that abdominal aortic surgery seems to be particularly associated with a significant risk of precipitating symptoms in patients with previously 'silent' stones. Why unrelated surgery should be associated with a short- to medium-term increase in the risk of symptom development in patients with asymptomatic gallstones remains a matter for conjecture. Clearly, changes in bile composition peri-operatively and bile stasis may play a role particularly in those patients in whom symptoms develop soon after operation. However, it is less clear as to why the apparent increased risk seems to carry over into the following number of years as well as in the immediate post-operative period.

Hormonal factors

A number of studies have suggested that women are more prone to develop symptoms from gallstones than men [20, 21, 35]. Hormonal factors have been considered to be the most likely explanation for these differences, with differences in bile composition and changes in biliary motility cited as possible mechanisms [24]. Similar factors may also be responsible for the apparent tendency for pregnancy to precipitate symptoms in women with pre-existing stones [24] (Table 2.2).

Choledocholithiasis

The prevalence of common bile duct stones in patients with gallbladder stones varies but is usually of the order of 10–15%. For example, in one study of common duct stones (both symptomatic and asymptomatic) detected by routine operative cholangiography in over 11 000 patients, the prevalence was found to be 13.3% [26]. Many of these stones are unsuspected and asymptomatic, and the clinical significance of such stones is disputed. Nevertheless, the key to the development of reliable guidelines for the management of such patients depends upon a knowledge of the natural history of such stones. There is increasing evidence that the majority of unsuspected stones (which are present in about 6% of patients undergoing cholecystectomy for gallstones [2, 26]) remain asymptomatic [2, 27]. It has been estimated that only one in ten of such stones will ever become symptomatic [27]. While many smaller stones may pass asymptomatically into the duodenum, it has also been pointed out that the incidence of unsuspected stones as detected by routine operative cholangiography closely approximates to the incidence of incidental common duct stones found at post-mortem examination [52].

Gallstone pancreatitis

Gallstone pancreatitis constitutes one of the most life-threatening complications of gallstone disease, and is believed to occur due to transient blockage of the ampulla of Vater by migrating gallstones

[53]. The majority of such stones pass spontaneously, and the incidence of detectable common duct stones in gallstone pancreatitis has been shown to be about 70% in the first 24 hours, 20% by the 3rd day, and to reach a plateau of about 14% by the 10th day [54]. Knowledge of this natural tendency towards spontaneous passage has guided surgeons in determining the optimum timing of gallbladder surgery in such patients and focussed attention on methods to allow early identification of patients with severe gallstone-associated pancreatitis who might benefit from urgent endoscopic sphincterotomy [55]. It is also of interest to note that a number of studies now suggest that biliary sludge, believed to be a precursor of gallstones [11, 14], is probably an important factor in the aetiology of many cases of what were hitherto considered to be idiopathic pancreatitis [12, 13].

Gallbladder carcinoma and gallstones

Carcinoma of the gallbladder is an uncommon neoplasm which occurs predominantly in elderly women. It is associated with a very poor prognosis with a 1 year survival rate of approximately 10% and less than 5% of patients are alive 5 years after diagnosis [56]. Seventy per cent of patients with gallbladder carcinoma have gallstones but only 1–2% of patients with gallstones subsequently develop carcinoma of the gallbladder. It has been calculated by Diehl and Beral [57] that one fewer death from gallbladder cancer occurs for every 100 cholecystectomies performed during the previous year. However, most authors agree that advocating cholecystectomy on the basis of preventing gallbladder carcinoma is not justified in patients whose stones are exhibiting no symptoms [1]. Whether or not factors in relation to the gallstones themselves may be associated with higher risks of carcinoma in some patients is not known. One report [58] suggested a significantly greater risk of gallbladder cancer in patients with larger stones but this finding remains to be confirmed.

Summary and conclusions

While much is now known about the factors which predispose to gallstone formation, we know considerably less about the factors which determine whether or not symptoms will develop. There is evidence to suggest that patients whose initial symptoms are mild, if left untreated, have a low risk of progression to severe symptoms, at least in the early years following diagnosis. Asymptomatic patients with gallbladder stones appear to have a low risk (about 10–20%) of symptom development in the 5–15 years after diagnosis, but diabetes mellitus, unrelated abdominal surgery, and female sex all increase the likelihood of symptoms developing. Many unsuspected common bile duct stones remain asymptomatic if left untreated, and the relationship between gallstones and gallbladder carcinoma is not sufficiently strong for the prevention of gallbladder carinoma to be considered an important factor in considering treatment options for patients with gallstones.

References

1 Gibney EJ. Asymptomatic gallstones. *Br J Surg* 1990; 77:368–72.
2 Gerber A, Apt MK. The case against routine operative cholangiography. *Am J Surg* 1982;143:734–6.
3 McEntee G, Grace PA, Bouchier-Hayes D. Laparoscopic cholecystectomy and the common bile duct. *Br J Surg* 1991;78:385–6.
4 Gardner AM, Holden WS, Monks PJW. Disappearing gallstones. *Br J Surg* 1966;53:114–20.
5 Gerber A. A requiem for the routine operative cholangiogram. *Surg Gynecol Obstet* 1986;163:363–4.
6 Bouchier IAD, Rhodes K, Brien M. A study of symptomatic and 'silent' gallstone. *Scand J Gastroent* 1968;3: 299–304.
7 Donaldson RM. Advice for the patient with 'silent' gallstones. *N Engl J Med* 1982;307:815–17.
8 Nahrwold DL. Chronic cholecystitis and cholelithiasis. In: Sabiston DC, ed. *Textbook of Surgery. The Biological Basis of Modern Surgical Practice.* 14th edn. Philadelphia: Saunders, 1991:1057–63.
9 Admirand WH, Small DM. The physicochemical basis of cholesterol gallstone formation in man. *J Clin Invest* 1968;47:1043–52.
10 Holzbach RT, Marsh M, Olszewski M, Holan K. Cholesterol solubility in bile with evidence that supersaturated bile is frequent in man. *J Clin Invest* 1973;52:1467–79.
11 Jennings WC, Drabek GA, Miller KA. Significance of sludge and thickened wall in ultrasound evaluation of the gallbladder. *Surg Gynecol Obstet* 1992;174:394–8.

12 Ros E, Navarro S, Bru C, Garcia-Puges A, Valderrama R. Occult microlithiasis in idiopathic acute pancreatitis: prevention of relapses by cholecystectomy or ursodeoxycholic acid therapy. *Gastroenterology* 1991;**101**:1701–9.

13 Lee SP, Nicholls JF, Park HZ. Biliary sludge as a cause of acute pancreatitis. *N Engl J Med* 1992;**326**:589–93.

14 Editorial. Biliary sludge. *Lancet* 1992;**339**:1087.

15 Paumgartner G, Sauerbruch T. Gallstones: pathogenesis. *Lancet* 1991;**338**:1117–21.

16 Godrey PJ, Bates T, Harrison M, King MB, Padley NR. Gallstones and mortality: a study of all gallstone related deaths in a single health district. *Gut* 1984;**25**:1029–33.

17 Bainton D, Davies GT, Evans KT, Gravelle IH. Gallbladder disease. Prevalence in a South Wales industrial town. *N Engl J Med* 1976;**294**:1147–9.

18 Wilbur RS, Bolt RJ. Incidence of gallbladder disease in 'normal' men. *Gastroenterology* 1959;**36**:251–5.

19 Barker DJP, Gardner MJ, Power C, Hutt MSR. Prevalence of gall stones at necropsy in nine British towns: a collaborative study. *Br Med J* 1979;**ii**:1389–92.

20 Rome Group for the Epidemiology and Prevention of Cholelithiasis (GREPCO). Prevalence of gallstone disease in an adult female population. *Am J Epidemiology* 1984;**119**:796–805.

21 Rome Group for the Epidemiology and Prevention of Cholelithiasis (GREPCO). The epidemiology of gallstone disease in Rome, Italy. Part I. Prevalence data in men. *Hepatology* 1988;**8**:904–6.

22 Bateson MC, Bouchier IAD. Prevalence of gallstones in Dundee: a necropsy study. *Br Med J* 1975;**iv**:427–30.

23 Tucker LE, Tangedahl TN, Newmark SR. Prevalence of gallstones in obese Caucasian American women. *Int J Obes* 1982;**6**:247–51.

24 Bennion LJ, Grundy SM. Risk factors for the development of cholelithiasis in man (Second of two parts). *N Engl J Med* 1978;**299**:1221–27.

25 Sampliner RE, Bennett PH, Comess LJ, Rose FA, Burch TA. Gallbladder disease in Pima Indians: Demonstration of high prevalence and early onset by cholecystography. *N Engl J Med* 1970;**283**:1358–64.

26 Gibney EJ. Operative cholangiography: selective or routine? *J Ir Coll Physicians Surg* 1989;**18**:259–64.

27 Starke ME, Loughry CW. Routine operative cholangiography with cholecystectomy. *Surg Gynecol Obstet* 1980;**151**:657–8.

28 Price WH. Gall-bladder dyspepsia. *Br Med J* 1963;**ii**:138–41.

29 Mok HY, Druffel ER, Rampone WM. Chronology of cholelithiasis. Dating gallstones from atmospheric radiocarbon produced by nuclear bomb explosions. *N Engl J Med* 1986;**314**:1075–7.

30 Ransohoff DF, Gracie WA, Wolfenson LB, Neuhauser D. Prophylactic cholecystectomy or expectant management for silent gallstones. A decision analysis to assess survival. *Ann Intern Med* 1983;**99**:199–204.

31 Newman HF, Northup JD, Rosenblum M, Abrams H. Complications of cholelithiasis. *Am J Gastroenterol* 1968;**50**:476–96.

32 Pickleman J, Gonzales RP. The improving results of cholecystectomy. *Arch Surg* 1986;**121**:930–4.

33 Diehl AK. Silent gallstones: the doctor's dilemma. *Comprehensive Therapy* 1982;**8**:62–8.

34 Truesdell ED. The frequency and future of gallstones believed to be quiescent or symptomless. *Ann Surg* 1944;**119**:232–45.

35 Lund J. Surgical indications in cholelithiasis: prophylactic cholecystectomy elucidated on the basis of long-term follow up on 526 nonoperated cases. *Ann Surg* 1960;**151**:153–62.

36 Thistle JL, Cleary PA, Lachin JM, Tyor MP, Hersh T. The natural history of cholelithiasis: the national cooperative gallstone study. *Ann Intern Med* 1984;**101**:171–5.

37 McSherry CK, Ferstenberg H, Calhoun WF, Lahman E, Virshup M. The natural history of diagnosed gallstone disease in symptomatic and asymptomatic patients. *Ann Surg* 1985;**202**:59–63.

38 Hoey J, Psihramis K. Cholelithiasis: a comparison of surgical and nonsurgical management strategies based on available evidence. *Clin Invest Med* 1979;**2**:75–81.

39 Vayda E. A comparison of surgical rates in Canada and in England and Wales. *N Engl J Med* 1973;**289**:1224–9.

40 Peterson R. Gall-stones during the course of 1 066 abdominal sections for pelvic disease. *Surg Gynecol Obstet* 1915;**20**:284–91.

41 Comfort MW, Gray HK, Wilson JM. The silent gallstone: a ten to twenty year follow-up of 112 cases. *Ann Surg* 1948;**128**:931–7.

42 Wenckert A, Robertson B. The natural course of gallstone disease. Eleven-year review of 781 nonoperated cases. *Gastroenterology* 1966;**50**:376–81.

43 Gracie WA, Ransohoff DF. The natural history of silent gallstones. *N Engl J Med* 1982;**307**:798–800.

44 Turrill FL, McCarron MM, Mikkelsen WP. Gallstones and diabetes: an ominous association. *Am J Surg* 1961;**102**:184–90.

45 Mundth ED. Cholecystitis and diabetes mellitus. *N Engl J Med* 1962;**267**:642–6.

46 Sandler RS, Maule WF, Baltus ME. Factors associated with postoperative complications in diabetics after biliary tract surgery. *Gastroenterology* 1986;**91**:157–62.

47 Ransohoff DF, Miller GL, Forsythe SB, Hermann RE. Outcome of acute cholecystitis in patients with diabetes mellitus. *Ann Intern Med* 1987;**106**:829–32.

48 Thompson JS, Philben VJ, Hodgson PE. Operative management of incidental cholelithiasis. *Am J Surg* 1984;**148**:821–4.

49 Ouriel K, Ricotta JJ, Adams JT, Deweese JA. Management of cholelithiasis in patients with abdominal aortic aneurysm. *Ann Surg* 1983;**198**:717–19.

50 Saade C, Bernard D, Morgan S, Tasse D, Rabbat A, Nadeau N. Should cholecystectomy be done en passant

for asymptomatic cholelithiasis? *Can J Surg* 1987;**30**: 350–3.

51 String ST. Cholelithiasis and aortic reconstruction. *J Vasc Surg* 1984;**1**:664–9.

52 Taylor FW. Routine operative cholangiogram. *Surg Gynecol Obstet* 1973;**136**:976–7.

53 Acousta JM, Ledesma CL. Gallstone migration as a cause of acute pancreatitis. *N Engl J Med* 1974;**290**: 484–7.

54 Schwesinger WH, Page CP, Sirinek KR, Levine BA, Aust JB. Biliary pancreatitis. Operative outcome with a selective approach. *Arch Surg* 1991;**126**:836–40.

55 Millat B, Fingerhut A, Gayral F, Zazzo JF, Brivet F. Predictability of clinicobiochemical scoring systems for early identification of severe gallstone-associated pancreatitis. *Am J Surg* 1992;**164**:32–8.

56 Piehler JM, Crchlow RW. Primary carcinoma of the gallbladder. *Surg Gynecol Obstet* 1978;**147**:929–42.

57 Diehl AK, Beral V. Cholecystectomy and changing mortality from gallbladder cancer. *Lancet* 1981;**i**: 187–9.

58 Diehl AK. Gallstone size and the risk of gallbladder cancer. *JAMA* 1983;**250**:2323–6.

Chapter 3
Ultrasonographic classification of gallstone structure

Y. Tsuchiya, S. Mikami & M. Ohto

Introduction

Oral bile salt dissolution therapy [1, 2] and extracorporeal shock wave lithotripsy [3, 4] have been performed worldwide for the non-invasive treatment of patients with gallbladder stones. The success of this therapy depends on correctly establishing the stone characteristics prior to treatment. We have demonstrated that stone characteristics [5, 6], and in particular stone structure can be determined from ultrasonographic patterns and this appears to be a decisive factor for achieving satisfactory fragmentation with gallstone lithotripsy [7, 8]. In this chapter we present a concise description of our ultrasonographic classification of gallstones.

In vitro analysis of echo patterns in gallstones

Ultrasonographic images of gallstones are characterized by a high echo region and distal shadowing [9], which may vary with the type of stone. The high echo represents the extent to which the ultrasound wave can penetrate the stone without strong attenuation. Distal shadowing results from the consumption of ultrasound energy in the gallstones.

The four basic echo patterns obtained from stones in our *in vitro* study are shown in Fig. 3.1. In pattern A (pure cholesterol stone), the stone echo on the B-mode display gradually attenuated and changed to distal shadowing. A corresponding pattern of ultrasound attenuation was also observed in the A-mode display. The cross-section of the stone indicated a radiate or homogeneous structure from the surface to the centre. In pattern B (combination stone), the stone echo in the B-mode display was sharp or arc-like with a clearly defined boundary, separating it from a distinct acoustic shadow. The A-mode display gave a high echo amplitude at the stone surface, followed by a sudden decline in echo level. The cross-sectional structure of the stone appeared layered near the stone surface. This type of stone was regarded as having a heterogeneous structure, with ultrasound energy being suddenly attenuated at the layer boundaries. In pattern C (mixed stone), there was a double stone echo in the B-mode, corresponding to a two-peak attenuation in the A-mode display. The stone structure appeared lamellated or heterogeneous. In pattern D (calcium bilirubinate stone), the whole image of the stone was delineated as of a weak acoustic shadow in the B-mode display. The A-mode display indicated that ultrasound attenuation occurred in the stones only to a very small extent. The stone structure was finely lamellated.

Sonographic features of gallstones

We studied the gallstones of 148 patients who underwent cholecystectomy. Of these, 134 patients had stones in the gallbladder while 14 had stones in the common bile duct. The types of stones were determined according to the gross structural classification of the Japanese Society of Gastroenterology [10]. In our study, the gross cross-sectional structures were divided into three basic patterns: radiate; lamellated; and finely lamellated or amorphous (Fig. 3.2).

The stones were categorized into large stones (10 mm or greater in the largest diameter) and small stones (less than 10 mm in diameter) by

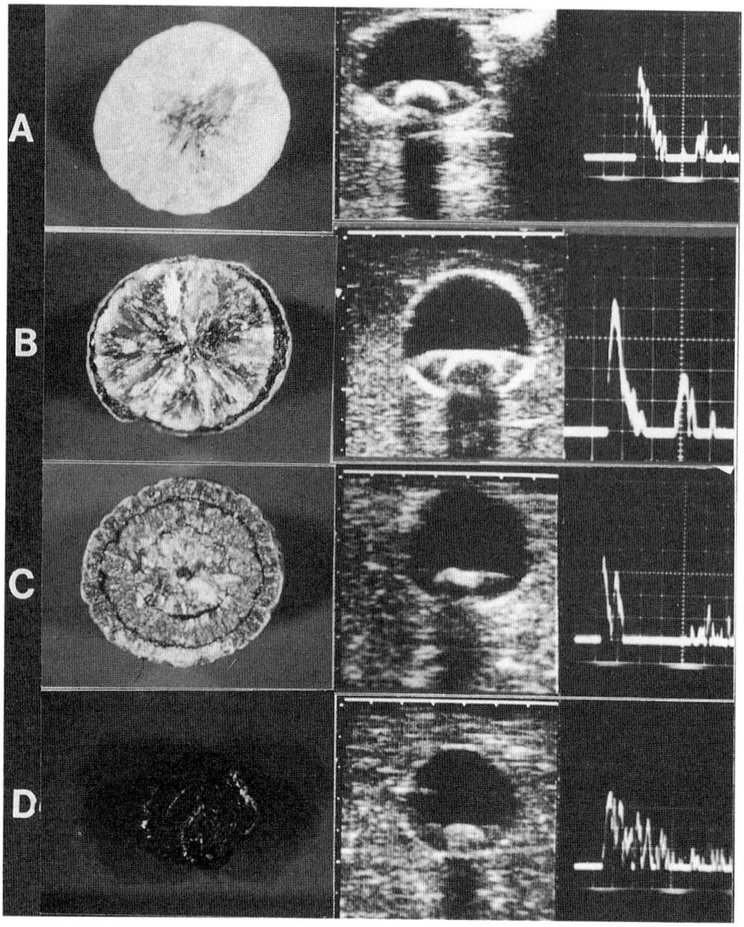

Fig. 3.1 Four basic echo patterns and their stone structures seen in *in vitro* study. (A) pure cholesterol stone; (B) combination stone; (C) mixed stone; and (D) calcium bilirubinate stone.

ultrasonographic analysis [5, 6]. Sonographic analysis was performed using a linear-array probe (3.75 MHz, SAL 90A, 77A; 5.0 MHz, 50A; Toshiba, Japan) with a 1.5 enlargement of the section, in which the acoustic shadow was most prominent.

Large stones

Three echo patterns were identified with large stones, and each pattern had two or three subpatterns (Fig. 3.3). In type I, the strong surface echo gradually changed to a distal shadowing. In type Ia, the echo from the stone was typically seen beyond the stone itself, or more rarely the stone echo occupied more than the anterior half of the stone. In type Ib, the stone had a half-moon shape and in type Ic, the stone was crescentic in appearance. Type I stones reflected high echoes, with much stronger distal shadowing than the liver parenchymal echo at the same depth from the skin. The typical type Ia stone, however, did not conform to this pattern.

In type II, the strong thin or arced stone echo changed to distal shadowing. Type IIa gave no internal echo while type IIb had a spotty or linear echo in the stones (double echo). Some stones exhibited multiple echo reflection behind the linear-double echo, indicating gas-containing stones. In type II stones, both stone echo and distal shadowing were strong.

In type III, the whole or most of the stone image was delineated by ultrasonography. In type IIIa, the parenchymal echo was similar to that of liver

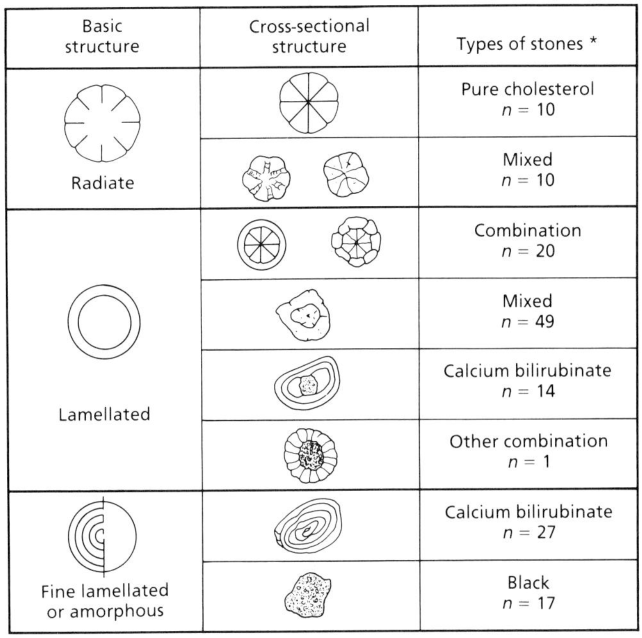

* According to the gross structural classification of the Japanese Society of Gastroenterology

Fig. 3.2 Basic structures in cross-section of the stones in 148 patients who had undergone operations.

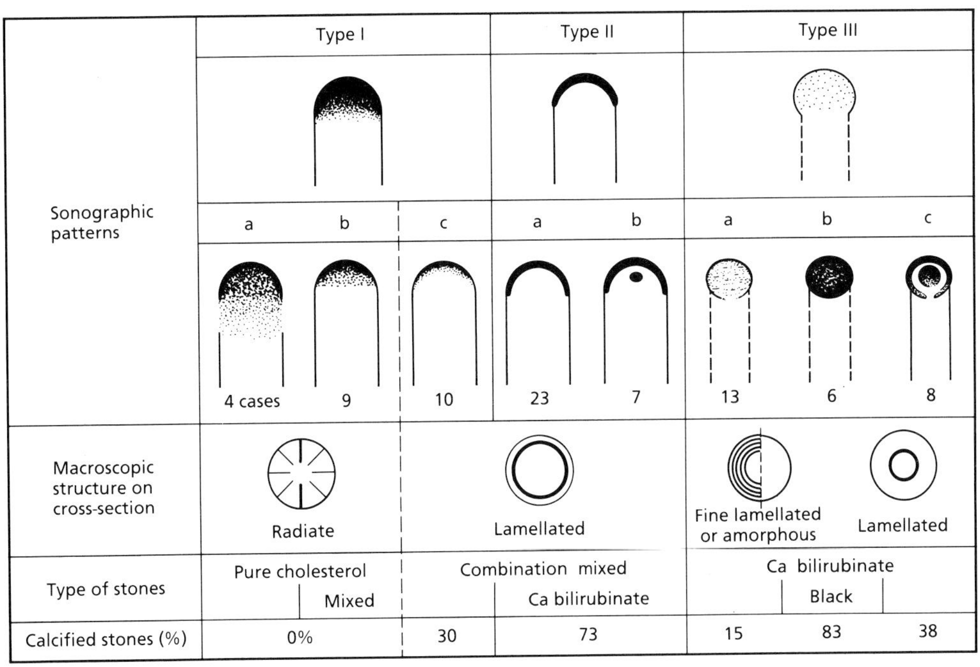

Fig. 3.3 Sonographic patterns and classification of large stones that were more than 10 mm in diameter in relation to cross-sectional anatomy. Calcification was assessed by soft X-ray roentgenography.

parenchyma, and both the stone echo and the acoustic shadow were weak. In type IIIb, there was a homogeneous high echo. The stone echo was high, and the distal shadowing weak. Type IIIc stones gave rise to a lamellar echo. The stone echo and acoustic shadow were somewhat stronger than those of type IIIa.

Small stones

Stones smaller than 10 mm in diameter were classified according to their sonographic features into the filling, piling, separate, floating, and sludge types (Fig. 3.4). In the filling type, high echoes followed by distal shadowing were seen in the gallbladder fossa with no visible gallbladder lumen. Piling type stones accumulated in the gallbladder leaving some gallbladder lumen. In the subtype piling-a stones, there were high echoes reflected from the stone surface, and the posterior wall of the gallbladder was hidden in the distal shadowing. In piling-b stones, the stones were seen in their entirety as high echoes, while the posterior wall of the gallbladder or the lowest layer of the stones were obscured, probably by the so-called comet-tail artefact. In piling-c stones, the stones were seen in their entirety with the posterior wall of the gallbladder or the lowest layer of the stones recognizable. The distal shadowing appeared strong in piling-a and piling-b, but weak in piling-c. Separate type stones smaller than 5 mm in diameter were seen as separate high-echo spots, commonly without shadowing. These were recognized as the stones because they moved when the patient was changed from a supine to a prone position. Separate type stones of 5–9 mm in diameter were estimated using the classification of the large stones. Floating type stones were seen as high-echo spots with distal shadowing, and appeared to be floating. The stone echo was seen as a double echo, showing no layer formation, with some stones in contact with the posterior gallbladder wall. Sludge type stones had a parenchymal echo similar to that of the liver parenchyma. They had the appearance of a coherent mass, with a weak acoustic shadow.

Discussion of factors influencing echo patterns in gallstones

The following three basic factors appear to account for the characteristic echo patterns of gallstones: physical structure; chemical composition; and artefact (Table 3.1).

The cross-sectional structure of gallstones cor-

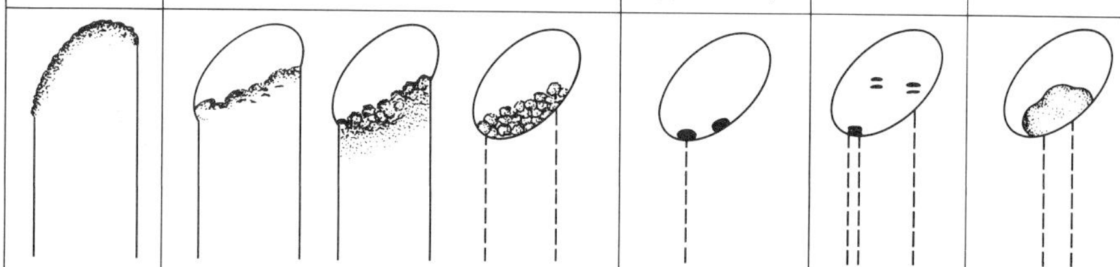

	Filling type	Piling type			Separate type ($\phi < 5$ mm)	Floating type	Sludge type
		a	b	c			
Sonographic pattern	10 Cases	19	4	15	13	3	3
Stones	Mixed	Mixed		Ca bilirubinate Black Mixed	Ca bilirubinate Black	Mixed	Ca bilirubinate (accumulation of small gallstones)
Calcified stones (%)	20%	15	0	46	50	0	0

Fig. 3.4 Sonographic patterns and classification of small stones that were less than 10 mm in diameter in relation to patterns of their existence in the gallbladder. Calcification was assessed by soft X-ray roentgenography. Separate type stones of 5–9 mm in diameter were estimated according to the sonographic classification of the large stones.

Table 3.1 Basic factors causing characteristics of the echo patterns of gallstones

Physical structure
Continuity of stone structure
→ Absorption of ultrasound energy
Chemical composition
Cholesterol, calcium, water, etc.
→ Echo level
Artefacts
Cholesterol crystals
→ Comet-tail artefact → pure cholesterol stone
Gas
→ Multiple reflection → gas-containing stone

relates closely with the consumption of ultrasound energy by the stones. When the stones have a homogeneous or continuous structure from the stone surface to the centre, they can be observed as a whole echo image because of the almost non-attenuated ultrasound in the stones. They included pure cholesterol stones, black stones, and some calcium bilirubinate stones. When stones have a heterogeneous structure near the surface, a distinct attenuation of ultrasound may occur at the discontinuous part in the stone structure, resulting in a narrow stone echo and strong distal shadowing. These images were typical of rimmed calcified combination stones. Our lithotripsy study has demonstrated that after a small amount of shock-wave discharge, type Ia stones changed to type Ic stones just before disintegration (Fig. 3.5). Simultaneously, the weak distal shadowing of the stone observed before lithotripsy changed to strong shadowing thereafter. This phenomenon can be explained on the assumption that the shock waves may change the homogeneous structure of the stones into a heterogeneous one, at least near the stone surface (Fig. 3.6). It seems very improbable that the shock waves can change the chemical composition of the stones. These findings demonstrate that the physical nature of the stones is critical for producing the various echo patterns [11].

The chemical composition of stones appears to be related to their echogenicity, regardless of distal shadowing [12, 13]. Components such as cholesterol and calcium can produce a high echogenicity as can be seen with pure cholesterol stones and black stones (Fig. 3.7). Their water content can lead to a low echogenicity, usually seen with calcium bilirubinate stones in the common bile duct.

There are two artefacts related to gallstone

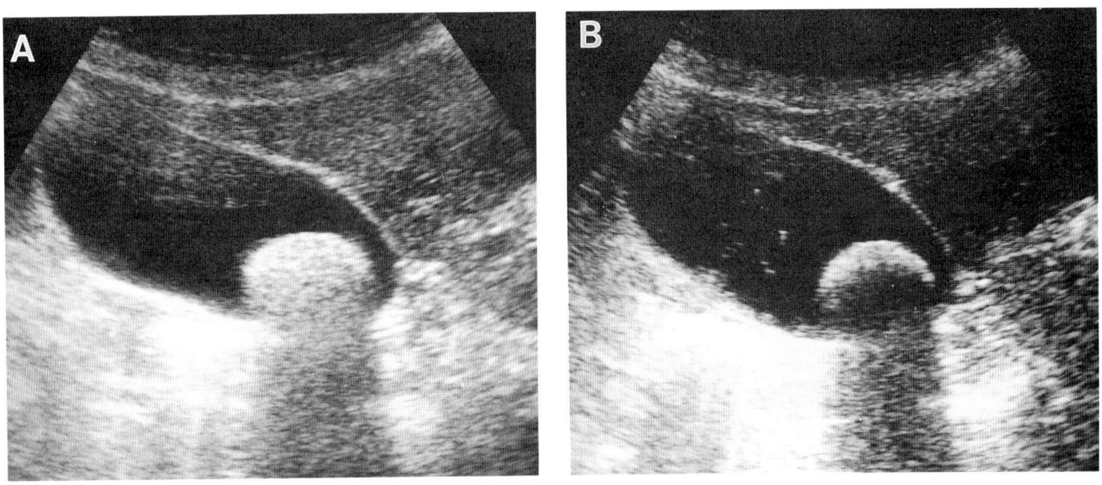

Fig. 3.5 Change of the stone echo pattern from type Ia (A) to type Ic (B) after a 15 minute shock wave application, using a piezoelectric lithotripter (LT-01, EDAP, France). Before lithotripsy, the stone showed a typical type Ia pattern, accompanied with the comet-tail artefacts beyond the stone itself, characteristic of pure cholesterol stones. Note after lithotripsy, the echo pattern changed to type Ic with a strong distal shadowing.

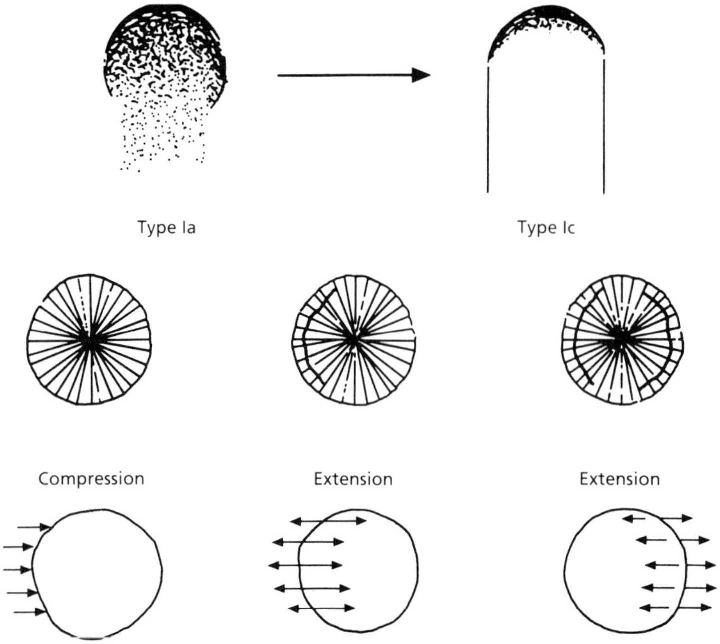

Fig. 3.6 Consideration of the reasons why shock wave application made the echo pattern change from type Ia to type Ic before stone disintegration.

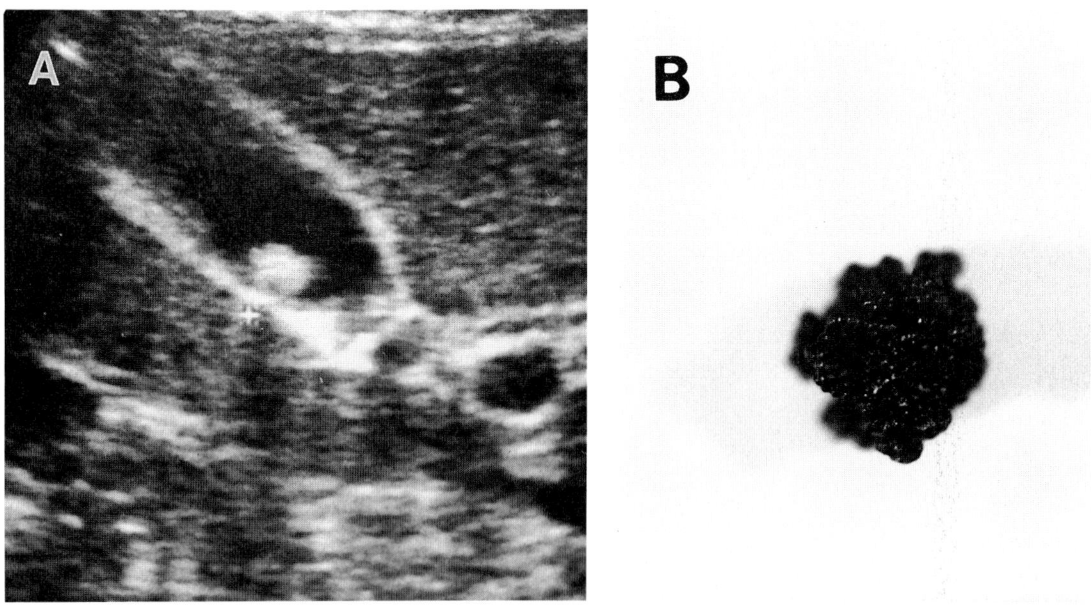

Fig. 3.7 Echo pattern of type IIIb stone. A hyperechoic stone is delineated as a whole image with a weak distal shadowing (A). Note the clear posterior wall of the gallbladder just behind the stone, because of the absence of the comet-tail artefact. After lithotripsy had failed to disintegrate the stone, the patient underwent an operation. (B), specimen of a typical black stone.

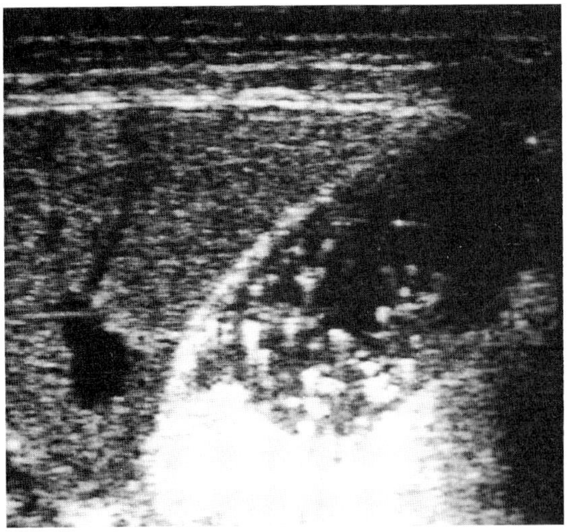

Fig. 3.8 The comet-tail artefacts caused by cholesterol crystals, seen after a successful disintegration of type Ia pure cholesterol stone.

echo patterns: the comet-tail artefact [14] and multiple echo reflection. Pure cholesterol stones gave echoes which were seen beyond the stones themselves. This is probably caused by the comet-tail artefact, characteristic of cholesterol crystals [15] (Fig. 3.8). The echo pattern of black stones was quite similar to that pure cholesterol stones, but these never present the comet-tail artefact. Some mixed stones are known to contain gas in which the fissure formation can be seen on the cross-section. Some of the stones with type IIb (linear-double echo) [16] showed a distal linear-multiple echo reflection [17], which is probably produced by gas in the stones (Fig. 3.9). The artefacts, characteristic of the ultrasound properties, seem to play an important role in the diagnosis of the stone characteristics.

References

1 Soenfield LJ, Lachin JM. Steering Committee, National Cooperative Gallstone Study Group. Chenodiol (chenodeoxycholic acid) for dissolution of gallstones: the National Cooperative Gallstone Study; a controlled trial of efficacy and safety. *Ann Intern Med* 1981; 95:257–82.
2 Fromm H, Roat JW, Gonzalez V *et al.* Comparative efficacy and side effects of ursodeoxycholic and chenodeoxycholic acids in dissolving gallstones: a double blind controlled study. *Gastroenterology* 1983;85: 1257–64.
3 Suerbruch T, Delius M, Paumgartner G *et al.* Fragmen-

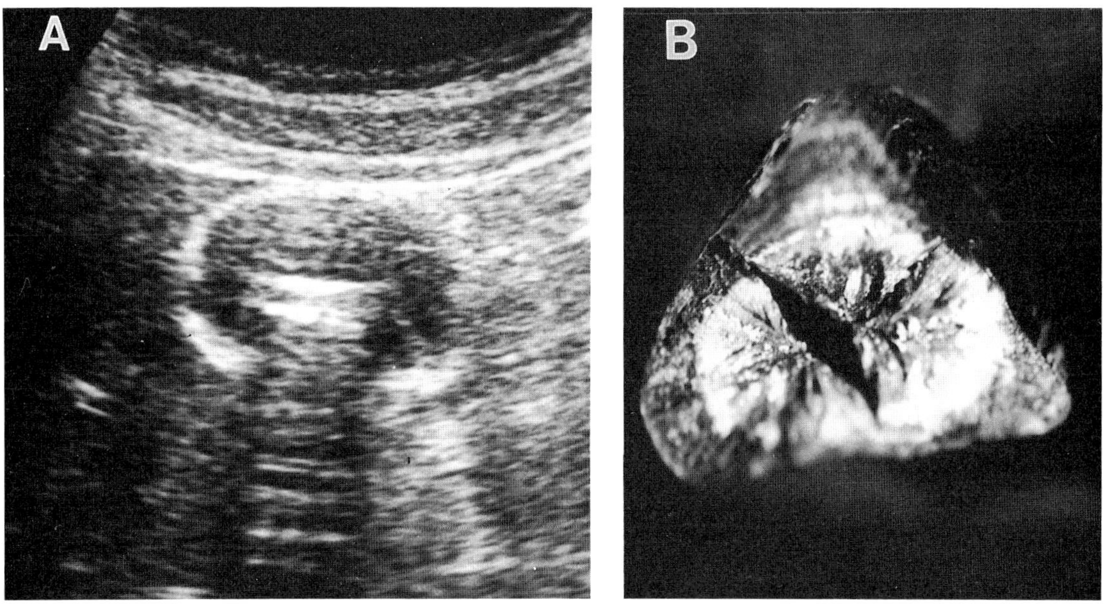

Fig. 3.9 Type IIb linear-double echo stone (A), showing a distal linear-multiple echo reflection, indicative of gas-containing mixed stones. (B), stone obtained at operation having a fissure formation in the cross section. The mean computed tomography (CT) value of this stone was −444 Hounsfield units (HU).

tation of gallstones by extracorporeal shock waves. *N Engl J Med* 1986;**314**:818–22.
4 Sackmann M, Delius M, Sauerbruch T *et al.* Shock-wave lithotripsy of gallstones. The first 175 patients. *N Engl J Med* 1988;**318**:393–7.
5 Tsuchiya Y, Ohto M, Yazawa T. Ultrasonic properties of gallstones. Differentiation between cholesterol stones and pigment stones. *Biliary Tracts and Pancreas* 1986;7:1483–91 (in Japanese).
6 Tsuchiya Y, Yazawa T, Ohto M, Okuda K. Sonographic diagnosis of gallstones. In: Speranza T, Barbara L, eds. *Problems in General Surgery. Changing Concepts in Biliary Stone Management.* Philadelphia: Lippincott, 1991;8:541–57.
7 Tsuchiya Y, Haniya K, Takanashi H, Nishiarai H, Ohto M. Piezoelectric shock-wave lithotripsy of gallbladder stones. A clinical evaluation of its efficacy and safety. *Stomach and Intestine* 1989;**24**:755–61 (in Japanese).
8 Dyrska H, Patel S, Saghavi B *et al.* Sonographic gallstone patterns are of value in predicting the outcome of biliary lithotripsy. *Am J Gastroenterol* 1991;**86**: 1626–8.
9 Gonzalez L, MacIntyre WJ. Acoustic shadow formation by gallstones. *Radiology* 1980;**135**:217–18.
10 Yamagata K, Maki T, Osuga T *et al.* The Gallstone Study Committee of Japanese Gastroenterology. A new classification of gallstones in Japan. *Jap J Gastroenterol* 1986;**83**:309–16.
11 Purdon RC, Thoma SR, Kereiskes JG *et al.* Ultrasonic properties of biliary calculi. *Radiology* 1980;**136**:729–32.
12 Carroll BA. Gallstones: *in vitro* comparison of physical, radiographic, and ultrasonic characteristics. *Am J Roentgenol* 1978;**131**:223–6.
13 Good LI, Edoll SL, Soloway RD *et al.* Ultrasonic properties of gallstones: effect of stone size and composition. *Gastroenterology* 1979;**77**:258–63.
14 Ziskin MC, Thickman DI, Goldberg NJ *et al.* The comet tail artifact. *J Ultrasound Med* 1982;**1**:1–7.
15 Shapiro RS, Winsberg F. Comet-tail artifact from cholesterol crystals: observation in the postlithotripsy gallbladder and an *in vitro* model. *Radiology* 1990;**177**: 153–6.
16 Mitchell DG, Needleman L, Frauenhoffer S *et al.* Gas-containing gallstones. The sonographic 'double echo sign'. *J Ultrasound Med* 1988;**7**:39–43.
17 Becker C, Vock P. Appearance of gas-containing gallstones on sonography and computed tomography. *Gastrointest Radiol* 1984;**9**:323–8.

Chapter 4
Extracorporeal shock wave lithotripsy for gallstones

A. Darzi, F.B.V. Keane & W.A. Tanner

Introduction

Ten years ago it would have been difficult to predict the changes and innovations that have occurred in the management of biliary lithiasis. One might wonder why these innovations did not occur earlier, but most of them are dependent on new technologies, which could only recently have been applied to gallstones. The rapidity of application of these new technologies has been fuelled by competition between the various proponents but most still require critical, short-term, and long-term evaluation.

Gallstones are common. The high prevalence of gallstones has become more apparent since the introduction of ultrasonography. An overall frequency of 8.2% was found amongst male civil servants in Rome, with an increase with age from 2.3% in the second decade to 14.4% in the 7th decade [1]. The incidence is thought to be higher in women in whom stones also occur at an earlier age.

As well as identifying the frequency of gallstones, ultrasonography has also helped to emphasize that gallstones are often harmless. Up to a few years ago prophylactic cholecystectomy for asymptomatic gallstones was performed routinely, especially for those under 50 years of age, in the expectation that they would soon develop symptoms, and some of these might be serious or life threatening. William Mayo suggested that there was no such thing as an 'innocent' gallstone. However, recent data has shown this practice and philosophy to be incorrect. In 1983, Ransohoff *et al.* summarized the outcome of 123 patients with asymptomatic gallstones with a follow-up ranging from 11–24 years [2]. They found that only 13% developed biliary pain, while complications developed in 2%. By subjecting these and other data to decision analysis, they suggested that the burden of disease was insufficient to warrant surgical intervention in patients with silent gallstones.

Nor does the threat of developing gallbladder cancer alter the conclusion that prophylactic cholecystectomy should not be performed for silent gallstones. It has been calculated that cholecystectomy would have to be performed on 200 Caucasian women, with gallstones, to prevent one gallbladder cancer [3]. The risk is even less in black races, and only in American Indians is there a particular risk.

Until further data becomes available, conventional wisdom would dictate, therefore, that only symptomatic gallstones should be treated by whatever modality, be it surgery or otherwise.

Open cholecystectomy has enjoyed a largely unchallenged supremacy as the treatment of choice in cholelithiasis since it was first performed by Carl Langenbuch, in 1882 [4]. The risk of complications (7% or less) or death (0.5% or less) in the average case is low, and those deaths that do occur, do so, usually, in those who display risk factors, particularly elderly patients with cardiopulmonary disease. Open cholecystectomy, however, does inflict considerable discomfort on the patient, requires hospitalization for about one week, and loss of work for up to one month. This has considerable cost implications for both the patient and the health-providing system.

The effort to reduce cholecystectomy to its least invasive form has led to the recent development of laparoscopic cholecystectomy [5, 6]. This development has continued the widening spectrum of laparoscopic procedures that can now be performed, including many gynaecological operations, division of adhesions, and appendicectomy. The rationale of laparoscopic cholecystectomy is based on the good cosmetic result, rapid resolution of postoperative pain, and a reduction of hospitalization, with the ability to return to work soon after surgery.

Laparoscopic cholecystectomy has developed in different centres with minor variations. Its advocates are excited by its early promise and suggest that over 90% of patients coming to cholecystectomy are suitable for this procedure. However, a unified approach has not yet been developed to cope with the 10–15% of patients coming to cholecystectomy, who have stones in the common bile duct. One approach is to perform intravenous cholangiography, pre-operatively, in any patients coming to surgery, and if choledocholithiasis is confirmed, then a formal open operation is performed. Whilst, if bile duct stones are found at a laparoscopic operation, on cholangiography, then either this procedure can be abandoned and an open operation with bile duct exploration can be performed, or an endoscopic retrograde cholangiopancreatography and stone removal can be carried out at a later date.

Because open operation might be required at any time during a laparoscopic cholecystectomy, the procedure should always be performed by biliary surgeons. There are many potential hazards, particularly if there has been previous surgery with adhesion formation. Surgeons require to learn and develop the necessary hand to eye coordination skills that are required in laparoscopic surgery carried out on a video screen.

Extracorporeal shock wave lithotripsy

The initial attempts to disintegrate human calculi by sound energy used a setup without direct contact between the transducer and the stone surface. All experimenters used continuous wave ultrasound. The first report on fragmentation of biliary calculi appeared already in 1950 from Lamport and Newman [7]. A 400 kHz transducer was able to destroy gallstones in water-filled cellophane bags within 5–60 seconds. The two ideas behind the application of ultrasound for stone destruction was either that '... the disruptive force exceeds the molecular attractive bond' (of the stone) [8] or that '... ultrasonic energy could produce vibrations within the calculus which would be great enough to overcome the adhesive power' [9].

This new technology was greeted with, perhaps, exaggerated enthusiasm, and a number of lithotripters were developed (Table 4.1). All of these lithotripters fragment stones, using shock waves that are generated under water and transmitted to the stones through a water bath or water-filled cushion, and then through the soft tissues of the abdominal wall. Shock waves are generated in three ways.

1 The spark-gap lithotripters create their shock waves using a high voltage spark between two electrodes. The resulting shock wave is then focussed by a semi-ellipsoid reflector so that the peak pressure is concentrated on a focal zone, several centimetres in front of the generator.

2 The piezoelectric lithotripters generate shock waves by applying an electrical current to many ceramic crystals set in a semi-elipsoid fixed array. The crystals expand instantaneously, producing a shock wave that is tightly focussed on a small high pressure zone in front of the generator.

3 Finally, electromagnetic lithotripters are constructed rather like a loudspeaker, in which the shock wave is set up by rapidly repelling a metal plate. The resulting shock wave is then focussed by an acoustic lens.

Each of these devices produce shock waves that differ in many respects, and this makes their comparison difficult. Not only are there differences in the pressure produced, but also in the configuration of the pressure wave, as well as the size and shape of the peak pressure zone. All lithotripters can fragment stones and most now do not require the patient to have either anaesthesia, intravenous analgesia or sedation. However, the differences in the machines will probably influence the kind of stones that can be treated, and the number of re-treatments that will be required.

Targeting of the shock waves is done, either by ultrasound or fluoroscopy. Ultrasound is the most satisfactory for gallbladder stones, while

Table 4.1 Second generation extracorporeal lithotripters (After Ferruci 1987)

Manufacturer	Model	Shock-wave	Focussing generation	Target	Coupling imaging	Suitability
Wolf (Germany)	Piezolith 2300	PE	Spherical array	US	Mini-tank	GB
Technomed Int. (France)	Sonolith 3000	SGE	Ellipsoid	US	Mini-tank	GB
EDAP (France)	LT-01	PE	Spherical array	US	Waterbag	GB
Siemens (Germany)	Lithostar	EM	Acoustic lens	X-ray	Waterbag	CBD
	Lithostar Plus	EM	Acoustic lens	X-ray + US	Waterbag	GB
Medstone Int. (USA)	1050 ST	SGE	Ellipsoid	X-ray ± US	Waterbag	CBD
Nitech (Denmark)		SGE	Ellipsoid	US	Waterbag	GB
Dornier Medizin (Germany)	HM4	SGE	Ellipsoid	X-ray	Waterbag	CBD
	MPL 9000	SGE	Ellipsoid	US	Waterbag	GB
	MFL 5000	SGE	Ellipsoid	X-ray	Waterbag	CBD
Direx (Israel)	Tripter XI	SGE	Ellipsoid	X-ray + US	Waterbag	GB
Northgate (USA)	SD 3	SGE	Ellipsoid	US	Waterbag	GB
Diasonics (USA)	Therasonic	PE	Spherical array	X-ray + US	Waterbag	GB
Storz Medical (Germany)	Modulith SL 10	PE	Spherical array	US	Waterbag	GB
	Modulith SL 20	PE	Spherical array	X-ray + US	Waterbag	GB

PE, piezoelectric; SGE, spark-gap electrode; EM, electromagnetic; US, ultrasound; GB, gallbladder stones; CBD, common bile duct stones.

fluoroscopy appears to be necessary when treating bile duct stones.

Cavitation, induced by the negative rebound of the shock wave, is probably responsible for stone fragmentation during extracorporeal shock wave lithotripsy (ESWL), but this process may also cause tissue damage. The balance between efficacy and safety has, therefore, to be established for each kind of lithotripter.

We addressed this question prospectively by first examining soft tissue changes following ESWL in an animal model and secondly in a series of patients receiving ESWL prior to cholecystectomy. Piezoelectric lithotripsy using the EDAP LT-01 has the capacity to produce significant soft tissue injury and the amount of injury is directly related to the number of shock waves delivered. Although our data is limited, the expression of injury appeared to be independent of the frequency in the range we used (2.5–20 shock waves/second). But, despite the pathological effects of a large number of shock waves in both the human and the animal studies, no untoward clinical effects were sustained. Furthermore, healing appeared to be complete in the guinea-pigs treated with 48 000 shock waves after 4 weeks with no evidence of residual damage of a macroscopic or microscopic nature. However, we should stress that the extrapolation of results from guinea-pigs to large species, such as the human must be interpreted with extreme caution, given the difference in abdominal wall thickness.

Low dose lithotripsy of 6 000 shock waves appears to produce insignificant tissue damage and it appears safe to use this dose when using the EDAP lithotripter at a single session. It is particularly gratifying to find that there was no cumulative injury after repeated episodes (up to six, at weekly intervals) at this dose. This has important management implications for patients with gallstones as it allows more than one attempt to fragment a solitary stone or group of gallstones.

Piezoelectric lithotripsy, because of its small focal region, should not affect relatively distant organs such as the lungs and kidneys in humans provided accurate targeting is maintained by the operator during lithotripsy. However, our experience at the Meath hospital in Dublin demonstrated distal haematomas such as in the duodenum and falciform ligament but these occurred early in our experience and may represent inaccurate gallbladder localization. However, drifting of the shock wave beam during therapy is possible and should be constantly monitored. The histological features that we have described appear to be specific lithotripsy-induced injuries. The changes that were found in patients at cholecystectomy were quite distinct from those that are associated with either acute or chronic cholecystitis.

Clearance of gallstone fragments after ESWL should theoretically be achieved either by mechanical ejection during gallbladder contraction or by the dissolution of fragments in surrounding bile.

The Munich group chose to treat patients with both modalities who traditionally would have been considered suitable candidates for bile acid therapy alone [10]. It would appear that bile acid therapy had a major influence on their results, in that only 30% of all their patients had achieved complete stone clearance at 2 months following lithotripsy whereas the corresponding figure at 18 months was 93% [11].

We examined the part played by lithotripsy and dissolution therapy either alone or in combination, and to establish: (1) whether gallstone fragments following lithotripsy could be cleared without the use of oral dissolution therapy; and (2), whether the combination of the two treatments is better than either treatment alone.

Early results suggest that mechanical ejection alone plays little part in emptying the gallbladder of fragments and that lithotripsy must be combined with dissolution therapy to achieve effective clearance. Indeed, no patient who received lithotripsy alone achieved significant clearance of their gallstone mass.

The selection criteria for gallstone lithotripsy are arbitrary and appear to be based on those that have become established for bile salt therapy alone [10, 12]. While this form of therapy requires a functioning gallbladder the physical characteristics of the gallstones selected for treatment are open to question. The stone characteristics defined by Sackmann *et al.* for inclusion into their study include solitary radiolucent stones with a diameter of up to 30 mm, or up to three radiolucent stones with a similar total stone mass [11].

Such strict criteria may reduce the number of patients suitable for this type of therapy and therefore limit its potential in management [13]. In order to extend the application of this treatment we broadened our criteria to include a wider range of gallstone morphology than has been previously suggested. We calculated that we would include up to 60% of patients who might otherwise be treated by cholecystectomy.

Over half of our patients, who have achieved total clearance, would not have been deemed suitable according to the Munich criteria [18]. Of particular note has been the success rate achieved in patients with more than three stones. Forty per cent of our patients who have achieved complete clearance had more than three stones. We have also achieved some success with calcified stones.

Although the clearance rates reported by Sackmann *et al.* [11] are better than ours, when the stone-free rates of patients with stone profile similar to those employed by the Munich group are compared the results are similar. However, we anticipate that the long-term future of ESWL will to a large extent depend upon its ability to treat a greater percentage of gallstone sufferers than the Munich group.

The complications of ESWL and dissolution therapy may relate to either aspect of the treatment. Some lithotripters give more discomfort than others, and require analgesia or sedation and there may be occasional mild post-treatment discomfort, some skin ecchymosis, and haematuria. The incidence of acute pancreatitis is surprisingly low during follow-up, at 1–2%. However, the incidence of episodes of biliary colic occurring during post-lithotripsy dissolution therapy, is high, often being greater than 30%. Our own experience has been lower than this, at around 13%, which we feel may be related to the spasmolytic properties of Rowachol, which we include in our dissolution regime, together with bile acids.

It is difficult to assess the exact role for ESWL and dissolution therapy in the future management of patients with gallstones. Patient acceptability is high as the treatments give little or no discomfort. Costs of treatment in our hands would compare favourably with those of cholecystectomy and the complications are few. However, the late costs particularly in terms of stone recurrence and their possible complications are, as yet, unknown.

Complete stone clearance is the end-point of most published studies, but so far, there is little data on symptomatic relief after ESWL, with or without dissolution therapy. It may be that acalculous gallbladder pain may persist after stone clearance or, indeed, it may be that a small amount of tiny particulate matter, detectable only by ultrasonography, may be of no clinical relevance.

Gallstone recurrence and its prevention

Prevention of gallstone formation has been considered under the headings of primary, secondary, or tertiary prevention. Primary prevention would be the inhibition of the formation of stones in those who have not previously had gallstones. Secondary prevention might be considered as the successful management of silent gallstones, either by clearing them or by preventing them from becoming symptomatic. Tertiary prevention is the prevention of gallstone recurrence in those who have an intact gallbladder, but have already had their gallstones cleared or dissolved, either by cholecystolithotomy or by oral dissolution therapy, with or without ESWL or by contact dissolution therapy. It is tertiary prevention that we are most concerned with here.

Previously reported high recurrence rates after cholecystolithotomy are difficult to interpret, because neither the tools nor the radiological skills have been available to absolutely confirm complete gallbladder clearance. Most available information on gallstone recurrence comes, therefore, from studies carried out on patients after dissolution therapy. These suggest that the recurrence rate in patients followed for 2–12 years after confirmed complete gallstone dissolution, is between 30 and 65% [14]. However, few patients have been followed for more than 5 years, and so the most reliable data are based on studies conducted over this period of time, and it is in these studies that recurrence rates range from 30 to 50%.

Early reports, and our own experience, suggest that the frequency of gallstone recurrence after successful lithotripsy and dissolution therapy, is similar to the recurrence rate after dissolution therapy on its own. It is, however, too early to assess the frequency of recurrence after cholecystolithotomy, using endoscopic procedures. Arguably, these procedures offer the most accurate means of confirmation of complete gallstone clearance, and this in itself might lead to a lower incidence of recurrence. Nevertheless, the incidence of gallstone recurrence appears to be high if the gallbladder is left *in situ*. This raises a number of issues to which, so far, there are no clear answers. For example, do these recurrent stones, like their forebears, cause symptoms? Should patients be followed up, and if so, for how long? Finally, can these recurrences be prevented, and if so, is prevention more cost-effective than retreating stones when they recur?

As in primary gallstone formation, the development of recurrent stones probably requires two, or maybe, even three abnormalities. Predominantly, there is the development of supersaturated bile. When bile acid therapy is withdrawn, there is a rapid and inevitable rebound of biliary cholesterol saturation. But as this does not always lead to gallstone recurrence, other factors may be involved. These include nucleation defects and impaired gallbladder motor function.

To date, efforts to prevent cholesterol gallstone recurrence have largely been based on attempts to, pharmacologically, modify the rebound in biliary cholesterol saturation. However, few trials have been designed scientifically as prospective, random allocation studies, and most have only included small numbers of patients which make it difficult to identify at-risk subgroups. Despite this, there is evidence to suggest that ursodeoxycholic acid probably reduces the incidence of gallstone recurrence, when taken at a dose of about 300 mg per day, particularly, in young patients [14].

An alternative pharmacological approach to the prevention of gallstone recurrence may be by the manipulation of nucleation factors. Patients with solitary primary stones are less likely to develop recurrences than those who, initially, had multiple stones, perhaps because of differences in the propensity to induce 'seeding' of stones from supersaturated bile. Non-steroidal anti-inflammatory drugs (NSAIDs) are thought to inhibit prostaglandin-mediated stimulation of mucin secretion by the gallbladder, and mucin may, in turn, act as a nucleating agent. In one study, which looked at patients' drug history, whilst assessing recurrence rates after gallstone dissolution, it was found that those taking NSAIDs had a significantly reduced incidence of recurrence [15]. Further evidence supporting NSAIDs, as candidates for preventative therapy, comes from animal studies, in which aspirin has been shown to prevent primary cholesterol gallstone formation in prairie dogs fed a lithogenic diet [16].

Cholecystolithotomy, by allowing access to the gallbladder, offers an alternative method for preventing stone recurrence. So-called, 'chemical' cholecystectomy requires two components: gallbladder mucosal ablation and cystic duct obstruction [17]. A number of chemicals have been shown to destroy gallbladder mucosa in the experimental animal, over short periods. However, in many instances re-epithelialization takes place from the cystic duct. Cystic duct occlusion, using a bipolar electrocoagulation catheter has overcome this and has been successfully described in experimental animals. Thus, chemical cholecystectomy, in combination with stone removal, offers a theoretical option for managing gallbladder stones, and preventing their recurrence using a minimalist one-stage technique. But this procedure is still experimental and anxiety must remain that such an ablative iatrogenic process may possibly increase the likelihood of gallbladder cancer.

References

1 GREPCO The Rome Group for Epidemiology and Prevention of Cholelithiasis (GREPCO) The epidemiology of gallstone disease in Rome, Italy Part 1 and Part 2. *Hepatology* 1988;8:904–913

2 Ransohoff DF, Gracie WA, Wolfenson LB *et al.* Prophylactic cholecystectomy or expectant management for silent gallstones. A decision analysis to assess survival. *Ann Int Med* 1983;**99**:199–204.

3 Hart J, Shani M, Modan B. Epidemiological aspects of gallbladder and biliary tract neoplasms. *Am J Public Health* 1972;**62**:36.

4 Langenbuch C. Einfall con Extirpation der Gallesblase wegen Chronischer cholelithiasis Heilung. *Berl Klin Wochenschr* 1882;**19**:725–9.

5 Reddick EJ, Olsen DO. Laparoscopic laser cholecystectomy. *Surg Endosc* 1989;**3**:131–3.

6 Dubois F, Icard P, Berthelot G, Levard H. Coelioscopic cholecystectomy. *Ann Surg* 1990;**211**:60–3.

7 Lamport H, Newman HF, Eichhorn RD. Fragmentation of biliary calculi by ultrasound. *Fed Proc* 1950;**9**:73–4.

8 Mulvaney WP. Attempted disintegration of calculi by ultrasonic vibrations. *J Urol* 1953;**75**:865–74.

9 Coats EC. The application of ultrasonic energy to urinary and biliary calculi. *J Urol* 1956;**75**:865–74.

10 Fromm H. Gallstone dissolution therapy: current status and future prospects. *Gastroenterology* 1986;**91**: 1560–7.

11 Sackmann M, Delius M, Sauerbruch T *et al.* Shock wave lithotripsy of gallstones. The first 175 patients. *New Eng J Med* 1988;**318**:393–7.

12 Fromm H. Ursodeoxycholic acid for adjuvant therapy with extracorporeal shock wave lithotripsy of gallstones. *J Clin Gastroenterol* 1988;10 (Suppl. 2): S18–S21.

13 Magnuson TH, Lillemoe KD, Pitt HA. How many Americans will be eligible for biliary lithotripsy? *Arch Surg* 1989;**124**:1195–2000.

14 Villanova N, Bazzoli F, Frabboni R *et al.* Gallstone recurrence after successful oral bile acid treatment: a follow-up study and evaluation of long term post-dissolution treatment (abstr). *Gastroenterology* 1987; **92**:1789.

15 Hood KA, Dowling RH, Keightley A *et al.* Piezoceramic lithotrispy of gallbladder stones: initial experience in 38 patients. *Lancet* 1988;**i**:1322–4.

16 Lee SP, Maher K, Nicholls JF. Origin and fate of biliary sludge. *Gastroenterology* 1988;**94**:170–6.

17 Becker GJ, Kopecky KK. Can the newer interventional procedures replace cholecystectomy for cholecystolithiasis? The potential role of percutaneous cystic duct ablation. *Radiology* 1988;**167**:275–9.

18 Darzi A, Monson JRT, Tanner WA *et al.* Current selection criteria of gallstone patients for extracorporeal shock wave lithotripsy are no longer valid. *Br J Surg* 1988;75:1246.

Chapter 5
Oral agents and contact dissolution of cholesterol gallstones

R. Sherry & T.R. Gadacz

Cholecystectomy has been and remains the unrivalled therapeutic option for the treatment of symptomatic gallstones. In 1882 Langenbuch first described elective cholecystectomy as a treatment for gallstones [1]. By 1891 Walker reported successful gallstone dissolution using ethyl ether infused into a cholecystostomy tube [2]. Interest in pharmacological approaches to eliminate gallstone disease expanded as the pathophysiology of stone formation came into perspective. In 1934 bile salt therapy was successfully used to reduce symptoms of biliary colic [3, 4] and in 1937 Rewbridge reported X-ray documentation of gallstone elimination with oral bile salt therapy in two patients [5].

Currently only two bile salts, chenodeoxycholate and ursodeoxycholate, are approved for use as oral dissolution agents. Monoctanoin (MO) is the only solvent approved for contact dissolution and methyl tert-butyl ether remains in use as an investigational drug. This chapter is focussed on the mechanism and clinical application of oral and contact dissolution of cholesterol gallstones. A prerequisite to understanding the pharmacological approach to gallstone disease is an understanding of the pathophysiology of cholesterol stone formation.

Pathogenesis of cholesterol gallstones

Hepatic cholesterol metabolism

Cholesterol metabolism is fundamental to cholesterol gallstone formation. The word 'cholesterol' is derived from Greek *chole* meaning bile and *stereos* meaning solid. Most mammalian cells synthesize cholesterol which is critical to cellular growth, differentiation, function, and regulation. Cholesterol is a key component of cell membranes and can be converted to steroid hormones, lipoproteins, bile salts, or excreted in bile. Cellular cholesterol content is affected by dietary intake and *de novo* hepatic synthesis. Lipoproteins in the serum serve as a source of cholesterol. This process is regulated by low density lipoprotein (LDL) receptors located on the cell membrane which binds and internalizes lipoproteins. Lysosomal enzymes can metabolize these lipoproteins to free cholesterol. This process is regulated by LDL receptor density which is responsive to cellular cholesterol requirements [6, 7].

De novo synthesis in the liver accounts for the majority of cholesterol production. Cholesterol is synthesized in a multi-step fashion from acetate. The rate-controlling enzyme in this process is hydroxy-methyl-gluteral CoA (HMG-CoA) reductase which reduces 3-hydroxy-3-methylglutaryl CoA to melalonate (Fig. 5.1). HMG-CoA reductase is an 888 amino acid with a half life of approximately 2 hours. HMG-CoA activity is controlled by its synthesis which is regulated by classic negative feedback control with cholesterol [8]. Melalonate is converted to intermediates which lead to cholesterol biosynthesis.

Free cholesterol can be stored in the form of cholesterol ester. This represents a metabolically inactive storage pool. Alternatively, free hepatic cholesterol can be used for a variety of synthetic purposes including catabolism to form bile salts or it can be eliminated by direct secretion into bile.

Bile salt metabolism

Bile salts are biological detergents synthesized in

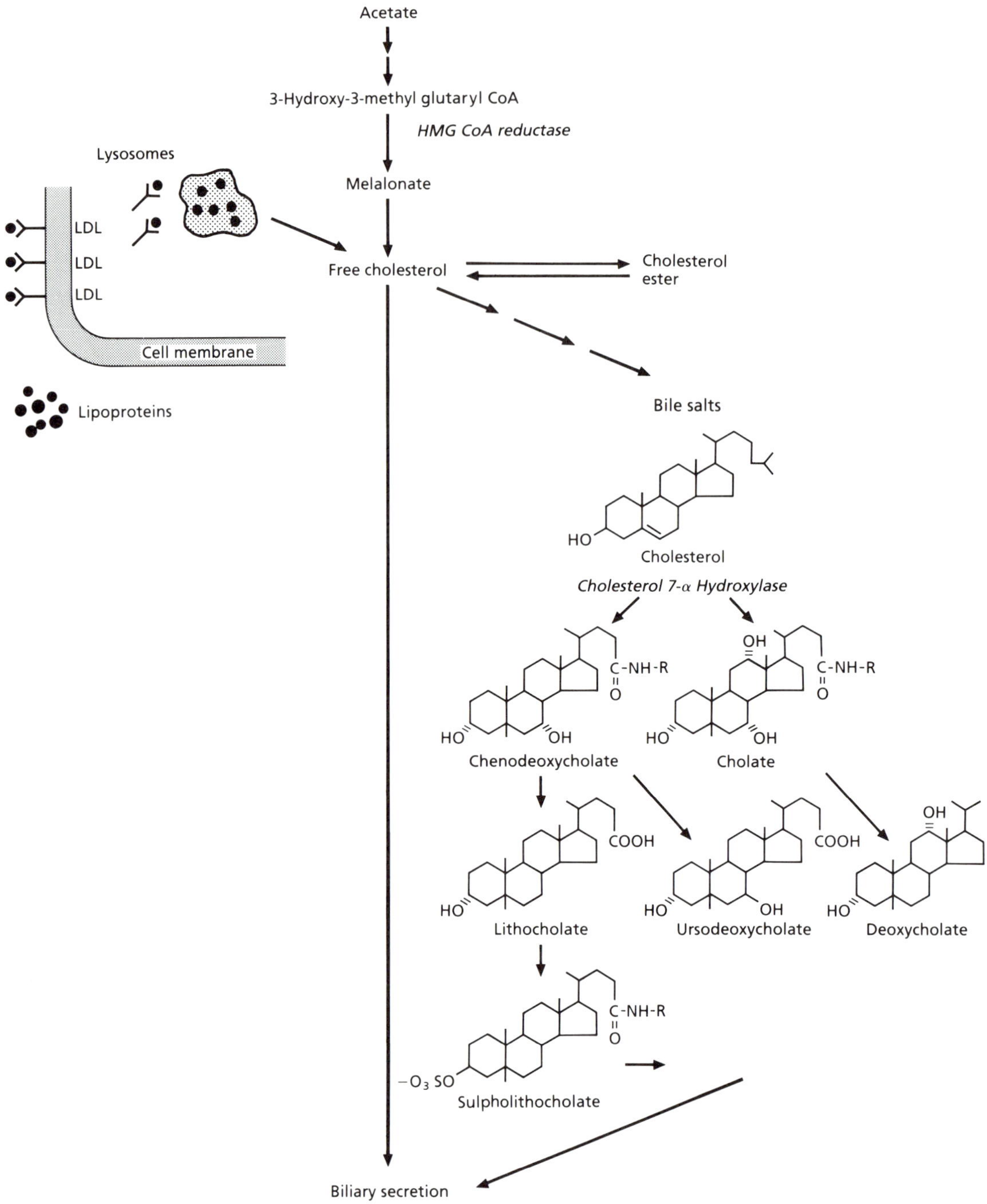

Fig. 5.1 Cholesterol content is maintained by a balance between synthesis and degradation including bile salt synthesis and biliary excretion.

the liver. They have multiple functions including the facilitation of cholesterol excretion in bile. Since bile salts are synthesized from cholesterol, they are also a major pathway for cholesterol elimination. Bile salts cycle between the intestine and liver in the enterohepatic circulation. The total amount of bile salts in the circuit is considered the bile salt pool. Bile, stored in the gallbladder during fasting, is released into the intestine following post-prandial release of cholecystokinin. In the small bowel bile salts facilitate intra-luminal solubilization and absorption of lipids. Ninety-five per cent of circulating bile salts are absorbed in the terminal ileum and returned to the liver while approximately 500 mg per day are lost in the stool and are replaced by newly synthesized bile acids [9]. The bile salt pool circulates eight to ten times per day [10].

The synthesis of bile salts from cholesterol is controlled by the rate limiting enzyme cholesterol 7-α-hydroxylase. Ultimately, chenodeoxycholate and cholate are produced. These primary bile salts are conjugated with taurine or choline. Bacterial transformation in the intestine results in the formation of the secondary bile salts deoxycholate, ursodeoxycholate, and lithocholate (see Fig. 5.1).

Regulation of cholesterol 7-α-hydroxylase is complex and incompletely understood. Hydrophobic bile salts (cholate, chenodeoxycholate, and deoxycholate) are potent inhibitors of bile salt synthesis. Hydrophilic bile salts have little effect on bile salt synthesis [11, 12]. Thus, bile salt synthesis is regulated in part by cycling hydrophobic bile salts which inhibit cholesterol 7-α-hydroxylase. This serves to emphasize the importance of the enterohepatic circulation.

It is noteworthy that there appears to be a relationship between cholesterol 7-α-hydroxylase and HMG-CoA reductase. The enzymatic activity of both is regulated in tandem under a variety of physiological conditions. Bile fistula [13], cholestryramine administration [13], glucocorticoids [14] and thyroid hormone [14] stimulate synthesis of both enzymes. Bile salt feeding inhibits both enzymes [15]. Ingestion of cholesterol [16] or melalonate [17] stimulates cholesterol 7-α-hydroxylase but inhibits HMG-CoA activity. The general parallel regulation of these two rate limiting enzymes illustrates and reflects the interrelationship between bile salts and cholesterol.

The size of the bile salt pool and the kinetics of the enterohepatic circulation are affected by bile salt synthesis, gallbladder emptying, transit time, and absorption in the terminal ileum. Abnormalities in any of these factors can interfere with bile salt function. Deficiencies can be compensated for by increased synthesis and increased recycling. For example, patients who have had resection of the terminal ileum have poor bile salt absorption and compensate with a high rate of bile salt synthesis and rapid recyling in the enterohepatic circulation. Normally an inverse relationship exists between the kinetics of the enterohepatic circulation and the size of the bile salt pool [18]. An interesting exception to this principle is seen in patients with chronic liver disease who have reduced synthesis and slow enterohepatic recycling of bile salts [19, 20].

Formation of cholesterol gallstones

Historically gallstone pathogenesis was con-

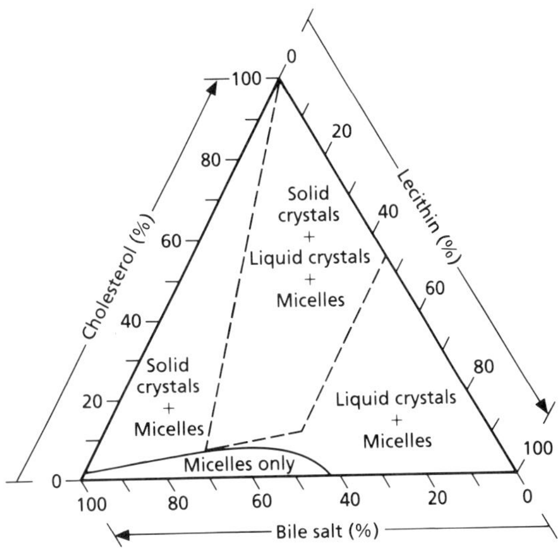

Fig. 5.2 Tricoordinate phase diagram illustrating the narrow range where cholesterol is fully solubilized in model aqueous solutions of bile salt, lecithin and cholesterol at a total liquid concentration of 10 g/dl (micelles only). All other regions represent bile solution in which cholesterol solubilization has been exceeded and crystallization occurs. (From *J. Clin. Invest* 1978;**61**:998).

sidered to be directly related to the fact that certain biliary lipids, inorganic salts, or organic salts exceeded their maximum solubility in bile. Bile is a heterogeneous product composed of cholesterol, bile salts, lecithin, pigments, electrolytes and water. Bile salts are the primary component of bile and together with cholesterol and lecithin account for 80% of its dry weight [21, 22].

Cholesterol is virtually insoluble in aqueous solution. Biliary solubilization of cholesterol is dependent on its interaction with lecithin and bile salts. Bile salts function as biological detergents and form micelles with hydrophobic groups removed from contact with water and with hydrophilic groups exposed to water molecules. Lecithin which is also water insoluble, is incorporated into bile salt micelles and allows the micelle to swell. Mixed lecithin–bile salt micelles can solubilize cholesterol and provide a vehicle for its excretion.

Once cholesterol exceeds its maximum solubility in bile, it can crystallize and precipitate to start a cascade which leads to gallstone formation. Admirand and Small [23] noted that the lipid composition of gallbladder bile in patients with cholesterol stones exceeded the limits of micellar cholesterol solubility. Normal patients showed a lipid composition within the micelle-only phase and showed no solid or liquid crystals. This relationship has been illustrated by a triangular coordinate plot which reflects bile salt, lecithin, and cholesterol equilibrium in aqueous solution (Fig. 5.2).

More recent data has challenged the mixed micelle concept of cholesterol solubilization and excretion. Somjen and Gilat [24, 25] have reported that a large portion of biliary cholesterol exists in a vesicular form. In this model the amphipathic molecules of bile salts and lecithin form a lipid bilayer similar to that found in cell membranes. Cholesterol can be solubilized in the non-polar portion of the bilayer.

In dilute bile or bile salt poor solution the vesicular bilayers are stable and can solubilize greater quantities of cholesterol than can micelles. Concentration of bile in the gallbladder destabilizes the vesicles and leads to a transfer of cholesterol and lecithin to micelles. This has led some authors to conclude that supersaturated bile becomes lithogenic only after it is concentrated in the gallbladder [18].

Nucleation and gallstone growth

Nucleation is a complex process that results in the formation of cholesterol monohydrate crystals. Cholesterol nucleation involves fusion of supersaturated vesicles [26, 27]. Nucleation occurs in the mucin gel which lines the gallbladder [22]. Mucin is a complex of glycoproteins secreted by gallbladder epithelial cells and is a key component of gallstones. Mucin glycoproteins accelerate cholesterol nucleation and serve as a matrix for stone growth [28, 29]. There is experimental evidence that this process can be promoted by calcium ions [30]. Moreover, calcium salts can serve as a nidus for cholesterol crystallization and nucleation [28, 31, 32].

The process of nucleation is affected by potent nucleating proteins. Multiple investigators have identified a heat labile protein in the bile of patients with cholesterol gallstones which reduces the time required for nucleation [33–35]. Antinucleating proteins have also been identified in the bile of normal patients. Kibe *et al.* [36] noted that apolipoprotein A-1 and A-2 prolonged nucleation time of cholesterol monohydrate crystals.

Clearly, nucleation is a critical process which is incompletely understood. Further investigation will undoubtedly lead to a better understanding of gallstone formation and perhaps suggest new pharmacological approaches to the disease.

The role of the gallbladder

The gallbladder plays a critical role in the pathogenesis of cholesterol gallstones. The importance of bile concentration in the gallbladder and the function of the mucin gel lining the gallbladder has been noted. Recent evidence suggests that defective acidification of bile by the gallbladder may reduce calcium solubility. Shiffman and Moore [37] found bile pH to be significantly elevated in 38 of 40 patients with gallstones. Heuman *et al.* [29] have suggested that excessive buffering by mucin glycoproteins reduces calcium solubility and promotes calcium salt nucleation. This hypothesis has been supported by the findings of Freston *et al.* [38], which have shown that gallbladder mucus hyper-secretion preceded the development of gallstones in a rabbit model.

Bile stasis in the gallbladder is associated with an increased frequency of gallstone formation and there is clear evidence from animal models that defects in gallbladder emptying precede development of stones [39–41]. In addition, cholecystokinin administration is known to reduce the incidence of gallstones [42]. The exact mechanisms by which bile stasis promotes gallstone formation is unknown although it is possible that it relates to the length of exposure of saturated bile to luminal components.

Oral agents for cholesterol gallstone dissolution

The treatment of cholesterol gallstones with litholytic agents is based on the assumption that cholesterol gallstone disease is a reversible process. In 1972, Danzinger *et al.* [43] published a report indicating that oral administration of the primary bile salt chenodeoxycholic acid (CDCA) successfully dissolved gallstones. In 1975 Makino *et al.* [44] reported that ursodeoxycholic acid (UDCA), a secondary bile acid, could also affect gallstone dissolution when taken orally. Both of these agents have been employed in controlled trials and our current understanding of oral agents for gallstone dissolution is based on an extensive basic science and clinical research experience.

Mechanism of action

Initially it was assumed that oral administration of any of the bile salts would be effective in dissolving gallstones. This assumption proved incorrect and highlighted the mechanisms of effective litholytic agents. Oral administration of CDCA, UDCA, cholate, or deoxycholate will expand the bile salt pool but only CDCA and UDCA dissolve gallstones *in vivo* [45–48]. Further investigation documented that despite the fact that they expanded the bile salt pool, both CDCA and UDCA caused a reduction in biliary cholesterol secretion [47]. It appears that reduced biliary cholesterol secretion plays a key role in gallstone dissolution during litholytic therapy.

The mechanism of CDCA reduction in cholesterol secretion is considered to be its suppression of hepatic HMG CoA reductase, the key enzyme for cholesterol synthesis [49]. In support of this is data documenting that bolus doses of HMG CoA reductase inhibitors profoundly reduce biliary cholesterol secretions in rats [50]. In addition, administration of competitive inhibitors of HMG CoA reductase reduces the cholesterol saturation of bile in humans [51]. The net result of CDCA administration is the production of bile less saturated with cholesterol which allows transfer of cholesterol from solid crystals to micelles.

The mechanism by which UDCA reduces biliary cholesterol secretion is less well understood. Unlike CDCA, UNCA does not inhibit HMG CoA reductase or alter cholesterol synthesis. UDCA does reduce intestinal absorption of cholesterol and this may account for the reduced biliary cholesterol secretion [52]. As noted earlier, oral administration of UDCA increases the bile salt pool and UDCA accounts for up to 50% of the bile salt pool composition in patients on therapy [53].

Chenodeoxycholate and UDCA differ fundamentally in their mechanism of gallstone dissolution. Ursodeoxycholate forms smaller micelles because of the differing orientation of a single hydroxyl group (see Fig. 4.1). As a result, UDCA accomplishes solubilization of cholesterol by a non-micellar mechanism. Another major distinction between CDCA and UDCA is that CDCA is known to inhibit endogenous bile acid production by suppression of cholesterol 7-α-hydroxylase the key enzyme of bile salt synthesis [54]. The clinical significance of this is unclear because in spite of this enzymatic inhibition, CDCA is associated with an increase in the bile salt pool.

Efficacy of bile salt therapy

The overall dissolution rate with litholytic bile salts varies from report to report depending on patient selection and bile salt dosage. In highly selected patients optimal treatment for 2 years has completely dissolved gallstones in 20–40% of cases. The National Cooperative Gallstone Study was a 24-month, three-arm trial consisting of patients placed on 700 mg/day of CDCA, 350 mg/day of CDCA, or placebo. This study documented complete dissolution of gallstones in 13.5% of patients receiving high dose CDCA [55].

Results from European trials using higher doses of CDCA showed better results. If CDCA was given at night and coupled with a low cholesterol diet, 75% of patients showed complete dissolution following 12 months of therapy [56, 57].

There is extensive experience with the efficacy of UDCA. Randomized studies from Europe suggest that UDCA and CDCA are equivalent in dissolving stones [58, 59]. Ursodeoxycholate accomplished dissolution in a shorter time and required a lower dose than CDCA.

Most patients who eventually achieved complete stone dissolution will show a partial response after 6 months of oral therapy. If partial stone dissolution does not occur following 12 months of treatment, the likelihood of success is considered to be low. Treatment with UDCA for 4 years showed no improvement in the rate of dissolution when compared to 2 years of therapy [60].

Because the mechanisms of CDCA and UDCA gallstone dissolution are different, combination therapy is theoretically attractive. A combination of 7.5 mg/kg/day of CDCA and 6.5 mg/kg/day of UDCA has been investigated [61–63]. The combination of the two drugs was not more effective than either alone but there were less side-effects associated with lower doses of CDCA. The cost of combination therapy was less expensive than that of CDCA alone.

Gallstone recurrence following cessation of therapy has been a major problem with bile salt therapy. Shortly after discontinuation of therapy lithogenic bile is again produced and stones can develop [64, 65]. Reported stone recurrence rates range from 11% to over 90%. Generally about 50% of patients develop stone recurrence and these typically occur in the first 5 years following therapy [66, 67]. Recurrent stones in patients who have had prior complete dissolution are composed of pure cholesterol and generally dissolve rapidly with repeat therapy [65].

Villanova *et al.* [68] reported patients not given long-term treatment after successful dissolution with UDCA had a recurrence rate of 69% at 5 years whereas those treated with UDCA after dissolution had a 32% recurrence rate at 7 years. Patients over age 50 showed no benefit from post-dissolution therapy. Patients under the age of 50 had a 15% recurrence rate when treated and a 69% recurrence rate when not treated. Patients with no post-dissolution therapy and solitary stones had a recurrence rate of 32% compared with a 77% recurrence rate in those with multiple stones. Although there is no agreement on the use of post-dissolution therapy, patients under 50 years of age with multiple stones are most likely to benefit.

Side-effects of bile salt therapy

The side-effects of CDCA therapy include diarrhoea, hepatotoxicity and altered cholesterol and lipoprotein levels. Diarrhoea is the most troubling clinical side effect of CDCA therapy. It is caused by CDCA induced secretion of water and electrolytes in the colon [69]. Patients on 700 mg/day had a 49% incidence of diarrhoea whereas those on 350 mg/day had a 22% incidence of diarrhoea. Temporary dose reduction improved the symptoms and no patients in the National Cooperation Gallstone Study had therapy discontinued as a result of diarrhoea [55].

Hepatotoxicity related to CDCA therapy tends to be mild and transient. In the National Cooperation Gallstone Study 39% of patients had elevated liver enzymes but only 3% of patients required early termination of therapy [55]. Finally, CDCA therapy is associated with increases in serum cholesterol and low density lipoprotein [70]. This is a result of inhibition of bile salt synthesis and reduced biliary cholesterol secretion which are both major routes of cholesterol elimination [52]. It is unclear as to whether these abnormalities alter the risk of atherosclerotic disease.

Bile salts are taken twice daily or as a single

dose at bedtime. The dose of CDCA is 12–15 mg/kg/day and UDCA is taken at a dose of 10 mg/kg/day [55, 58, 59]. Patients receiving CDCA must have hepatic enzymes monitored frequently while patients on UDCA do not require serial monitoring of liver function tests. Serum cholesterol levels should be periodically evaluated.

Both CDCA and UDCA reduce biliary cholesterol secretion [47]. Consequently, the therapeutic effects of bile salt therapy can be monitored by periodic sampling of bile by aspiration through a duodenal tube. Gallbladder contraction is stimulated by cholecystokinin administration and bile is collected [73]. A biliary cholesterol saturation index can be calculated and serially monitored during therapy [74, 75]. This allows for optimal dose titration while minimizing side-effects.

Ultrasonography, obtained 9–12 months after the initiation of litholytic therapy, is critical to assess the progress of gallstone dissolution. Schoenfield and Marks [76] have suggested that if this ultrasound shows no evidence of dissolution, therapy should be discontinued. If partial shrinkage is documented, therapy can be continued for another 9–12 months. In the event that complete gallstone dissolution has occurred, they recommend that bile salt therapy be continued for an additional 3 months. Following cessation of a successful course of therapy, yearly gallbladder ultrasonography is indicated.

The cost of UDCA therapy for a 70 kg patient is estimated to be $1 400/year. This estimate does not include the cost of follow-up, laboratories, or any radiological tests.

In contrast to CDCA, UDCA has less toxicity and is well tolerated by most patients. There is no increase in serum cholesterol and no evidence of hepatic enzyme elevation [71, 72]. Diarrhoea occurs in less than 1% of patients on UDCA therapy. Because of the lower incidence of toxicity, UDCA is considered to be the litholytic agent of choice.

Patient selection and follow-up

The ideal candidate for litholytic therapy is a patient with minimal symptoms from cholelithiasis and a prohibitive operative risk for surgery. Patients with significant frequent symptoms are not suitable candidates because a long duration of therapy is often required. Symptomatic patients with acceptable operative risk are better served with open or laparoscopic cholecystectomy. The role of medical therapy for asymptomatic gallstones is unclear although these patients are generally not candidates for either medical or surgical treatment.

Identification of patients with gallstones likely to respond to bile salt therapy can be challenging. Only non-calcified cholesterol gallstones can be dissolved. Patients with chronic liver disease or with hemolytic disease are likely to have pigment stones. Gallstones which show calcification on plain film, oral cholecystogram or computed tomography are generally refractory to bile salt therapy. Patients having gallstones with a diameter of over 20 mm are not proper candidates because of the slow rate of dissolution. Finally, cystic duct occlusion is an absolute contraindication to litholytic therapy. Historically, this has been established by gallbladder visualization on oral cholecystogram. Radionuclide scanning should also be satisfactory to document cystic duct patency and gallbladder function.

Future directions

Bile salt therapy has proved to be safe and effective in dissolving cholesterol gallstones in some patients. Current research is focussed on developing more potent agents. The combination of UDCA and extracorporeal shock wave lithotripsy has demonstrated promise and appears to be more effective than either therapy alone [77]. Investigators have reported that litholytic agents show synergism with other cholesterol lowering medications in reducing biliary cholesterol [75]. Ursodeoxycholic acid has proven to be useful in preventing gallstone formation in patients undergoing rapid weight loss [78]. The clinical promise of litholytic therapy may be realized in its use as prophylactic treatment for patients at high risk for developing cholelithiasis.

The use of HMG CoA reductase inhibitors in combination with UDCA represents another promising field of investigation. Lovastatin and simvastatin, both HMG CoA reductase inhibitors used for treatment of hypercholesterolemia, lower the cholesterol saturation index of gallbladder bile [51]. Recently Logan and Duane [75] reported that lovastatin given in combination with UDCA significantly reduced the cholesterol saturation index when compared to UDCA therapy alone. Interestingly, those subjects that had the greatest additive effect of lovastatin were those with less than optimal reduction in saturation indices during treatment with UDCA. The ability of lovastatin to lower total and LDL cholesterol levels was not impaired by UDCA. The benefit of this combination therapy needs to be confirmed in clinical trials.

Contact dissolution of cholesterol stones

Potent organic solvents are available for contact dissolution of cholesterol gallstones. Monoctanoin and methyl tert-butyl ether are the most familiar and well studied agents. Both solvents require direct biliary access via percutaneous gallbladder catheterization or infusion into an indwelling T-tube. Neither agent is suitable for oral ingestion. Patients with stones likely to respond to contact dissolution are very similar to those who will respond to bile salt therapy. Only non-calcified cholesterol stones can be dissolved by these organic solvents. Unlike bile salt therapy, stones of any size may be effectively treated with contact dissolution.

Monoctanoin

Monoctanoin is a medium chain diglyceride of capric and caprylic acids which is an excellent *in vitro* and *in vivo* cholesterol solvent. Monoctanoin has been used primarily to dissolve retained common duct stones. In 1986 Palmer and Hofmann [79] reported on 343 patients who had intraductal MO for the dissolution of bile duct stones. Complete dissolution was noted in 26% of patients while another 8% were considered to have benefited from therapy as an adjunct to interventional treatment. In 36% of patients MO infusion was totally ineffective. Low cholesterol stone content was considered to be the major factor which accounted for treatment failures.

In this same study 9% of patients had therapy terminated because of side-effects or complications. Minor side-effects such as abdominal pain, nausea, vomiting and diarrhoea were common and occurred in a dose dependent fashion. No treatment related deaths were reported but life threatening sequellae including sepsis, pulmonary oedema, intestinal bleeding, and pancreatitis were detected in 5% of patients [79]. Although clearly effective in many patients, MO infusion requires 4 to 21 days of continuous therapy [80–82].

Postoperatively, MO can be infused into the common bile duct as soon as there is no leak from the choledochotomy site. The solution can be infused with a battery powered pump and at a rate of 3–7 ml/hour. A manometer which communicates with the pump prevents excess infusion pressure (>30 cm of solution) in the bile duct. Increased bile duct pressure can result in cholangitis. The infusion rate should be tailored to minimize the sequella of pain, vomiting, nausea and diarrhoea.

Stones in the proximal bile duct present a special problem because of poor contact with the solvent. For stones in the proximal duct or obstructing the distal common bile duct, a catheter should be placed near the stone for direct infusion while allowing adequate drainage through the T-tube.

Monoctanoin is the only solvent approved for contact dissolution of cholesterol stones and has proven to be safe and effective in experienced hands. The best results are obtained when the retained stone is known to have a high cholesterol content. This can be established by incubating other stones obtained at surgery in MO at 37°C. In this highly selected group the rate of dissolution has been reported to be as high as 91% [81]. In selected patients it can be used on an outpatient basis.

Although effective for dissolution of gallbladder stones, its slow rate of dissolution makes it more attractive as for use in the therapy of retained cholesterol common bile duct stones. Its use has been limited by its prolonged dissolution time and rapid improvement in alternative invasive techniques.

Methyl tert-butyl ether

Methyl tert-butyl ether (MTBE) is an aliphatic ether which may be the best clinical solvent for cholesterol gallstones and is certainly more potent than MO [82]. It is used for gallbladder stones and not for common bile duct stones. Thistle *et al.* [83] reported on 75 patients that had MTBE administered by percutaneous transhepatic infusion into the gallbladder. Treatment consisted of catheter insertion under local anaesthesia followed by continuous manual infusion and aspiration 4–6 times per minute for an average of 5 hours a day for 1–3 days. MTBE caused no deaths, few side-effects, and no patients had therapy discontinued for side effects or complications. Complete stone dissolution occurred in 37% of treated patients. By the end of the study 72 of 75 patients had 95% of stones dissolved. Six of the 75 patients required surgery during a follow-up period of 6–42 months. Other reports have confirmed that MTBE infusion into the gallbladder has few significant toxic effects [82]. Automatic infusion pumps which eliminate the need for manual infusion and aspiration are now available.

Methyl tert-butyl ether infusion for treatment of bile duct stones is associated with frequent side-effects [84]. Neoptolemos [85] reported that bile duct stones were completely dissolved in approximately 50% of patients treated with MBTE infusion. In the British experience 79% of patients suffered complications which included drowsiness, transient elevation of liver enzymes, pain, anorexia, and hypotension. The use of MBTE to dissolve common duct stones has been less than satisfactory because it is more difficult to prevent the escape of the solvent and because common duct stones are less likely to be high in cholesterol. The use of MTBE to dissolve common bile duct stones is contra-indicated.

Future directions

Current research is focussed on the development of more potent and less toxic organic solvents. In addition, less invasive delivery techniques are necessary. Interest in contact dissolution of cholesterol stones has diminished as the safety and effectiveness of laparoscopic cholecystectomy, endoscopic sphincterotomy and basket stone extraction have become evident. Currently the use of contact dissolution agents is limited to patients who have failed non-operative approaches for retained common duct stones or to patients with symptomatic gallstones who will not safely tolerate cholecystectomy. It is possible that combinations of organic solvents or direct enzymatic dissolution may be more effective and less toxic.

References

1 Langenbuch C. Ein Fall von Extirpation der Gallenblase wegen chronischer cholelithiasis. Heilung. *Berl Klin Wochenschr* 1882;19:725–7.
2 Walker JW. The removal of gallstones by ether solution. *Lancet* 1891;1:874.
3 Rosenak BD, Kohlstaedt KG. Bile salt therapy in liver and gall bladder disease. *Am J Dig Dis Nutrit* 1936; 3:577–80.
4 Lyon BV, Swalm WA. Therapeutic effectiveness of dehydrocholic acid in liver and biliary disease. *Med Rec* 1934;139:123.
5 Rewbridge AG. The disappearance of gallstone shadows following the prolonged administration of bile salts. *Surgery* 1937;1:395–400.
6 Goldstein JL, Brown MS, Anderson RGW *et al.* Receptor-mediated endocytosis: Concepts emerging from the LDC receptor system. *Annu Rev Cell Biol* 1985;1:1–9.
7 Cooper AD. Metabolic basis of cholesterol gallstone disease. *Gastroenterol Clin N Am* 1991;20(1):21–46.
8 Cooper AD. Hepatic lipoprotein and cholesterol metabolism. In: Zakim D, Boyer TD, eds. *Hepatology: A Textbook of Liver Disease.* Philadelphia: Saunders, 1990:96–123.
9 Vlahcevic ZR, Heuman DM, Hyleman PB. Physiology and pathophysiology of enterohepatic circulation of bile acids. In: Zakim D, Boyer TD, eds. *Hepatology: a Textbook of Liver Disease.* Philadelphia: Saunders, 1990:341–77.
10 Brunner H, Northfield TC, Hofmann AF *et al.* Gastric emptying and secretions of bile acids, cholesterol, and pancreatic enzymes during digestion: duodenal perfusion studies in health subjects. *Mayo Clin Proc* 1974;49:851–60.
11 Heuman DM, Hernandez CR, Hylemon PB *et al.* Regulation of bile acid synthesis: I. Effects of conjugated urso deoxycholate and cholate on bile acid

synthesis in chronic bile fistula in the rat. *Hepatology* 1988;8:358–65.
12 Heuman DM, Vlahcevic ZR, Bailey ML *et al.* Regulation of bile acid synthesis: II. Effect of bile acid feeding on enzymes regulating hepatic cholesterol and bile acid synthesis in the rat. *Hepatology* 1988;8:892–7.
13 Danielsson H, Einarsson K, Johansson G. Effects of biliary drainage on individual reactions in the conversion of cholesterol to taurocholic acid. *Eur J Biochem* 1967;2:44–9.
14 Balasubramaniam S, Mitropoulos KA, Myant NB. Hormonal control of the activities of cholesterol 7 a-hydroxylase and hydroxy-methyl-gluteryl-CoA-reductase in rats. In: Matern S, Hackanschmidt J, Back P, eds. *Advances in Bile Acid Research III*. Bile Acid Meeting, Freiburg. Stuttgart, Verlag, 1974:61.
15 Shefer S, Hauser S, Lapar V *et al.* Regulatory effects of sterols and bile acids on hepatic 3-hydroxy-3-methyl glutoryl CoA-reductase and cholesterol 7-α-hydroxylase in the rat. *J Lipid Res* 1973;**14**:573–80.
16 Raicht RF, Cohen BI, Shefer S *et al.* Sterol balance studies in the rat. Effects of dietary cholesterol and B-sitosterol on sterol balance and rate limiting enzymes of sterol metabolism. *Biochim Biophys Acta* 1975;**388**: 374–84.
17 Mok HYI, von Bergmamm K, Grundy SM. Kinetics of enterohepatic circulation during fasting: biliary lipid secretion and gallbladder storage. *Gastroenterology.* 1980;**78**:1023–33.
18 Carey MC, Cahalane MJ. The enterolepatic circulation. In: Arias I, Popper H, Schachter D *et al.*, eds. *The Liver: Biology and Pathobiology*. New York: Raven Press, 1988:573–616.
19 Vlahcevic ZR, Buhac I, Farrar JT *et al.* Bile acid metabolism in patients with cirrhosis. I. Kinetic aspects of cholic acid metabolism. *Gastroenterology* 1971;**60**: 491–8.
20 Vlahcevic ZR, Judijudata P, Bell CC Jr. *et al.* Bile acid metabolism in patients with cirrhosis. II. Cholic and chemodeoxy cholic metabolism. *Gastroenterology* 1972;**62**:1174–81.
21 Saunders KD, Cates JA, Roslyn JL. Pathogenesis of gall stones. *Surg Clin N Am* 1990;**70**(6):1197–1216.
22 Donovan JM, Carey MC. Physical-chemical basis of gallstone formation. *Gastroenterol Clin N Am* 1991;**20**(1):47–66.
23 Admirand WH, Small DM. The physicochemical basis of cholesterol gallstone formation in man. *J Clin Invest* 1968;**47**:1043–52.
24 Somjen GJ, Gilat T. A non-micellar mode of cholesterol transport in human bile. *FEBS Lett* 1983;**156**:265–8.
25 Somjen GJ, Gilat T. Contribution of vesicular and micellar carriers to cholesterol transport in human bile. *J Lipid Res* 1985;**26**:699–704.
26 Halpern Z, Dudley MA, Lynn MP *et al.* Vesicle aggregation in model systems of supersaturated bile: Relation to crystal nucleation and lipid composition of the vesicular phase. *J Lipid Res* 1986;**27**:295–306.
27 Halpern Z, Dudley MA, Kibe A *et al.* Rapid vesicle formation and aggregation in abnormal human bile. A time-lapsed video-enhanced contrast microscopy study. *Gastroenterology* 1986;**90**:875–85.
28 Gallinger S, Taylor RD, Harvey PRC *et al.* Effect of mucous glycoprotein on nucleation time of human bile. *Gastroenterology* 1985;**89**:648–58.
29 Heuman DM, Moove EW, Vlahcevic ZR. Pathogenesis and dissolution of gall stones. In: Zakim D, Boyer TD, eds. *Hepatology: a Textbook of Liver Disease*. Philadelphia: Saunders, 1990:1480–1516.
30 Kibe A, Dudley MA, Halpern Z *et al.* Factors affecting cholesterol monohydrate crystal nucleation time in model systems of supersaturated bile. *J Lipid Res* 1985;**26**:1102–11.
31 Craven BM. Crystal structure of cholesterol monohydrate. *Nature* 1976;**260**:727–9.
32 Westbrook P, DeJong EW. *Biomineralization and Biological Metal Accumulation: biological and Geological.* Dordrecht Netherlands: Reidel, 1982:1.
33 Burnstein MJ, Ilson RG, Petrunka CN *et al.* Evidence for a potent nucleating factor in the gallbladder bile of patients with cholesterol gallstones. *Gastroenterology* 1983;**85**:801–7.
34 Gallinger S, Harvey PRC, Petrunka CN *et al.* Biliary proteins and the nucleation defect in cholesterol cholelithiasis. *Gastroenterology* 1987;**92**:867–75.
35 Groen AK, Stout JPJ, Drapers J *et al.* Isolation of cholesterol nucleating activating activity in gallbladder bile. *J Hepatol* 1986;**3**:S59.
36 Kibe A, Holzbach RT, Lakusso NF *et al.* Inhibition of cholesterol crystal formation by apolipoproteins in supersaturated model bile. *Science* 1984;**225**:514–16.
37 Shiffman ML, Moore EW. Acidification of gallbladder bile is defective in patients with all types of gallstones. *Gastroenterology* 1988;**94**:A591. (Abstract).
38 Freston JW, Bouchier IAD, Newman J. Biliary mucous substances in dihydro cholesterol induced cholelithiasis. *Gastroenterology* 1969;**57**:670–8.
39 Gurll NJ, Meyer PO, Denbesten L. Effect of cholesterol crystals on gallbladder function in cholelithiasis. *Surg Form* 1977;**28**:412–13.
40 Pitt HA, Doty JE, DenBesten L *et al.* Stasis before gallstone formation: Altered gallbladder compliance or cystic duct resistance? *Am J Surg* 1982;**143**:144–9.
41 Doty JE, Pitt HA, Kuchenbeckar SL *et al.* Impaired gallbladder emptying before gallstone formation in the prairie dog. *Gastroenterology* 1983;**85**:168–74.
42 Roslyn J, Denbesten L, Pitt HA *et al.* Effects of cholecystokinin on gallbladder stasis and cholesterol gallstone formation. *J Surg Res* 1981;**30**:200–204.
43 Danzinger RG, Hofmann AF, Schoenfield JL *et al.* Dissolution of cholesterol gallstones by chenodeoxycholic acid. *N Engl J Med* 1972;**286**:1–8.
44 Makino I, Shinozaki K, Yoshino K *et al.* Dissolution of cholesterol gall stones by ursodeoxycholic acid. *Jap J Gastroenterol* 1975;**72**:692–700.
45 Thistle JL, Schoenfield JL. Induced alterations in

composition of bile of persons having cholelithiasis. *Gastroenterology* 1971;**61**:488–96.
46 LaRusso NF, Hoffman NE, Hofmann AF *et al.* Effect of primary bile acid ingestion on bile acid metabolism and biliary lipid secretion in gallstone patients. *Gastroenterology* 1975;**69**:1301–14.
47 Nilsell K, Angelin B, Leijd B *et al.* Comparative effects of ursodeoxycholic acid and chemodeoxycholic acid on bile acid kinetics and biliary lipid secretion in humans. *Gastroenterology* 1983;**85**:1248–56.
48 LaRusso NF, Szczepanik PA, Hofmann AF. Effect of deoxycholic acid ingestion on bile acid metabolism and biliary lipid secretion in normal subjects. *Gastroenterology* 1977;**72**:132–40.
49 Salem G, Nicolau G, Shefer S. Chenodeoxycholic acid inhibits elevated hepatic HMG-CoA reductase activity in subjects with gallstones. *Clin Res* 1973;**21**:523 (Abstract).
50 Kempen HJ, deLange J, Vos Van Holstein MP *et al.* Effect of ML-236B (compactin) on biliary excretion of bile salts and lipids and on bile flow in the rat. *Biochim Biophys Acta* 1984;**794**:435–43.
51 Duane WC, Hunninghake DB, Freeman ML *et al.* Simvastatin, a competitive inhibitor of HMG CCA reductase lowers cholesterol saturation index of gallbladder bile. *Hepatology* 1988;**8**:1147–50.
52 Hardison WG, Grundy SM. Effect of ursodeoxycholate and its taurine conjugate on bile acid synthesis and cholesterol absorption. *Gastroenterology* 1984;**87**: 130–85.
53 Talamini MA, Gadacz TR. Gallstone dissolution. *Surg Clin N Amer* 1990;70(6):1217–30.
54 Salem G, Tint GS, Shefer S. Treatment of cholesterol stones with litholytic bile acids. *Gastroenterol Clin of N Amer* 1991;20(1):171–82.
55 Schoenfield LJ, Lachin JM. Chenodiol (chenodeoxycholic acid) for dissolution of gallstones. The National Cooperative Gallstone Study: A controlled trial of efficacy and safety *Ann Intern Med* 1981;**95**:257–82.
56 Maudgal DP, Kupfer RM, Northfield TC. Factors affecting gallstone dissolution rate during chenic acid therapy. *Gut* 1983;**24**:7–10.
57 Maudgal DP, Bird R, Blackwood WS *et al.* Low cholesterol diet enhancement of effect of CDCA in patients with gallstones. *Br J Med* 1978;**2**:851.
58 Erlinger S, Go AL, Husson JM *et al.* Eranco-Belgian cooperative study of ursodeoxycholic acid in the medical dissolution of gallstones: A double blind, randomized, dose response study and comparison with chenodeoxycholic acid. *Hepatology* 1984;**4**:308–14.
59 Roda E, Razzoli F, Labate AM *et al.* Ursodeoxycholic acid vs chenodeoxycholic acid as cholesterol gallstone dissolving agents: A comparative randomized study. *Hepatology* 1982;**2**:804–10.
60 Gleeson D, Ruppin C, Saunders A *et al.* Final outcome of ursodeoxycholic acid treatment in 126 patients with radiolucent gallstones. *Quart J Med* 1990;**76**: 711–29.
61 Podda M, Zuin M, Diogurardi ML *et al.* A combination of chenodeoxycholic acid and ursodeoxycholic acid is more effective than either in reducing biliary cholesterol saturation. *Hepatology* 1982;**2**:334–9.
62 Podda M, Zuin M, Battezat PM. Non-surgical treatment of gallstones: cheno vs ursodeoxycholic acid. In: Northfield T, Jazrawi R, Zentler-Munro P, eds. *Bile Acids in Health and Disease.* Boston, Dordrecht Kluwen, 1988:87.
63 Stiehl A, Raedsch R, Lzygam P *et al.* Effects of biliary bile acid composition on biliary cholesterol saturation in gallstones patients treated with chenodeoxycholic acid and/or ursodeoxycholic acid. *Gastroenterology* 1980;**79**:1192–8.
64 Ruppin DC, Dowling RH. Is recurrence inevitable after gallstone dissolution by bile acid treatment? *Lancet* 1982;**1**:181–5.
65 Thistle JL, Pu PYI, Hofmann AF *et al.* Prompt return of bile to supersaturated states followed by stone recurrence after discontinuation of chenodeoxycholic acid therapy. *Gastroenterology* 1974;**66**:789. (Abstract).
66 Lanzini A, Jazrawi RP, Kupfer RM *et al.* Gallstone recurrence after medical dissolution. An over threat? *J Hepatol* 1986;**3**:241.
67 O'Donnell LDJ, Heaton KW. Recurrence and re-recurrence of gallstones after medical dissolution: A long term follow-up. *Gut* 1988;**29**:655–8.
68 Villanova N, Bazzoli F, Taroni F *et al.* Gallstone recurrence after successful oral bile acid treatment. *Gastroenterology* 1989;**97**:726–31.
69 Mekhjian HS, Phillips SF, Hofmann AF. Colonic secretion of water and electrolytes induced by bile acids: Perfusion studies in man. *J Clin Invest* 1971;**50**: 1569–77.
70 Albers JJ, Grundy SM, Cleary PA *et al.* National Cooperative Gall Stone Study: The effect of chenodeoxycholic acid on lipoproteins and apoliopoproteins. *Gastroenterology* 1982;**82**:638–46.
71 Tint GS, Salem G, Coladlillo A *et al.* Ursodeoxycholic acid: A safe and effective agent for dissolving gallstones. *Ann Intern Med* 1982;**97**:351–6.
72 Bachrach WH, Hofmann AF. Ursodeoxycholic acid in the treatment of cholesterol lithiasis. *Dig Dis Sci* 1982;**27**:333–56.
73 Duane WC, Ginsberg RL, Bennion LJ. Effects of fasting on bile acid metabolism and biliary lipid composition in man. *J Lipid Res* 1976;**17**:211–9.
74 Carey MC, Small DM. The physical chemistry of cholesterol solubility in bile: Relationship to gallstone formation and dissolution in man. *J Clin Invest* 1978;**61**:998–1026.
75 Logan GM, Duane WC. Lovastatin added to ursodeoxycholic acid further reduces biliary cholesterol saturation. *Gastroenterology* 1990;**98**:1572–6.
76 Schoenfield LJ, Marks JW. Oral agents to dissolve gallstones. *Semin Gastrointest Dis* 1991;**2**:204–11.
77 Shoenfield LJ, Berci G, Carnovale RL *et al.* The effect of urosodiol on the efficacy and safety of extracorporeal

shock-wave lithotripsy of gallstones. *N Engl J Med* 1990;**323**:1239–45.
78 Broomfield PH, Chopera R, Sheinbaum RC *et al.* Formation and prevention of lithogenic bile and gallstones during weight loss. *N Engl J Med* 1988;**319**:1567.
79 Palmer KR, Hofmann AF. Intraductal mono octanoin for the direct dissolution of bile duct stones: Experience in 343 patients. *Gut* 1986;**27**:196–202.
80 Thistle JL, Carlson GL, Hofmann AF *et al.* Mono octanoin, A dissolution agent for retained cholesterol bile duct stones: Physical properties and chemical application. *Gastroenterology* 1980;**78**:1016–22.
81 Gadacz, TR. The effect of mono octanoin on retained duct stones. *Surgery* 1981;**89**:527–31.
82 Hofmann AF, Schteingart CD, van Sonnenberge *et al.* Contract dissolution of cholesterol gallstones with organic solvents. *Gastroenterol Clin N Am* 1991;**20**(1): 183–99.
83 Thistle JL, May GR, Bender CE *et al.* Dissolution of cholesterol gallstones by methyl tert-butyl ether administration by percutaneous transhepatic catheter. *N Engl J Med* 1989;**320**:633–9.
84 Brandon JC, Teplick SK, Haskin P *et al.* Common bile duct calculi: Updated experience with dissolution with methyl tert-butyl ether. *Radiology* 1988;**166**:665–7.
85 Neoptolemos JP, Hall C, O'Conner HJ *et al.* Methyl tert-butyl ether for treating bile duct stones: The British experience. *Br J Surg* 1990;**77**:32–5.

Chapter 6
Methyl tert-butyl ether dissolution of cholesterol gallstones

J.L. Thistle

For patients at high-risk for general anaesthesia who have symptomatic gallstones, a minimally invasive, well tolerated method for clearing the gallbladder and bile ducts of stones is optimal. For example, patients with severe cardiovascular disease are at particular risk for peri-operative myocardial infarction or life-threatening cardiac dysrhythmia [1]. Patients with severe pulmonary insufficiency also may not tolerate general anaesthesia well. Alternatively, patients with extensive upper abdominal adhesions from previous surgery, inflammatory conditions, or trauma may be more safely managed by non-operative techniques. About 80% of patients have cholesterol stones and most of these are soluble in methyl tert-butyl ether (MTBE) [2]. This solvent will dissolve even large stones (4–6 cm in diameter) within hours and has been highly effective and safe in experienced hands [3, 4]. A direct contact solvent can be delivered most effectively by percutaneous transhepatic catheter although endoscopic retrograde placement via the cystic duct is often successful and can be utilized in selected patients.

Methods

At the Mayo Clinic all percutaneous transhepatic catheter procedures are performed by interventional radiologists. The importance of a team approach with focussed expertise is reflected in their 100% success in placing dissolution catheters into the gallbladder in more than 140 patients without significant complications. We have not observed clinically significant bleeding, bile leakage requiring surgical interventional procedures or other major complications. Percutaneous transhepatic catheterization requires adequate analgesia and prophylaxis for vasovagal reactions is prudent.

We prefer fluoroscopic targeting of the gallbladder using oral cholecystographic contrast media. Oral administration for 2 consecutive days preceding the procedure enhances opacification of the gallbladder. If non-opacification occurs or if the cystic duct is known to be obstructed, ultrasonography has been utilized for initial placement of a needle in the gallbladder to infuse radiopaque contrast material. Adequate analgesia is important with appropriate precautions in patients with severe respiratory insufficiency. Local infiltration of the catheter entry tract as well as infusion of a long-acting analgesic at the hepatic peritoneal surface is combined with a variable amount of sedation and analgesia intravenously. Blood pressure and oximeter monitoring are routinely employed but we have not used electrocardiogram (ECG) monitoring or required the participation of an anaesthetist except in one or two extremely fragile patients with an unusually unstable cardiopulmonary status. Patients with a thick-walled gallbladder, especially if it has less than the usual attachment to the liver, may require some gentle persistence and application of maximum skill to achieve entry of the sheath then catheter into the lumen. By entering the gallbladder through the area of hepatic attachment, usually high on the gallbladder body or neck and using a variety of equipment and techniques, we have not yet encountered a gallbladder in which the catheter could not be placed in satisfactory position to allow dissolution therapy to proceed [4, 5] (Figs 6.1–6.3). We have most commonly used a 5 F pigtail catheter designed for this purpose (Cook Inc., Bloomington, Ind. USA).

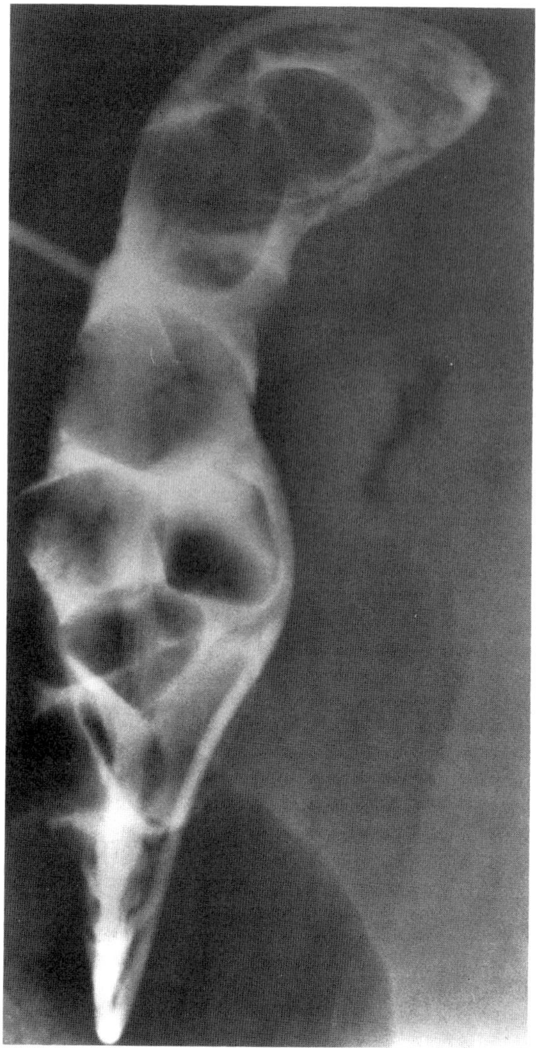

Fig. 6.1 The percutaneous transhepatic catheter has been placed with at least one full loop in the gallbladder for stability and with the pigtail in the fundus. Multiple radiolucent stones fill the gallbladder.

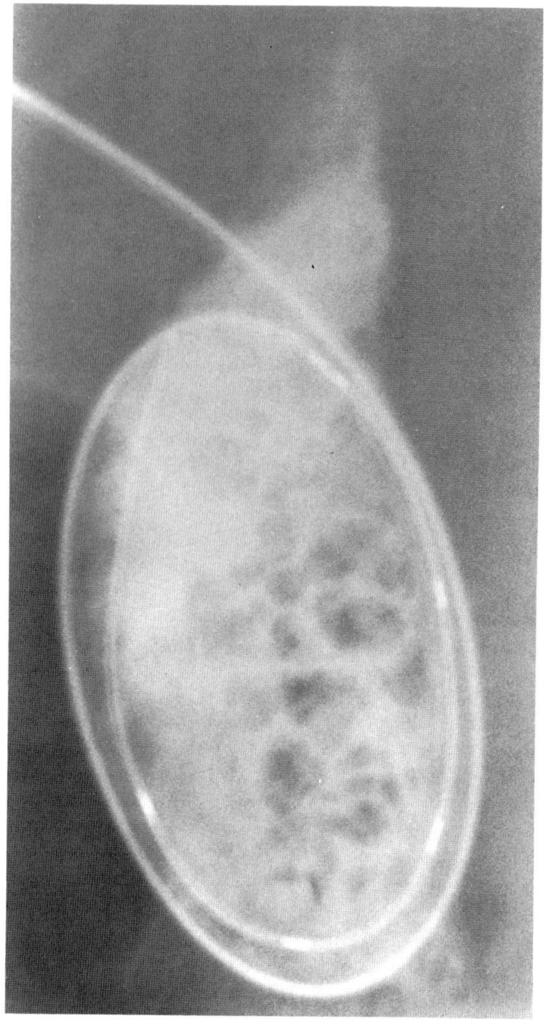

Fig. 6.2 As stone dissolution progresses, residual stone material is corralled into the fundus within the region of the pigtail using a guidewire.

Occasionally, a 7 F catheter is employed especially if we anticipate a substantial amount of insoluble debris to be released during cholesterol dissolution, for example for stones containing some calcium detectable by computed tomography (CT) scan.

Occasionally patients present with important contraindications to transhepatic catheter placement such as marked ascites or a coagulopathy. In the absence of cystic duct obstruction, a nasobiliary catheter can usually be placed retrograde via the cystic duct as has been described by a number of other investigators [6, 7]. We have utilized this technique in several patients successfully (Fig. 6.4). This approach is most likely to be effective if the stones are completely radiolucent on CT scan because the nasobiliary placement does not allow manipulation of stones into the optimal dissolution focus within the confines of the pigtail. Consequently, dissolution may be

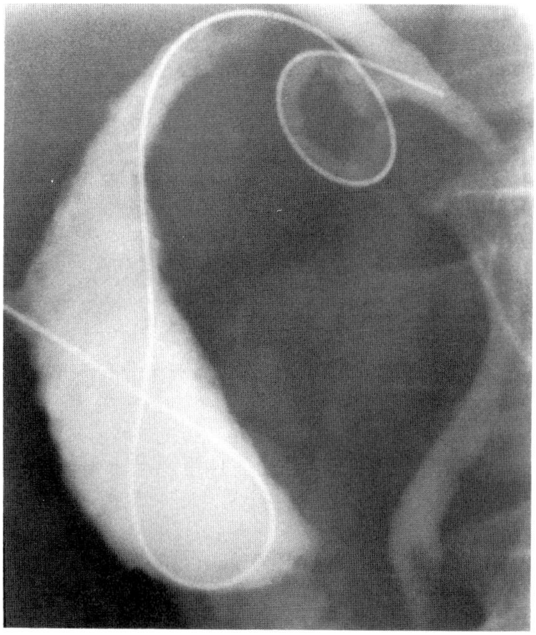

Fig. 6.3 Following complete stone dissolution, the gallbladder is almost completely collapsed then swept with loops of guidewire to search for any residual fragments. Any stones in the cystic duct system can usually be approached using this access route but may require extraction back into the gallbladder or dissolution *in situ* using a catheter placed into the cystic duct adjacent to the stone.

much more prolonged if the gallbladder is filled with mixed stones, many of which are outside of the pigtail region. Nevertheless, the endoscopic placement may be well tolerated and in some patients achieved without a papillotomy. An endoscopic procedure, however, may not be as easily tolerated in certain patients, for example those with severe pulmonary insufficiency.

At least one full loop of catheter is placed in the gallbladder to ensure that the pigtail does not migrate out into the hepatic parenchyma or completely out of the gallbladder because of respirations or patient movement, especially during the night (see Fig. 6.1). Although it is not uncommon for several centimetres of catheter to move from the gallbladder to the peritoneal interface, we have not lost gallbladder access when at least a loop of catheter has been placed in the gallbladder. Optimal location of the pigtail is in the fundus of the gallbladder away from the cystic duct and preferably away from the catheter entry site. As many stones as possible are corralled to within the confines of the pigtail which is the region toward which all of the infusion ports of the catheter are directed. Stone dissolution is much more rapid in this area than elsewhere in the gallbladder demonstrating the major enhancing effect of stirring of the solvent. Before leaving the radiology suite, the filling volume of the gallbladder is assessed with radioopaque contrast media as is the minimum volume which envelopes the stones. Often only 2 or 3 mL thoroughly encompasses the stone burden at least in the fundus including within the pigtail. Occasionally, extravasation at the catheter entry site can be demonstrated especially as the gallbladder is filled with contrast. To avoid traumatizing the fresh entry site, only minimal contrast is

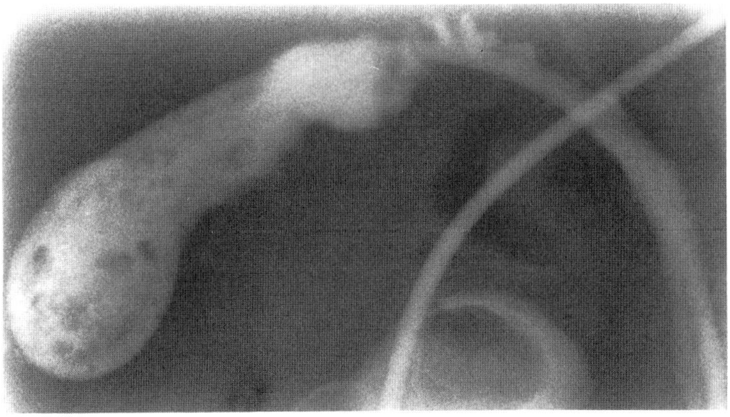

Fig. 6.4 Endoscopic retrograde placement of a 7 F catheter was utilized in this patient with ascites secondary to congestive heart failure allowing flushing of his mucopurulent bile and dissolution of the stones.

allowed to extravasate. Whenever demonstrated, this extravasation has always sealed spontaneously within 1–3 days.

Dissolution therapy is almost always initiated immediately following catheter placement although rarely, in a very fragile patient, this might be delayed until the following day. The volume of MTBE used for stone dissolution is at least several millilitres less than the demonstrated overflow volume of contrast and also less than the volume which might be seen to extravasate. Indeed, rapid stone dissolution can be achieved using only 0.5–1.0 mL of MTBE greater than the deadspace of the catheter which in the case of the Cook 5 F 70 cm catheter is 0.7 mL. When well tolerated and in the absence of extravasation, however, 3–7 mL is more commonly used. Patients often experience discomfort on the introduction of MTBE into the gallbladder. This discomfort resolves usually within the first few hours or by the second day. Discomfort can be minimized by using smaller volumes, for example, 1.5 or 2 mL and low doses of IV analgesia. We usually use butorphanol (Stadol®) 0.5–1.0 mg intravenously which is infrequently associated with nausea or other side-effects. While initial discomfort is common, we have never been asked to discontinue the treatment because of the discomfort. The mechanism of the discomfort seems most likely to be migration of MTBE along the fresh catheter entry tract since it is not a universal phenomenon and almost always resolves within a few hours. Persistence of pain suggests significant extravasation or overflow of MTBE from the gallbladder and should lead to radiological reassessment and reconsideration of treatment volume or adjustment of pigtail location rather than just completely masking it with analgesia.

The dissolution procedure can be well managed by an experienced paramedical person who understands the objectives and potential risks. The procedure is labour-intensive, however, and requires the full-time attention of one individual. Two or more paramedical participants allow continuous treatment with appropriate respite. Automatic pump systems have been developed and appear to be safe and effective [8, 9, 10]. These are not yet commercially available in the USA. Manual administration, however, is quite effective and practical. Optimal dissolution is achieved with continuous slow infusion and aspiration manually using a glass syringe. As the stone(s) dissolves, inflowing hepatic bile and released insoluble stone debris are removed with each aspiration at which time the gallbladder is completely emptied. A few millilitres of MTBE are then infused and either stirred back and forth for a few minutes or immediately reaspirated and reinfused. Inflowing bile will displace ether (which floats) from the stones and should not be allowed to accumulate. Moreover, if bile accumulates in the gallbladder, the overflow volume of the gallbladder (bile plus ether) may be exceeded. Overflow of more than a few millilitres of MTBE down the duct system may cause nausea, vomiting, discomfort, and potentially, if persistent over a period of hours, might cause duodenitis and, in sufficient concentration, even intravascular hemolysis [11]. These complications are easily prevented and we have not observed clinically significant evidence of these complications in more than 150 patients treated.

Confirmation of rapid dissolution of cholesterol can be observed by flooding a microscopic slide with MTBE after 10–15 minutes of continuous infusion and aspiration of the gallbladder. The ether can then be evaporated leaving a layer of white waxy, sticky cholesterol on the slide. This proves beyond doubt that the stones are indeed cholesterol and are dissolving and provides initial encouragement to the patient and family. Because MTBE is quite volatile even though liquid at body temperature (boiling point 55°C), we have installed a spark-free exhaust fan with a flexible hood under which MTBE can be evaporated from microscopic slides and the supply of MTBE filled syringes kept. Although neither patients, families, nor paramedical assistants have found the odour of MTBE in the treatment room a concern, this solvent is a potentially explosive general anaesthetic in very high concentrations. These conditions might occur with a large volume spill. Our individual syringes are usually filled with 10 mL and do not represent a significant risk providing reasonable and minor precautions are observed.

Progressive dissolution is often reassessed at 3–4 hour intervals so as to manipulate additional stones into the pigtail region or to document complete stone dissolution (see Fig. 6.2 and 6.3). Loops of guidewire are swept throughout the gallbladder in the presence of a thin layer of contrast while the gallbladder is collapsed around the loop of catheter. This allows detection of any small residual which can then be corralled into the pigtail. When no stone material can be detected fluoroscopically, an additional hour or two of treatment is preferred to minimize the possibility of any residual soluble material.

Catheter removal can usually be performed within 1–3 days of placement although deferring removal for 7–10 days is optimal and can be utilized in patients who can conveniently return to the medical centre the following week. A small soft catheter is very well tolerated in almost all patients especially after the first few hours. The catheter is not removed if extravasation of contrast can be demonstrated by distending the gallbladder sufficiently to overflow and fill the entire duct system. The absence of stones in the duct system and free duodenal runoff is always documented before catheter removal. Patients who have had contrast extravasation freely into the peritoneal cavity rather than contained within the hepatic interface should have catheter removal deferred for a day or two. In patients whose catheters are removed within the first week (almost all patients), we have placed a 2–3 cm cylinder of compressed sterile gelatin (Gelfoam®) in the transhepatic tract at the time of catheter removal using a sheath placed over the catheter. We have designed and manufactured a small device for preparing 1.7 mm diameter (5 F) compressed Gelfoam® cylinders from strips of Gelfoam®.

Patients are asked to stay overnight following catheter removal. An ultrasound examination of the gallbladder is performed the following morning (after the gallbladder has filled with bile) so that an accurate assessment of any residual debris can be made as a baseline for assessing stone regrowth or recurrence. Follow-up ultrasound examinations in 6 and 12 months then annually are routinely recommended.

Efficacy

Patient selection

Successful stone dissolution is predominantly determined by stone composition. Black bilirubin polymer stones are insoluble, and diffusely calcified cholesterol stones are difficult to dissolve with currently available direct contact solvents. Stone composition can best be determined by radiodensity. Stones which are radiopaque on plain abdominal X-ray films are not candidates for dissolution. Computed tomography is much more sensitive, however, and about half of the stones which are radiolucent on plain film will have calcification detectable by CT scan [12]. Our experience *in vitro* and *in vivo* suggests that most stones which have only surface (rim) calcification can be successfully treated with MTBE [8] (Figs 6.5–6.8). Stones with diffuse radiopacity or central calcification may dissolve very slowly, incompletely, or both. Pigment stones in the gallbladder are often radiolucent on plain film but are radiodense on CT scan [13]. Pigment stones,

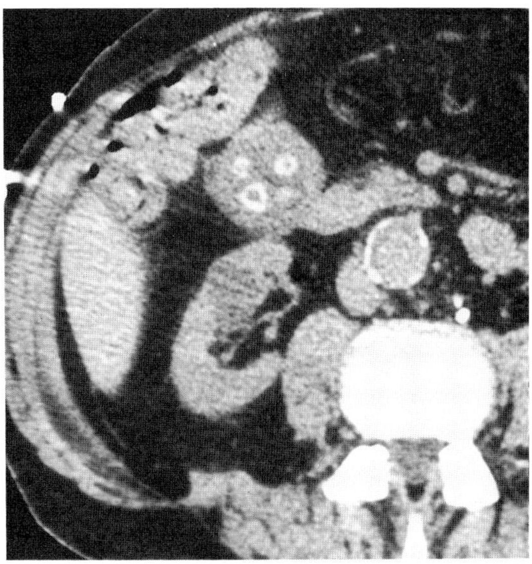

Fig. 6.5 CT scan demonstrates multiple rim calcified gallstones. This calcification was not apparent on abdominal plain films. The stones dissolved completely as illustrated in Figs 6.6–6.9.

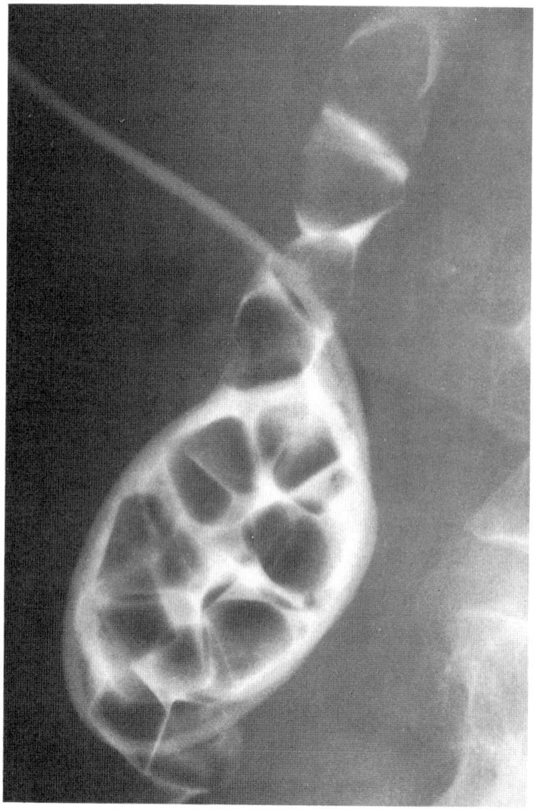

Fig. 6.6 In this patient, the percutaneous transhepatic catheter loops are all within the lower half of the gallbladder. The stones in the neck will be manipulated into the fundus after the stones in that area have been dissolved.

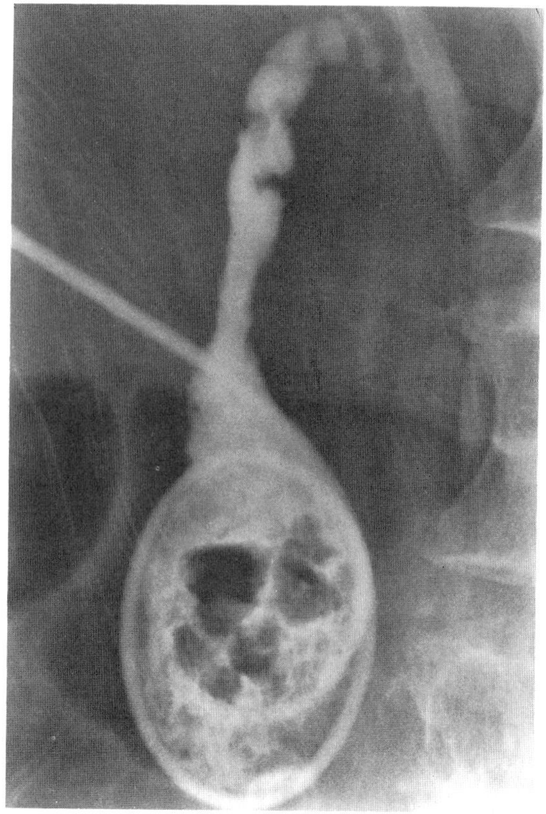

Fig. 6.7 The stones previously in the gallbladder neck have now been manipulated into the pigtail region of the catheter.

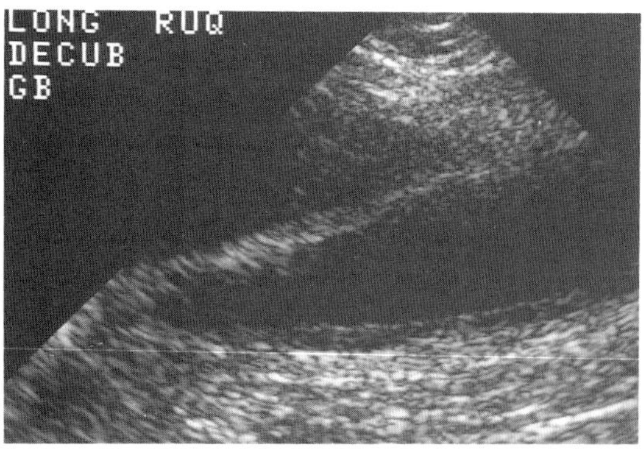

Fig. 6.8 Ultrasonography the day after catheter removal demonstrated no residual echogenic material. Mild gallbladder wall thickening is commonly observed and resolves without clinical sequelae.

however, are often less than 5 mm in diameter and if the stone burden is small, they may be missed by the CT scanner. A slice or two of the gallbladder may be omitted from scanning if the patient inspires to varying depths between slices. The gallbladder usually moves several centimetres per respiration. To minimize this artefact, we have used 3 mm slices through the gallbladder and prefer fast scanning technique which usually allows complete scanning of the gallbladder with a single breath hold [13]. It should be obvious that any contrast in the gallbladder will mask stone calcification and even oral contrast sequestered in the duodenum adjacent to the gallbladder may be difficult to differentiate from a small collection of radiopaque stones. It is, therefore, important to avoid either intravenous or oral contrast at the time of the CT scan. Moreover, if oral cholecystography is performed to ascertain cystic duct patency, the contrast may not be completely cleared from the gallbladder for 7–10 days.

Oral cholecystography is useful in documenting cystic duct patency although ultrasonography, radionuclide, or endoscopic retrograde radiocontrast methods will suffice. Oral cholecystography has the advantage of better demonstrating stone contour and possible buoyancy in the presence of radiopaque contrast. Cholesterol stones are usually smooth and often round, oval, or faceted. A family of high cholesterol content stones are also often similar in size and shape. In contrast, pigment stones are infrequently larger than 5 mm in diameter and are often much more irregular in surface contour and tend to be variable in size and shape. Mixed cholesterol-pigment stones may share some of the characteristics of both types of stones. If stones float in a layer in the presence of dense radiopaque contrast, they are high cholesterol content stones which will dissolve rapidly in MTBE.

Most patients have their diagnosis of gallstones made by ultrasonography. Although patency of the cystic duct can also be demonstrated with acceptable confidence if a stimulus to the gallbladder is administered and a convincing reduction in gallbladder volume (e.g., 50%) is documented, ultrasonography is a poor method for establishing stone composition. One can sometimes infer that stones are cholesterol stones based on some of the criteria described above, for example a large ovoid solitary stone is virtually always cholesterol. It may, however, be a heavily calcified cholesterol stone. Stone calcification can be suspected by ultrasonography especially if an inner ring of echodensity can be detected but CT scan is much more accurate. Unfortunately, the composition of multiple small stones cannot be reliably determined by ultrasonography.

Magnetic resonance imaging demonstrates stones in the gallbladder but has not been found to provide useful information about their composition. Duodenal drainage during cholecystokinin stimulation of gallbladder contraction provides gallbladder bile for examination microscopically. The demonstration of cholesterol crystals strongly supports a cholesterol component of the stones but does not guarantee that they do not have a substantial proportion of even an impenetrable layer of insoluble material.

The ideal patient for MTBE gallstone dissolution is one with cholesterol stones completely radiolucent by CT scan and a patent cystic duct with no specific risk factors for percutaneous transhepatic catheter placement. Most patients with an obstructed cystic duct can be treated successfully but the impacted stone(s) may require some additional manipulation or placement of a dissolution catheter directly into the cystic duct. A remote possibility which we have not encountered is a completely stenosed cystic duct. It is very rare to have so much bowel surrounding the liver so as to prevent a safe placement of a percutaneous transhepatic catheter but this would be one instance in which an endoscopic retrograde catheter placement would be useful. Patients at high risk for cholecystectomy presenting with acute cholecystitis are often successfully treated emergently by percutaneous transhepatic drainage of the gallbladder. After the inflammation has resolved, these patients are often excellent candidates for MTBE stone dissolution if their stones are soluble. Under these circumstances, the catheter tract does not need to be enlarged and the procedure is very well tolerated. When cystic, intrahepatic or extrahepatic duct stones are present, these can usually be successfully dissolved or extracted either via the percutaneous transhepatic catheter tract or by the endoscopic retrograde approach. A variety of single and double balloon catheters stable in MTBE are available to retain and retrieve MTBE and to optimize stone–solvent contact in the duct system by either access route [14].

The predominant contraindications to dissolution therapy are: insoluble stones; suspicion of gallbladder neoplasm; an acute inflamed gallbladder (which may be gangrenous or otherwise at risk for perforation); and inability to safely place a catheter into the gallbladder. However, pigment or heavily calcified cholesterol stones can be mechanically extracted. Stones may be fragmented by extracorporeal or direct contact lithotripsy techniques then either dissolved or extracted or a combination of both.

Results

Our experience in treating more than 150 patients with MTBE has demonstrated that cholesterol stones radiolucent by CT scan can be completely and rapidly dissolved with MTBE in almost all patients [3]. About 5% of patients have some residual material usually 5 mm or less in diameter detectable by fluoroscopy but insoluble in MTBE. Patients with multiple mixed stones are often left with one or more echogenic fragments of insoluble sludge detectable only by ultrasonography. Solitary CT radiolucent stones often contain little MTBE insoluble material and usually do not leave residual sludge. We have never had a patient come to cholecystectomy or require endoscopic papillotomy because of symptoms or complications from residual sludge. Some patients do develop stone regrowth which may or may not become symptomatic and require treatment. Although stone size and number influence the number of hours of treatment required, stone composition is a much more important variable. Stones of 4–6 cm in diameter have dissolved within 1 day of treatment whereas multiple 5 mm stones have required 3 or 4 days of treatment (Figs 6.9 and 6.10). When all stones can be encompassed by the pigtail, dissolution is more rapid than if the gallbladder body and neck are filled with stones. Unless very high in cholesterol content, the stones in the neck may not be effectively treated until the stones in the fundus are dissolved to make room for those in the upper half of the gallbladder to be brought into the pigtail. Cholesterol stones in the intrahepatic or extrahepatic duct system can be as effectively treated as gallbladder stones providing adequate stone-solvent contact is achieved. However, excessive exposure of MTBE to the duodenum and systemic absorption must be avoided.

Side-effects

Techniques for minimizing the discomfort of catheter placement and appropriate analgesia during initial treatment have been addressed above. Almost all patients are sufficiently comfortable to sleep the first evening without analgesia or only propoxyphene-acetominophen and by the second day of treatment, many patients require no analgesia during treatment. This ether is an anaesthetic but little is absorbed from the biliary tract. If substantial airflow from the gallbladder is permitted, patients may become drowsy and exhale MTBE easily detectable on their breath. The ether is rapidly exhaled and any sedation is transient. Neither bleeding nor bile leakage have been a problem during treatment. Following catheter removal, bile leakage can develop within minutes and cause quite severe pain. This usually stops spontaneously, and we have not recommended surgical intervention for any patients under these circumstances. As described above, we do not remove the catheter in the presence of extravasation at the gallbladder entry site and a Gelfoam® plug is placed when the catheter has been in position for less than a week. If a bile leak is suspected, patients are

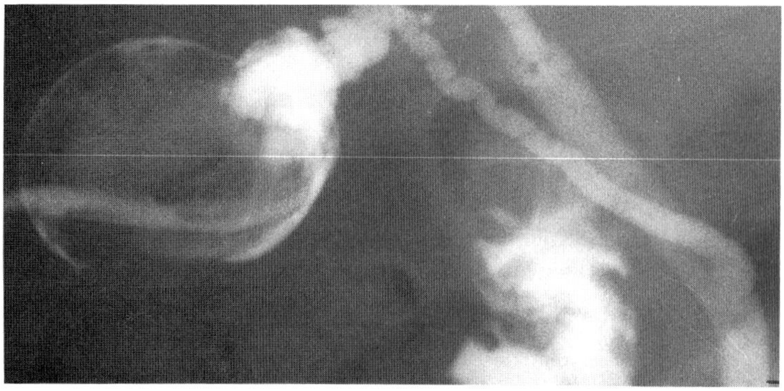

Fig. 6.9 A 6 cm solitary gallstone radiolucent on abdominal plain film and CT scan was associated with acute cholecystitis in a patient with severe cardiomyopathy. A percutaneous cholecystostomy was placed for initial decompression.

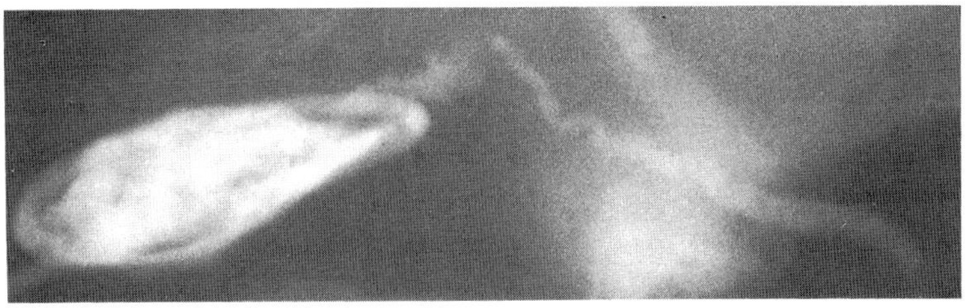

Fig. 6.10 After resolution of acute cholecystitis, a pigtail catheter was placed around the large solitary stone and MTBE therapy initiated. After 1 day of treatment, no definite residual was apparent. The gallbladder mucosa was irregular because of the severe chronic and recently acute inflammatory process.

treated with analgesia and prophylactic antibiotics. If discomfort persists for more than 2 or 3 days, persistent bile leakage can be documented by a radionuclide biliary scan and treated by a percutaneous transhepatic catheter inserted into the gallbladder via a new entry tract or a nasobiliary catheter placed endoscopically into the common hepatic duct.

Gallstone recurrence

Gallstone recurrence following MTBE dissolution is probably similar in frequency to that following other treatments which leave the gallbladder and cystic duct intact, for example after extracorporeal shock wave lithotripsy, oral bile acid therapy, or percutaneous cholecystolithotomy. Specifically, solitary cholesterol stones recur in 10–20% of patients and multiple stones in 50–70% of patients within 2–5 years. Our initial observation suggests that the presence of slight residual debris does not enhance the potential for stone regrowth. Other factors are probably more important, for example the balance of cholesterol nucleating and antinucleating factors. Moreover, cholesterol supersaturation and possibly abnormal motility must also be present. These three factors probably predominately determine whether stones recur independently of the presence or absence of a few fragments of calcium bilirubinate.

If stones recur they may be observed, as generally recommended for asymptomatic stones. Alternatively, these small new cholesterol stones may be treated with ursodiol for 3–6 months. Another option is to attempt to prevent stone recurrences in these high risk often elderly patients with prophylactic ursodiol, 6–8 mg/kg daily. The cholesterol synthesis inhibitors which are now available (lovastatin, simvastatin, and pravistatin) decrease biliary cholesterol secretion and prevent cholesterol stone formation in animal models. It remains unclear whether these will be effective in humans but for patients with hypercholesterolemia, these agents would be a logical choice and may also prevent gallstone formation.

Summary

Dissolution of soluble stones by MTBE introduced either by percutaneous or endoscopically placed catheters, has been very well tolerated and safe when performed by experienced clinician investigators. Patients with severe cardiovascular and pulmonary disease have been treated without compromising their multiple major medical problems. Alternatives are available including placement of cholecystostomy catheters under local anesthesia or using interventional radiology techniques. These approaches usually require larger catheters and are most safely performed in multiple stages. They may be associated with more discomfort and risk than placement of a 5 F catheter into the gallbladder. Nevertheless, these more invasive approaches may be preferable for an inexperienced physician or surgeon. For these infrequent patients, however, referral to a biliary treatment centre where direct contact dissolution can be performed with a high level of efficacy, safety, and comfort may be the optimal approach.

References

1 Mangano DT. Perioperative cardiac morbidity. *Anesthesiology* 1990;**72**:153–84.
2 Nelson PE, Moyer TP, Thistle JL. Gallstone dissolution *in vitro* using methyl tert-butyl ether: radiologic selection criteria. *Gastroenterology* 1990:**98**:1280–3.
3 Thistle JL, May GR, Bender CE *et al.* Dissolution of cholesterol gallbladder stones using methyl tert-butyl ether administered by percutaneous transhepatic catheter. *N Eng J Med* 1989:**320**:633–9.
4 Leuschner U, Hellstern A, Guldutuna S, Gatzen M, Leuschner M. Direct contact dissolution of gallbladder stones with methyl tert-butyl ether: experience in 209 patients. *Z Gastroenterol Verh* 1991;**26**:199–201.
5 vanSonnenberg E, Casola G, Zakko SF *et al.* Gallbladder and bile duct stones: percutaneous therapy with primary MTBE dissolution and mechanical methods. *Radiology* 1988;**169**:505–9.
6 Soehendra N, Schulz H, Nam VC *et al.* ESWL and gallstone dissolution with MTBE via a naso-vesicular catheter. *Endoscopy* 1990;**22**:176–9.
7 Foerster EC, Buhler H, Domschke W. Direct dissolution of gallbladder stones. *Lancet* 1989;**1**:954.
8 Ridgway TM, Stadheim, LM, Gray JE *et al.* Complete dissolution of cholesterol gallstones radiopaque on CT scan by methyl tert-butyl ether (MTBE) using an automatic pump system (APS) in vitro. *Gastroenterology* 1990;**98**:A259. (Abstract).
9 Poterucha JJ, Ridgway TM, Petersen BT *et al.* Dissolution of cholesterol gallstones (CGS) with methyl tert-butyl ether (MTBE) using an infusion-aspiration pump: phase I clinical studies. *Gastroenterology* 1991;**100**: A334. (Abstract).
10 Zakko SF, Hofmann AF. Microprocessor-assisted solvent-transfer system for gallstone dissolution. In vitro and in vivo validation. *Gastroenterology* 1990;**99**: 1807–13.
11 Ponchon T, Baroud J, Pugol B *et al.* Renal failure during dissolution of gallstones by methyl tert-butyl ether. *Lancet* 1988;**2**:176–7.
12 Ell C, Schneider T, Benninger J *et al.* Significance of computed tomography for shock-wave therapy of radiolucent gallbladder stones. *Gastroenterology* 1991; **101**:1409–16.
13 Poterucha JJ, Ridgway TM, Petersen BT *et al.* Patient selection for gallstone dissolution: differentiating soluble from insoluble gallstones. *Gastroenterology* 1991; **100**:A334. (Abstract).
14 Hurwich DB, Bender CE, LeRoy AJ *et al.* Direct contact dissolution of biliary duct and impacted gallbladder neck stones. *Hepatology* 1992;**16**:263A. (Abstract).

Chapter 7
Percutaneous cholecystolithotomy

R.C.G. Russell

Introduction

During the mid-1970s the concept of interventional radiology in biliary tract disease was explored, and percutaneous puncture of intra-abdominal structures either under fluoroscopy or ultrasound guidance became commonplace. These techniques were developed by urologists to drain the kidney. Subsequently, dilatation of the needle track to gain access to the pelvis of the kidney and remove renal stones proved possible. Recently, several similar non-invasive and minimally invasive techniques have been pioneered for the management of gallbladder stones [1].

The ability to puncture the gallbladder percutaneously under radiological control has resulted in the development of new diagnostic and therapeutic techniques. Transhepatic puncture of the gallbladder has been used for cholecystography and cholangiography, for aspiration of bile or pus, for culture in suspected cases of acute cholecystitis or empyema, and for biopsy of lesions within the gallbladder [2]. Direct percutaneous access to the gallbladder allows non-operative management of gallstone disease and this technique is being increasingly used, particularly in elderly and high-risk patients, for the treatment of acute cholecystitis, and empyema of the gallbladder as well as the perforated gallbladder with localized abscess formation [3]. Other therapeutic options made possible by percutaneous puncture of the gallbladder include contact dissolution of gallstones with solvents [4] and percutaneous cholecystolithotomy.

Percutaneous extraction of gallstones was first described in 1985 for treatment of high risk patients with acute cholecystitis, and was performed in up to five stages using a percutaneous transhepatic tract [5, 6]. The technique evolved from the introduction of percutaneous cholecystostomy as an alternative to surgical cholecystostomy and utilized well established techniques for dilating percutaneous tracts and stone extraction. In 1988, Kellett *et al.* adapted the technique of percutaneous nephrolithotomy for the extraction of gallbladder stones [7]. The gallbladder is accessed transperitoneally and not transhepatically, as large cannulae, which make stone extraction easier, cause unnecessary trauma to the liver.

Percutaneous cholecystolithotomy avoids the disadvantages of conventional cholecystectomy, namely: pain related to a large unsightly wound; a week of hospitalization; and 4–6 week's convalescence. Furthermore, there may be a place for preserving a functioning gallbladder in young patients [8] who have solitary or few stones and who may not have stone recurrence [9]. The main indications for this technique are the young and fit who may wish to preserve their gallbladders, the old and unfit who are not suitable for other methods of gallstone or gallbladder removal, and those who have a drain placed in the gallbladder to relieve an acute emergency [10].

Patient selection

Patients who have characteristic biliary disease should be carefully assessed by ultrasonography to determine: stone size; the number of stones; gallbladder wall thickness and position; and finally gallbladder function. The size of the common bile duct should be measured to determine the probability of a stone in the common bile duct

[11]. Gallbladder function (emptying) is best assessed by measuring the change in the fasting gallbladder volume after a fatty meal. Long axis and transverse images of the gallbladder are obtained and the volume calculated using the ellipsoid method [12], from the following formula

$$\text{Gallbladder volume (mL)} = \pi/6 \times \text{length} \times \text{width} \times \text{height}$$

A reduction in volume of 30% is regarded as satisfactory gallbladder function. Patients with stones of any composition, size and number contained in a thin-walled gallbladder with a fasting volume of greater than 15 mL are suitable for percutaneous cholecystolithotomy. Provided that there is a minimum gallbladder volume of 15 mL, neither an acute complication of gallbladder disease nor a non-functioning gallbladder (if caused by a stone impacted in Hartmann's pouch) are considered contraindications to treatment. Thus, patients with thick-walled contracted gallbladders are excluded because of the technical difficulty of puncturing and dilating a track through such a thickened, fibrosed gallbladder wall.

The procedure

Anaesthesia

The procedure can be performed under local or general anaesthesia. General anaesthesia is preferable as the procedure can be done in one stage with minimum discomfort. If local anaesthesia is used, a staged procedure is necessary with puncture of the gallbladder, dilatation of the track and then the stone extraction. The disadvantage of local anaesthesia is that some patients develop a profound acute vagal reaction with severe hypotension, bradycardia and diaphoresis during the puncture procedure [13]. Typical sedation under local anaesthesia includes intravenous morphine and midazolam hydrochloride or diazepam. Alternatively, an epidural anaesthetic may be used [14].

Approach

There are two general approaches to the gallbladder: transhepatic or transperitoneal. The advantage of the transhepatic approach is that bile leakage both at the time of the procedure and on removal of the tube should be minimal, and it should be possible to remove the tube earlier as the liver is said to seal the track more rapidly. The disadvantage of the transhepatic approach is that dilatation is more difficult, and dilatation is dangerous above 18 F. Further, the angle of approach to the gallbladder is inappropriate for a rigid choledochoscope. The advantage of the transperitoneal approach is that a fundal puncture can be achieved with a single stage dilatation up to 30 F and a good view of the whole gallbladder obtained with a rigid scope. The disadvantage of the transperitoneal approach is that access may be limited on account of overlying liver or colon.

Transhepatic approach

The gallbladder is first located with computed tomography (CT) or ultrasonography and a suitable pathway for the tract is identified. After CT localization, percutaneous cholecystostomy is performed with a combination of ultrasonic and fluoroscopic guidance. With the use of a Seldinger technique, an 8 or 10 F retention pigtail catheter is placed in the lumen of the gallbladder. Cultures of bile are obtained at initial aspiration, and patients are treated with the appropriate antibiotics. The following day, the tract is dilated with coaxial telescopic Teflon dilators (Dilators for Use with Stone Removal; Cook Inc., Bloomington, Ind., USA) to 18 F. An 18 F Teflon sheath is placed over an 18 F Teflon dilator, and all subsequent manipulations are performed through this sheath. A safety wire is coiled in the gallbladder lumen before the tract is dilated in order that the tract may be re-established if the Teflon sheath is displaced. On occasions the tract is difficult to dilate and the gallbladder rotates on the Teflon sheath. In such instances the gallbladder can be stabilized by removable T-fasteners (Cook).

Transperitoneal approach

Under ultrasound control the gallbladder is punctured with a Kellett needle (152 mm Longdwell

Sheathed Needle, Becton Dickinson, Ontario, Canada) or a spinal needle (Fig. 7.1). Contrast is injected into the gallbladder so that subsequent imaging is performed both by fluoroscopy and ultrasound. A suitable route for definitive puncture is chosen after screening. This is usually subhepatic, subcostal and transperitoneal, but occasionally an intercostal approach is more appropriate depending on the position of the liver relative to the costal margin. The aim is to puncture the gallbladder at the fundus optimizing access and visualization for the endoscopist. A 1 cm incision is made in the skin and the fundus punctured with the Kellett needle. A 0.89 mm wire with a floppy tip [Lunderquist; Cook, Europe] is introduced into the gallbladder (Fig. 7.2) with the tip placed in the cystic duct. The needle is removed and the track dilated with Teflon dilators, followed by rigid telescopic metal dilators [Olympus, Southend, UK] introduced in a coaxial fashion. The tract is dilated to 30 F and a Teflon sheath of the same dimension is introduced coaxially (Fig. 7.3). The metal dilators are removed. A 0.89 mm wire with a J formation (3 mm in diameter) [William Cook, Europe] is introduced so that its distal (5–10 cm) is curled up within the gallbladder and the Lunderquist wire is removed. The J wire is left in place and is held in position by an assistant to prevent displacement during stone extraction.

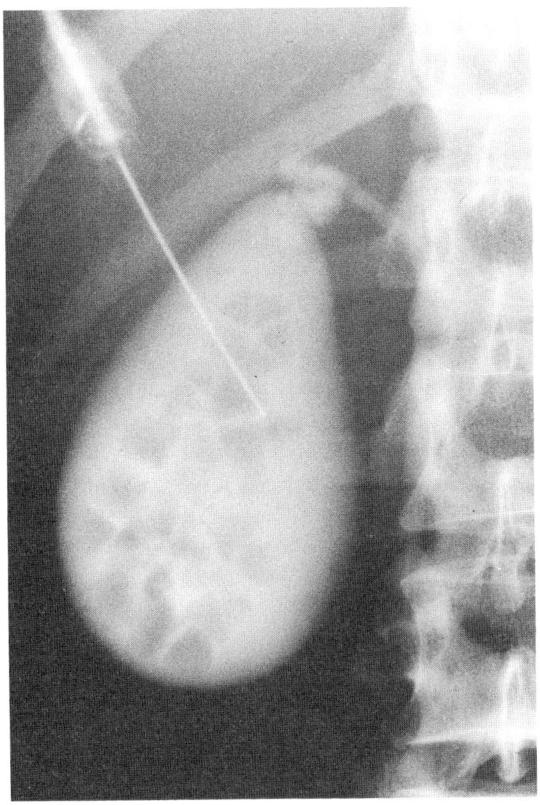

Fig. 7.1 Opacification of the gallbladder by injection of contrast via a transhepatically placed needle.

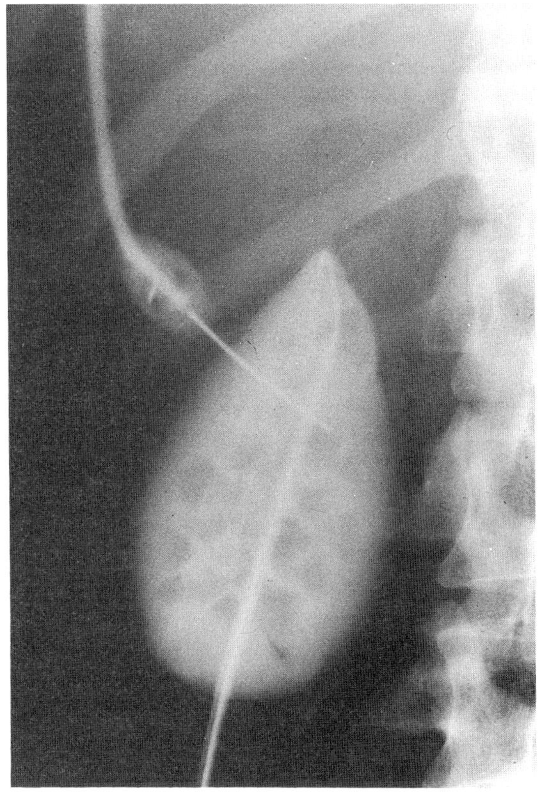

Fig. 7.2 A 0.89 mm guidewire with a floppy tip has been introduced into the lumen of the gallbladder by the transperitoneal fundal route.

Endoscopic techniques

The recent advances in both flexible endoscopes and rigid videoendoscopes have enabled changes to take place at this stage of the procedure. With the transhepatic approach stone extraction is

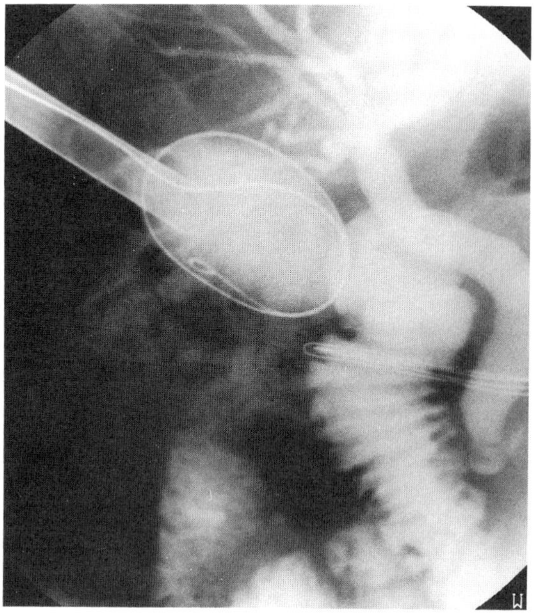

Fig. 7.3 A Teflon sheath has been placed into the gallbladder with a flexible guidewire to ensure that access is maintained.

performed by a combination of fluoroscopic guidance and direct visualization with a flexible choledochoscope (model CHF-4B; Olympus, Southend, UK). The flexible choledochoscope is 15 F in diameter and has a 2 mm working channel. With use of the working channel, stones are removed from the gallbladder with baskets and graspers. However, often the most efficient method of stone removal is irrigation of the gallbladder with a small catheter passed directly through the sheath to flush out the small stones. Prototype cholecystoscopes of 10 or 12 F (XCHF, Keymed, Olympus, Southend, UK) with a 3 F working channel are available and will enable the procedure to be performed through smaller Amplatz sheaths.

With the transperitoneal route large tracks can be achieved enabling the use of large instruments for more effective gallstone retrieval. The standard rigid straight viewing 26 F nephroscope with an 8 F working channel (Keymed, Olympus, Southend, UK) is ideal for the larger stones. Continuous saline irrigation via the nephroscope is necessary to maintain a clear field of view. Careful manipulation of the Amplatz sheath enables examination of the whole gallbladder.

Removal of gallstones

Stones larger than 1 cm have to be broken prior to removal either by means of direct contact lithotripsy or using crushing baskets or forceps. Lithotripsy is performed under direct vision with the lithotripter probe on the stone, using either electrohydraulic, ultrasound or laser medium to shatter the stone (Fig. 7.4). Ideally, the stone is broken up into larger fragments which can be picked out with the triradiate forceps. Once all the fragments are removed, clearance is assessed radiographically; a 14 or 16 F Foley catheter is introduced through the Amplatz sheath, the J wire removed, and the balloon of the Foley catheter inflated (Fig. 7.5). Gentle traction is applied to the

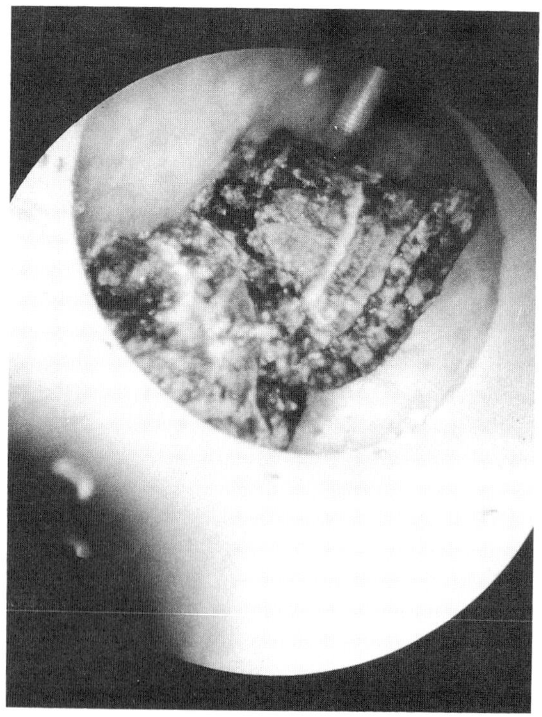

Fig. 7.4 The lithotripter probe in contact with a stone causing stone disruption.

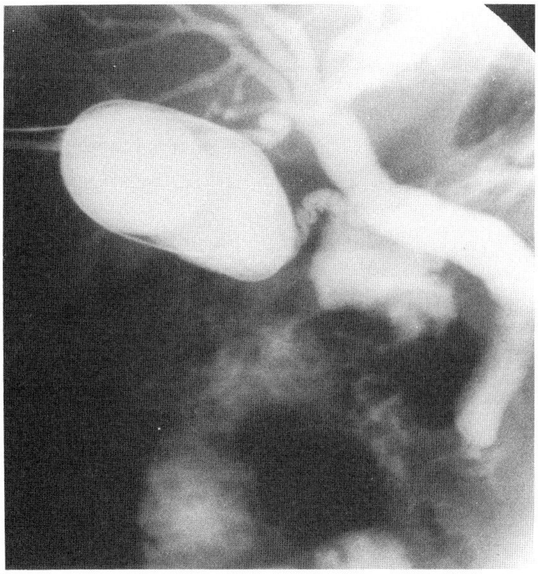

Fig. 7.5 Foley catheter in the gallbladder prior to removal of the guidewire.

catheter as the Teflon sheath is removed to minimize bile leakage. Contrast is then injected to ascertain the clearance of all the stones. If stone clearance is confirmed the Amplatz sheath is removed.

Patient management

The Foley catheter is attached to a drainage bag and the patient returned to the ward. The patient is discharged on the 2nd day and returns on the 14th day as an outpatient to have a contrast examination of the biliary tree. If no stones are seen, the Foley catheter is removed; while if stones are noted, removal using the flexible choledochoscope is undertaken.

Cholecystoscope

As an alternative to localizing the gallbladder under ultrasound control, a cholecystoscope can be used. This instrument consists of two concentric tubes sealed at one end. Suction applied to the space between the tubes creates a ring vacuum which fixes the instrument to the gallbladder fundus. Under epidural anaesthesia a 2.5 cm incision is made in the right upper quadrant of the abdomen and the peritoneal cavity is entered. The cholecystoscope is introduced, the gallbladder fundus identified, and the cholecystoscope fixed to the fundus by a vacuum created to ensure a seal between the instrument and the gallbladder. The gallbladder is incised under direct vision, and the stones removed either with the aid of a scope or by direct vision using grasping forceps. When the gallbladder is clear of stones, a Foley catheter is left in the gallbladder. Only Johnson's group [15] have experience with this instrument. The authors contend that this procedure is safe, inexpensive and requires minimal training. It is ideal for those who do not have access to good interventional radiology. It is yet another technique of value in the sick elderly person for whom operative intervention is inappropriate.

Laparoscopic cholecystolithotomy

Unfortunately, many of those undertaking laparoscopic cholecystectomy do not remember the option of laparoscopic cholecystolithotomy; for its intelligent use could save many patients a laparotomy and prevent inexperienced laparoscopists from getting into problems with which they are unable to deal. If at laparoscopy one unexpectedly encounters an acutely inflamed pus-filled gallbladder with multiple adhesions such that the anatomy around the porta hepatis is obscured, and thus cholecystectomy would be unsafe, the fundus of the gallbladder should be exposed, and the right lateral trocar inserted into the gallbladder and the contents aspirated. Two courses of action are now open, either a drainage catheter is inserted into the gallbladder and the operation concluded or the stones are removed immediately with a nephroscope. Perissat and his group used this technique during his early experience with laparoscopic cholecystectomy and treated 17 patients with biliary colic with minimal morbidity [16]. It still has value if there is a large stone load which makes grasping the gallbladder difficult or obscures important anatomical landmarks. Removal of the stones with a nephroscope and lithotripsy can transform a difficult operation into a straightforward procedure.

Results of percutaneous cholecystolithotomy

There is an initial learning curve with percutaneous cholecystolithotomy. However, stone clearance can be achieved in approximately 90% of patients. Chiverton *et al.* achieved clearance of the gallbladder in 56 of 60 patients [17]; in 4 patients there was a failure of access which necessitated cholecystectomy. Seven of the patients had complications postoperatively, none of which were major. In another series, Cheslyn-Curtis *et al.* [18] successfully performed percutaneous cholecystolithotomy in 100 of 113 patients. Complications, usually biliary collections, developed in 15 patients and all were managed conservatively. In a further series, Picus *et al.* [19] were successful in removing all the stones in 56 of 58 patients, including cystic duct calculi in 15 patients.

The long-term results of patients following percutaneous cholecystolithotomy are as yet poorly documented. Burhenne's group followed 63 patients who had undergone successful cholecystolithotomy [20]. Follow-up examinations in 48 of these patients at a mean of 18 months after the procedure, showed a recurrence of gallstones in 13 patients (27%). Our own experience is similar with a 31% recurrence rate at a mean of 2 years.

Comment

Percutaneous cholecystolithotomy is a feasible technique, successful in achieving stone clearance, but associated with a high incidence of recurrent stone formation. Thus, its role is limited, and should be reserved for the elderly sick patient who is unsuitable for laparoscopic cholecystectomy. It has been my experience that recurrence can be managed by laparoscopic cholecystectomy, which is the first line of treatment. This type of radiological treatment should not be undertaken in the young fit patient, unless reasons for preservation of the gallbladder are shown to be of greater advantage.

References

1 Cheslyn-Curtis S, Russell RCG. New trends in gallstone management. *Br J Surg* 1991;78:143–9.
2 van Sonnenberg E, D'Agostino HB, Casola G, Varney RR, Ainge GD. Interventional radiology in the gallbladder: diagnosis, drainage, dissolution, and management of stones. *Radiology* 1990;**174**:1–6.
3 McGahan JP, Lindfors KK. Percutaneous cholecystostomy: an alternative to surgical cholecystostomy for acute cholecystitis. *Radiology* 1989;**173**:481–5.
4 Leuschner U, Hellstern A, Schmidt K *et al.* Gallstone dissolution with methyl tert-butyl ether in 120 patients —efficacy and safety. *Dig Dis Sci* 1991;**36**:193–9.
5 Akiyama H, Nagusa Y, Fujita T *et al.* A new method for nonsurgical cholecystolithotomy. *Surg Gynecol Obstet* 1985;**161**:73–4.
6 Kerlan RK, LaBerge JM, Ring EJ. Percutaneous cholecystolithotomy: preliminary experience. *Radiology* 1985;**157**:656–6.
7 Kellett MJ, Russell RCG, Wickham JEA. Percutaneous cholecystolithotomy. *Br Med J* 1988;**296**:453–5.
8 Walsh TN, Russell RCG. Cholecystectomy and gallbladder conservation. *Br J Surg* 1992;**79**:4–5.
9 Dowling RH. Medical treatment of gallbladder stones: good news and bad news. In: Paumgartner G, Stiehl A, Gerok W, eds. *Trends in Bile Acid Research*. Dordrecht: Kluwer Academic, 1988:283–305.
10 Ainley CC, Williams SJ, Smith AC *et al.* Gallbladder sepsis after stent insertion for bile duct obstruction: management by percutaneous cholecystostomy. *Br J Surg* 1991;78:961–3.
11 Gillams A, Cheslyn-Curtis S, Russell RCG, Lees WR. Can cholangiography be safely abandoned in laparoscopic cholecystectomy? *Ann R Coll Surg Engl* 1992; **74**:248–51.
12 Dodds WJ, Groh WJ, Darweesh RMA, Lawson TL, Kishk SMA, Kern MK. Sonographic measurement of gallbladder volume. *Am J Radiol (Roentenol)* 1985;**145**:1009–10.
13 vanSonnenberg E, D'Agostino HB, Goodacre BW, Sanchez RB, Casola G. Percutaneous gallbladder puncture and cholecystostomy: results, complications, and caveats for safety. *Radiology* 1992;**183**:167–70.
14 Cope C, Burke DR, Meranze SG. Percutaneous extraction of gallstones in 20 patients. *Radiology* 1990:**176**: 19–24.
15 Majeed AW, Reed MWR, Watkin DFL, Smart JG, Johnson AG. Sheffield cholecystoscope: new instrument for minimally invasive gallbladder surgery. *Br J Surg* 1991:78:557–8.
16 Perissat J, Collet DR, Belliard R. Gallstones: Lapar-

oscopic treatment, intracorporeal lithotripsy followed by cholecystostomy or cholecystectomy – a personal technique. *Endoscopy* 1989;21:373–4.

17 Chiverton SG, Inglis JA, Hudd C, Kellett MJ, Russell RCG, Wickham JEA. Percutaneous cholecystolithotomy: the first 60 patients. *Br Med J* 1990;300: 1310–12.

18 Cheslyn-Curtis S, Gillams A, Russell RCG *et al.* Selection, management and early outcome of 113 patients with symptomatic gallstones treated by percutaneous cholecystolithotomy. *Gut* 1992;33:1253–9.

19 Picus D, Hicks ME, Darcy MD *et al.* Percutaneous cholecystolithotomy: Analysis of results and complications in 58 consecutive patients. *Radiology* 1992;183: 779–84.

20 Gibney RG, Chow K, So CB, Rowley VA, Cooperberg PL, Burhenne HJ. Gallstone recurrence after cholecystolithotomy. *Am J Roentgenol* 1989;153:287–9.

Chapter 8
Open cholecystolithotomy

A.L. Leahy

The first effective surgical treatment for symptomatic gallstones was, in fact, discovered by accident! In 1743 Jean-Louis Petit, the leading French surgeon reported three patients in whom the gallbladder was inadvertently opened during operations to incise abscesses in the upper abdomen. Despite the fact that only one of these patients survived, Petit recommended the operation of cholecystolithotomy for gallstones [1]. Subsequently, the operation became widely practised, even after the introduction of cholecystectomy by Carl Langenbuch in 1882.

In the 1920s the operation was largely abandoned because of the high incidence of retained and recurrent calculi. The incidence of recurrent stones may be as high as 50% over 3 years [2] and 83% at 15 years follow-up [3]. Many of these recurrences are likely to have resulted from fragments or stones overlooked at the initial operation.

Current indications for cholecystolithotomy

Planned mini-cholecystostomy

Increasingly, elderly infirm patients are presenting for treatment of symptomatic gallstones, and surgical mortality is higher in this group. The mortality rate for patients over 80 years of age is 7% for elective cholecystectomy and 14% if the operation is performed after acute cholecystitis [4]. Consequently, mini-cholecystostomy with stone removal, under local anaesthesia and as a planned procedure, offers a therapeutic option in high-risk elderly patients with symptomatic gallstones.

Laparotomy or laparoscopic cholecystostomy

Cholecystostomy is an important surgical strategy when attempted cholecystectomy is found to be too dangerous. The commonest indication for cholecystostomy in these circumstances is 'difficult dissection' and occasionally patients may be deemed unstable or unfit for completion of a cholecystectomy [5].

Technique of mini-cholecystostomy

Many patients considered for this procedure will be over 60 years of age and have concomitant disease, so adequate pre-operative medical preparation is essential. In obtaining informed consent the patients should be advised that general anaesthesia and full laparotomy may be occasionally required. Antibiotic prophylaxis is given and patients are fasted pre-operatively.

Immediately prior to operation the gallbladder is localized by real-time ultrasonography, paying particular attention to its relationship to overlying liver and colon. The surface marking of the gallbladder fundus is marked on the skin with an indelible pen (Fig. 8.1). The site of incision is infiltrated with 0.5% bupivicaine and adrenaline, and patients are sedated with intravenous opiate analgesia.

A 3 cm abdominal incision is made over the gallbladder. The gallbladder fundus is infiltrated with a 1% lignocaine subserosally and grasped with Babcock forceps. A 3.0 polyglyconate purse-string suture is inserted and bile is aspirated using an Ochsner gallbladder trocar and cannula. The gallbladder opening is widened and stones are removed using Desjardin's forceps and other im-

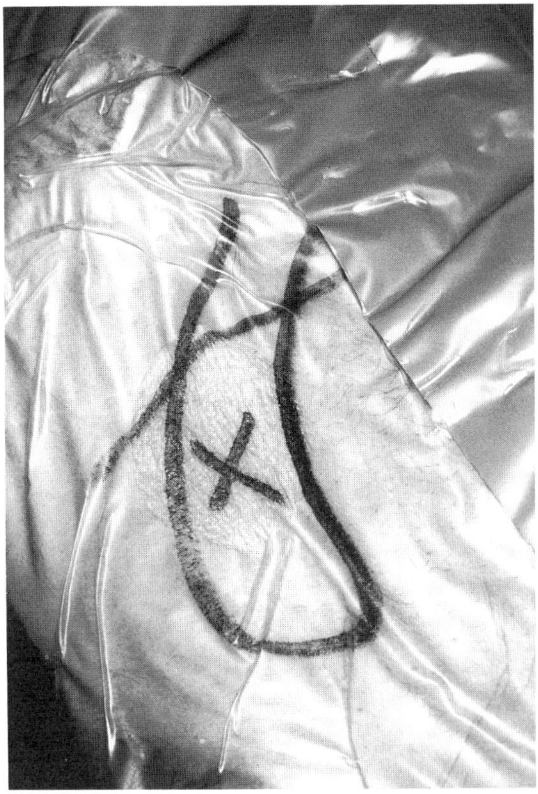

Fig. 8.1 The gallbladder fundus is located by real-time ultrasound and marked with indelible pen on the skin.

plements (Fig. 8.2). A cylindrical sheath is then secured in the gallbladder by a purse-string suture (Fig. 8.3). The gallbladder lumen is then examined using 24 F rigid nephroscope (Richard Wolf GmBH, Knittlingen, Germany) and residual stones are removed by forceps, or if large or impacted, they are fragmented using an ultrasonic contact lithotripter (Richard Wolf GmBH, Knittlingen, Germany) (Figs 8.4 and 8.5). When stone clearance is confirmed endoscopically a 24 F Foley catheter is secured in the gallbladder with monofilament polyglyconate sutures and the wound is closed (Fig. 8.6). Tube cholecystography is performed to confirm stone clearance (Fig. 8.7) and to outline the bile ducts, using 20–30 ml of 25% Hypaque contrast (Stirling Research Laboratories, Guildford, Surrey, UK).

Patients are allowed to mobilize, eat and drink on the same day, and are discharged the following day. Stone debris and mucus threads are discharged from the gallbladder for up to 5 days post-operatively. Once stone clearance is confirmed by cholecystography on day 7, the Foley catheter and sutures are removed.

Electromagnetic and laser lithotripsy can also be used as an adjunct to direct stone removal. The gallbladder epithelium can be damaged directly by the electromagnetic lithotripter probe so it must be used with caution. Pulsed dye laser is safer

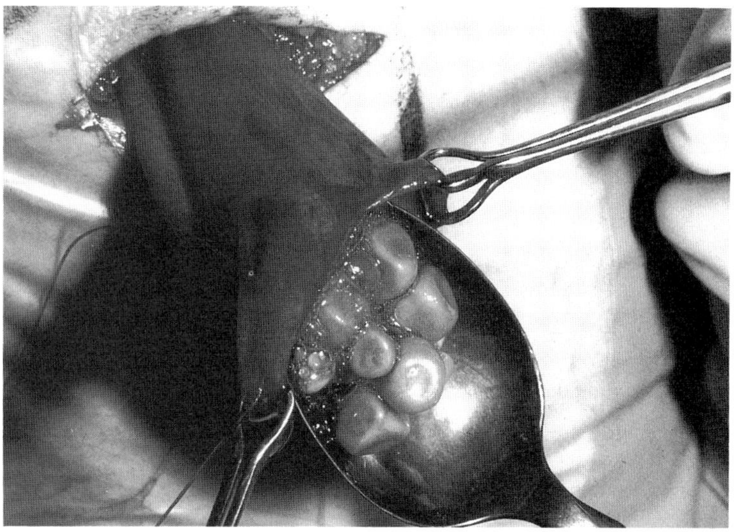

Fig. 8.2 Stones are removed through the cholecystostomy.

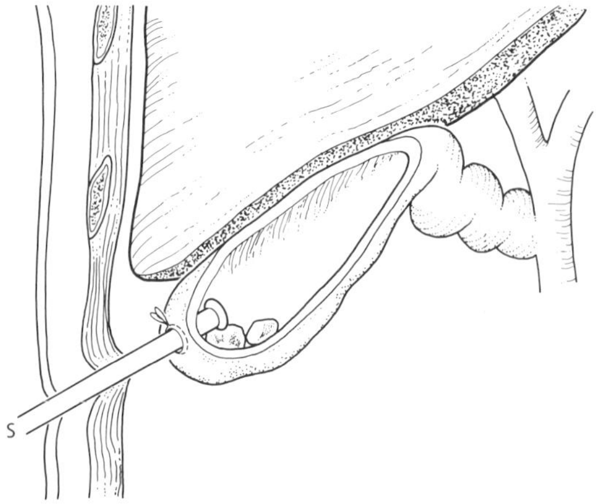

Fig. 8.3 Diagrammatic representation of a sheath (S) secured in the gallbladder by a purse-string suture. The sheath is used for introduction of a rigid endoscope.

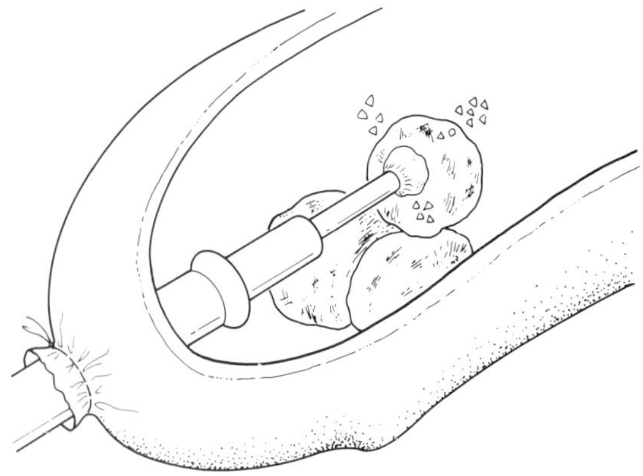

Fig. 8.5 Diagrammatic representation of ultrasound contact lithotripsy probe, introduced through a 24 F 'nephroscope', fragmenting gallstones.

to use, but expensive. Alternatively, Gibney and colleagues [6] have described the technique of mini-cholecystostomy combined with radiological techniques for stone extraction at a later date. Delaying stone extraction is inconvenient and unnecessary in most patients [7].

Technique of laparoscopic or laparotomy cholecystolithotomy

On occasions a planned cholecystectomy will need to be aborted and cholecystolithotomy performed. After preliminary aspiration of the gallbladder with an Ochsner gallbladder trocar and cannula at open operation, or a Veres needle at laparoscopy, stones are removed. Areas of necrotic gallbladder wall can be removed if necessary, and a large Foley or mushroom catheter is left in the gallbladder lumen. Cholecystectomy may be required at a later date.

Future role

Open cholecystostomy will continue to play an

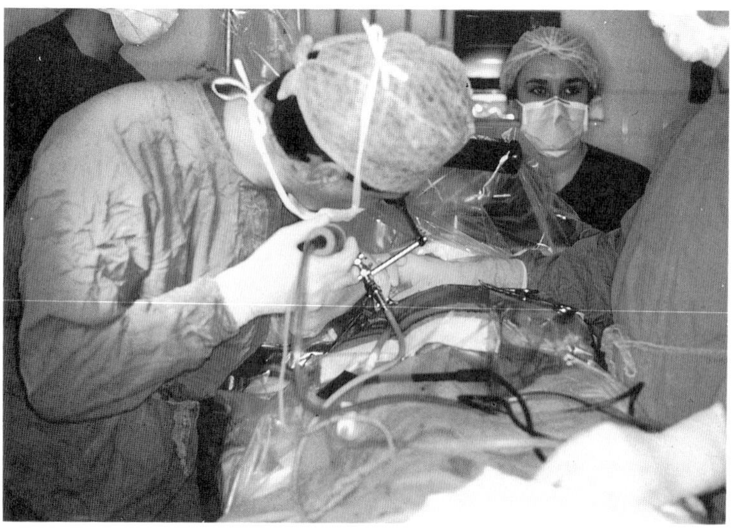

Fig. 8.4 The gallbladder is examined endoscopically and contact lithotripsy (in operator's right hand) is used to fragment larger calculi.

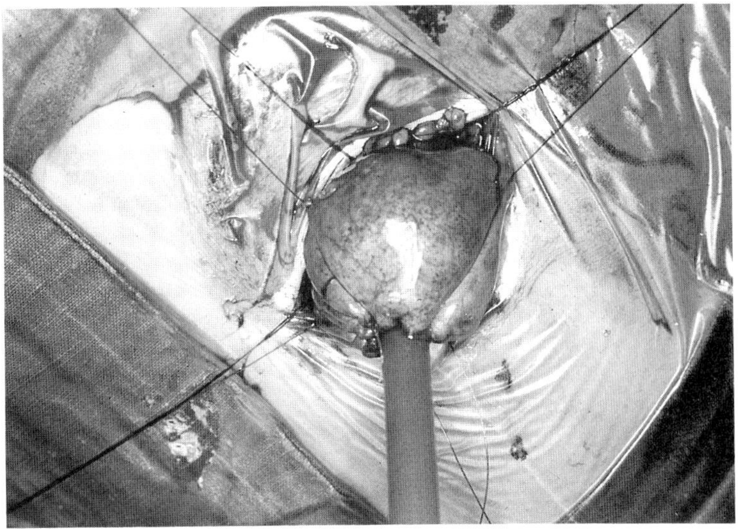

Fig. 8.6 A Foley catheter provides drainage postoperatively and access for tube cholecystography.

important, if limited, role in patients who are unfit for cholecystectomy, or in whom unclear anatomy precludes cholecystectomy. These indications have not been altered by the advent of laparoscopic cholecystectomy. Complete stone clearance can nowadays be achieved at minicholecystolithotomy using endoscopy and contact lithotripsy. This allows resolution of symptoms at a single operation and, in most suitable patients, given their age and intercurrent disease, there is little likelihood of stone recurrence becoming a problem in the future [8].

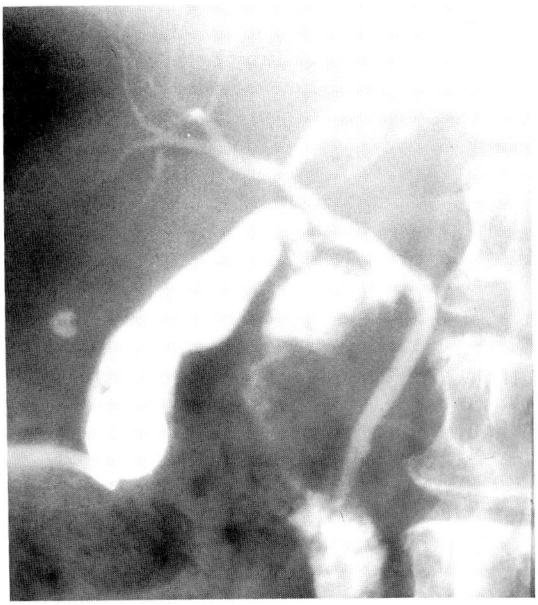

Fig. 8.7 Normal cholecystogram performed prior to removal of the Foley catheter on day 7.

Percutaneous cholecystolithotomy has been proposed as an alternative to open cholecystolithotomy. Kellett and colleagues [9] have reported successful removal of gallstones using percutaneous cholecystolithotomy under radiological guidance. This procedure usually requires general anaesthesia and has major complications including gallbladder rupture, bile peritonitis, bleeding, fatal vagal reactions, hypotension and acute respiratory distress [10, 11]. Percutaneous cholecystolithotomy is unlikely to replace open cholecystolithotomy under local anaesthesia in high-risk patients.

Finally, mini-cholecystostomy could be combined with chemical cholecystectomy in the future [8]. This could potentially obviate the need for laparoscopic or laparotomy cholecystectomy and extend the indications for mini-cholecystostomy.

References

1 Heager KHM. The triumph of complex operations. In: *The Illustrated History of Surgery*. London:

Starke, 1989:225–8.
2 Schild E. On cholecystolithotomy. *Acta Soc Med Uppsala* 1960;**65**:91–5.
3 Norrby F, Schonebeck J. Long-term results with cholecystolithotomy. *Acta Chir Scand* 1970;**136**:711–13.
4 Gutman H, Deutsch AA, Nudelmann IL, Reiss R. Cholecystectomy for octogenarians. *Dig Surg* 1988;**5**: 189–93.
5 Hawyard SJ, Walker SJ, Holt S. Cholecystostomy: a safe alternative? *Br J Clin Practice* 1990;**44**:593–5.
6 Gibney RG, Fache JS, Becker CD *et al.* Combined surgical and radiological intervention for complicated cholelithiasis in high risk patients. *Radiology* 1988;**165**: 715–19.
7 Leahy AL, Darzi AW, Murchan PM *et al.* A safe new procedure for high-risk patients with symptomatic gallstones. *Br J Surg* 1991;**78**:1319–20.
8 Leahy AL, McCollum PT, O'Gorman S *et al.* Cystic duct obliteration and gallbladder mucosal destruction: a feasible alternative to cholecystectomy. *Br J Surg* 1991;**78**:1321–4.
9 Kellett MJ, Wickham JE, Russell RC. Percutaneous cholecystolithotomy. *Br Med J (Clin Res)* 1988;**296**: 453–5.
10 van Sonnenberg E, D'Agostino HB, Goodacre BW *et al.* Percutaneous gallbladder puncture and cholecystostomy: results, complications, and caveats for safety. *Radiology* 1992;**183**:167–70.
11 LeBerge JM, Gordon RL, Kerlan RK, Ring EJ. Delayed gallbladder rupture following percutaneous cholecystostomy. *J Vasc Intervent Radiol* 1991;**2**:539–41.

Chapter 9
Laparotomy cholecystectomy

J.G. Geraghty & D.H. Osborne

Introduction

Cholecystectomy was first performed in 1882 and the operation remains the most commonly performed major abdominal procedure in the UK and the USA. However, the advent of laparoscopic cholecystectomy had resulted in a marked reduction in the numbers of patients having a laparotomy or open cholecystectomy. Within the next 5–10 years surgical trainees will have experience with laparoscopic cholecystectomy, but comparatively little exposure to the open procedure. Open cholecystectomy will probably remain a widely performed procedure in developing countries where the lack of technology dictates surgical practice.

Indications

First choice procedure

Some surgeons hold the view that open cholecystectomy via a traditional or mini-laparotomy incision is the preferred surgical treatment in the management of gallstone disease. Reports of the unacceptably high rates of common bile duct injury have been forwarded as the main reason for opting for open surgery (Table 9.1).

Failed laparoscopic cholecystectomy

Laparoscopic cholecystectomy may be converted to the open procedure for a number of different reasons: unclear ductal anatomy; an acutely inflammed gallbladder; obesity; and in patients who have had previous upper abdominal surgery. In the majority of patients it is usually possible to predict pre-operatively those in whom laparoscopic cholecystectomy may be difficult or unsuccessful.

Common bile duct stones

The use of endoscopic retrograde cholangiography with sphincterotomy as treatment for common bile duct stones has increased. However, many surgeons are concerned about the uncommon but occasionally fatal complications of endoscopic sphincterotomy, and also about bile duct damage at laparoscopic cholecystectomy. They would, therefore, recommend open cholecystectomy with common bile duct exploration as being a safer method of management.

Other surgery

Open cholecystectomy may be performed as part of other surgical procedures (e.g., Whipple's operation). If gallstones are found as an incidental finding during another open procedure then cholecystectomy may be indicated if there is evidence of previous gall bladder inflammation.

Operative technique

The gallbladder may be removed in one of two ways: either by starting the dissection from the fundus of the gallbladder (retrograde approach) or from the cystic duct (antegrade approach). The cystic duct approach is recommended unless there is difficulty in identification of the structures in Calot's triangle. In this case, the fundus-first approach is the method of choice. The fundus-first approach allows clear identification of the

Table 9.1 Bile duct injury (Laparoscopic cholecystectomy)

Author	Incidence (%)
Soper [19]	2.0
Cushieri *et al.* [18]	0.3
Peters *et al.* [16]	1.0
Deziel *et al.* [15]	0.6
Meyers [17]	0.5

cystic duct and common bile duct anatomy. Thus, common bile duct injury is less likely to occur, despite oozing from the gallbladder bed.

Antegrade cholecystectomy (cystic duct approach)

The approach to the gallbladder is through a vertical (right paramedian or midline) or right subcostal (Kocher's) incision. On opening the abdominal cavity, a hand should be passed over the top of the liver to abolish the vacuum which may exist between the liver and the right hemidiaphragm and to facilitate downward displacement of the liver. Two packs are then inserted. The first pack is to retract the hepatic flexure of the colon and small bowel. The assistant's hand is placed over this pack, thus retracting the second part of the duodenum away from the gallbladder. The second pack is placed over the antral region of the stomach and first part of the duodenum, keeping the stomach out of the operative field. The fundus of the gallbladder is grasped with a sponge-holding or a Duval forceps and the gallbladder retracted downwards and outwards by the operator. A second forceps is placed on Hartmann's pouch. This is also drawn caudally and laterally by the operator. These measures place the cystic duct on stretch so that Calot's triangle (where the cystic artery lies) may be identified. An incision is made over the peritoneum of the neck of the gallbladder and the fatty tissue in this region is dissected away from Hartmann's pouch towards the common bile duct. This technique will allow identification of the supraduodenal portion of the common bile duct. The junction of the cystic duct and the common bile duct should be carefully identified and further dissection towards the liver into Calot's space will display the cystic artery and the common hepatic duct. Care should be taken to ensure that the artery seen is not the right hepatic artery and it may be necessary to trace the cystic artery out into the body of the gallbladder. The cystic artery is a small vessel which should be handled gently and should be suture ligated. Operative cholangiography should be performed if there is a possibility of common bile duct stones or if the anatomy is difficult to define. A cannula is introduced and tied into the cystic duct and two films taken following injection with 3 mL and 8 mL of contrast material. When the films have been inspected the cystic duct should be divided after suture ligation of the distal cystic duct. The cystic artery should also be divided after suture ligature. Once the cystic duct and artery have been divided the gallbladder will come away from the liver bed. Careful dissection between gallbladder and liver bed will prevent perforation of the gallbladder or excessive bleeding from the liver. In those situations where there is a large tense gallbladder, finger dissection between liver and gallbladder may be a more suitable technique.

Retrograde cholecystectomy (fundus-first approach)

The gallbladder is approached through vertical or subcostal incisions. It may be necessary to decompress the gallbladder using a trochar and cannula following placement of a purse-string suture in the fundus. The gallbladder is then grasped with a suitable forceps and the organ is gradually dissected free from the liver bed using scissors or diathermy dissection. If there is a lot of oozing from the gallbladder bed it may be controlled by the placing of a pack. Careful dissection is required near Hartmann's pouch to allow accurate identification of the cystic artery. This is particularly true in patients with cholecystitis where the cystic artery is an extremely friable vessel. The cystic duct and common hepatic duct junction can usually be clearly identified using sharp and blunt dissection. Careful finger dissection of

Hartmann's pouch between index finger and thumb of the right hand will usually allow isolation of an inflammed cystic duct. Cholangiography at this stage is wise prior to cholecystectomy.

Discussion

The advent of laparoscopic cholecystectomy has focussed attention on the current indications for open cholecystectomy. It is clear from the results of many large series of open cholecystectomy that this is a safe operation [1–7]. It is also the standard against which other surgical and medical means of treating gallstones should be compared. McSherry [1] in an analysis of over 10 000 cholecystectomies carried out in the period 1932–84 showed that open cholecystectomy had a mortality rate of 0.6%. Although mortality rates vary (from 1.8% in 28 000 patients reported by Arnold [2] to 0% reported by Ganey and colleagues [3]) the overall mortality for elective cholecystectomy is less than 1% [4–9].

As well as a low mortality, open cholecystectomy is also associated with low morbidity. Bile duct injury following open cholecystectomy [7–14] is very low (Table 9.1) compared with reports of similar injuries after laparoscopic cholecystectomy (Table 9.2) [15–20]. There are a number of safety features of open cholecystectomy which contribute to the low incidence of bile duct injury. Most important is the ability to feel and isolate the cystic duct and to see the junction of the cystic duct and the common bile duct. If this is not possible there are two important procedures at open surgery which facilitate identification of this junction. The first of these is operative cholangiography which can be performed more easily at open surgery than during laparoscopy. Either the cystic duct may be cannulated or a butterfly needle may be used to inject contrast directly into the common bile duct. The second is the ability at open surgery to perform a retrograde or fundus-first cholecystectomy which is a valuable method of avoiding bile duct damage in technically difficult cases. This latter technique is difficult to perform using the laparoscope.

There are a number of risk factors which influence outcome after open cholecystectomy. Two factors which most commonly influence mortality after open cholecystectomy are age and the presence of acute cholecystitis at surgery. Meyer and colleagues [4] have shown that there is a stepwise increase in mortality with increasing age after open cholecystectomy. McSherry [21] reviewing 7 000 elective open cholecystectomies demonstrated that patients over 50 years of age had a 10-fold increase in mortality compared to those in the younger age group (0.8% versus 0.08%) figures which agree with a recent publication by Roslyn *et al.* [7]. Glenn [22] published a mortality rate of 4.6% in patients over 65 years and suggested cholecystostomy as an alternative to cholecystectomy in this age group. Although chronological age alone cannot in itself be used as a risk factor, most series agree that old age and associated concomitant disease are major risk factors in patients undergoing open cholecystectomy.

The influence of timing of open surgery for acute cholecystitis on outcome is more contentious. Many authors believe that surgery for acute cholecystitis/biliary colic should be performed during the same hospital admission. The results from Pickleman and Gonzales [23] show that major complications following surgery for acute cholecystitis are similar in patients undergoing immediate compared to interval surgery (6.6% versus 5.5%). They point out that immediate surgery reduces the risk of gallstone complications while patients await elective surgery. However, there is also a strong body of opinion demonstrating that immediate or early

Table 9.2 Bile duct injury (Open cholecystectomy)

Author	Incidence (%)
Borgstrom [12]	0.09
Rosenquist & Myrim [8]	0.2
Viikari [9]	0.2
Michie & Gunn [11]	0.3
Bismuth & Lazorthes [10]	0.15
Gilliland & Traverso [14]	0.2
Lennon [13]	0
Roslyn *et al.* [7]	0.2

cholecystectomy (next available operating list) is associated with a higher incidence of complications. Arnold [2] and Meyer *et al.* [4] both showed a greater than twofold increase in the mortality of patients undergoing immediate surgery for acute cholecystitis. Those authors in favour of acute surgery for cholecystitis are not clear which time is optimal for intervention. The consensus view is that surgery performed 5 days after the acute attack is more difficult [4, 24] but that this factor does not influence subsequent mortality [25, 26]. The one clear message emerging from this debate is that the combination of immediate surgery for acute cholcystitis and age are major risk factors.

Two other risk factors which deserve a mention in patients undergoing open cholecystectomy are diabetes and hepatic cirrhosis. It has been shown that there is an 11% mortality rate in diabetics on oral hypoglycaemics undergoing early cholecystectomy for acute cholecystitis [27, 28]. Furthermore, this incidence is as high as 47% in insulin-dependant diabetics [27, 28]. It should be pointed out however, that these articles were written 30 years ago and more recent publication could not demonstrate any increase in the incidence of complications of cholecystectomy associated with diabetes [23]. Most series agree that hepatic cirrhosis is a major risk factor in patients undergoing elective cholecystectomy. The two major causes of death associated with this condition are intra-operative bleeding and post-operative hepatic failure [29, 30].

Conclusion

Open cholecystectomy is a safe operation with acceptable morbidity and mortality figures in both acute and chronic cholecystitis. Laparoscopic cholecystectomy has largely replaced open cholecystectomy in many centres. The track record of open cholecystectomy is such that it is the gold standard against which each centre should audit its experience with laparoscopic cholecystectomy. The choice as to which procedure is preferable will depend largely on the incidence of bile duct injury associated with laparoscopic cholecystectomy. In the meantime, it is important for surgeons to recognize that the conversion from laparoscopic to open cholecystectomy is not a technical failure but an option which will result in a safer procedure. If this philosophy is adopted, long, hazardous laparoscopic dissections in Calot's triangle will be avoided and this approach should minimize the incidence of bile duct injury during laparoscopic cholecystectomy. Open cholecystectomy will retain its place as an important and effective means of treating patients with gallstone disease.

References

1 McSherry CK. Cholecystectomy: The gold standard. *Am J Surg* 1989;**158**:174–8.
2 Arnold DJ. 28,621 cholecystectomies in Ohio. *Am J Surg* 1970;**119**:714–17.
3 Ganey JB, Johnson PA, Prillaman PE, McSwain GR. Cholecystectomy: Clinical experience with a large series. *Am J Surg* 1986;**151**:352–7.
4 Meyer KA, Capos NJ, Mittlepunkt AI. Personal experiences with 12,661 cases of acute and chronic cholecystitis and cholelithiasis.
5 Bartlett MK, Quinby WC Jr. Mortality and complications of cholecystectomy and choledochostomy for chronic cholecystitis. *N Eng J Med* 1956;**254**: 154–8.
6 Colcock BP, MacManus JE. Experiences with 1,356 cases of cholecystitis and cholelithiasis. *Surg Gynec Obs* 1955;**101**:161–5.
7 Roslyn JJ, Binns GS, Hughes EFX. Saunders-Kirkwood K, Zinner MJ, Cates JA. Open Cholecystectomy. *Ann Surg* 1993;**218**:129–37.
8 Rosenquist H, Myrin SO. Operative injury to the bile ducts. *Acta Chir Scand* 1960;**119**:92–107.
9 Viikari SJ. Operative injuries to the bile duct. *Acta Chir Scand* 1960;**119**:83–92.
10 Bismuth H, Lazorthes F. *Les traumatismes operatoires de la voie biliaire principale*. Paris: Masson Cie, 1981, Vol 1.
11 Michie W, Gunn A. Bile duct injuries. A new suggestion for their repair. *Brit J Surg* 1964;**51**:96–9.
12 Borgstrom S. Operative injury of the choledochus. *Acta Chir Scand* 1959;**118**:25–9.
13 Lennon F. Laparoscopic cholecystectomy: a cautionary note (letter). *Br J Surg* 1991;**78**:1400.
14 Gilliland TM, Traverso W. Modern standards for comparison of cholecystectomy with alternative treatments for symptomatic cholelithiasis with emphasis on relief of symptoms. *Surg Gynec Obs* 1990;**170**: 39–44.
15 Deziel DJ, Millikan KW, Econonmou SG *et al.* Complication of laparoscopic cholecystectomy: Results of a national survey of 4,292 hospitals and analysis of 77,604 cases. *Am J Surg* 1993;**165**:9–14.

16 Peters JJ, Ellison GC, Innes JT *et al.* Safety and efficacy of laparoscopic cholecystectomy. *Ann Surg* 1991;**213**: 3–12.
17 Meyers WC. A prospective analysis of 1,518 laparoscopic cholecystectomies. *N Engl J Med* 1991;**324**: 1073–78.
18 Cuschieri A, Dubois F, Moniel J *et al.* The European experience with laparoscopic cholecystectomy. *Am J Surg* 1991;**161**:385–7.
19 Soper NJ. Laparoscopic cholecystectomy. *Cur Probl Surg* 1991;**28**:587–655.
20 Irish Laparoscopic Cholecystectomy Group. Early experience of laparoscopic cholecystectomy in 5 Irish hospitals. *Ir J Med Sci* 1992;**161**:410–13.
21 McSherry CK. The national co-operative gallstone study report. *Ann Int Med* 1981;**95**:379–80.
22 Glenn F. Surgical management of acute cholecystitis in patients 65 years of age and older. *Ann Surg* 1981; **193**:56–9.
23 Pickleman J, Gonzalez RP. The improving results of cholecystectomy. *Arch Surg* 1986;**121**:930–4.
24 Haff RC, Butcher HR, Ballinger W. Biliary tract operations. *Arch Surg* 1969;**98**:428–34.
25 Saltzstein EC, Peacock JB, Mercer CC. Early operation for acute biliary tract stone disease. *Surgery* 1983;**94**: 704–8.
26 Jarvinen HJ, Hastabacka J. Early cholecystectomy for acute cholecystitis. *Ann Surg* 1980;**191**:501–5.
27 Mundth ED. Cholecystitis and diabetes mellitus. *N Eng J Med* 1962;**267**:642–6.
28 Turnill F-L, McCarron MM, Mikkelsen WP. Gallstones and diabetes: an ominous association. *Am J Surg* 1961;**102**:188–93.
29 Castaing D, Houssin D, Lemoine J, Bismuth H. Surgical management of gallstones in cirrhotic patients. *Am J Surg* 1983;**146**:310–13.
30 Van Landingham S. Cholecystectomy in cirrhotic patients. *South Med J* 1984;**77**:38–40.

Chapter 10
Mini-cholecystectomy

P.J. O'Dwyer & A.J. McMahon

Introduction

Mini-cholecystectomy or small incision open cholecystectomy was first reported by Dubois and Berthelot in 1982 [1]. This modification to conventional cholecystectomy was made feasible by improvements in lighting, retraction and anaesthesia that have taken place in the century since Langenbuch described the first cholecystectomy in 1882. The indications for mini-cholecystectomy are the same as those for conventional cholecystectomy.

Technique

The preparation and positioning of the patient on the operating table is similar to that for conventional open cholecystectomy. Additional lighting may be provided by use of a headlight and mini-cholecystectomy is performed by an operator and two assistants. If the surgeon is left-handed the operation is more easily accomplished from the patient's left side. Although mini-cholecystectomy has been performed through an incision as small as 3 cm, a 5–10 cm transverse incision makes this operation technically easy and something that can be accomplished by any surgeon with experience in conventional cholecystectomy. The incision begins over the surface marking of the fundus of the gallbladder, about one finger's breadth below the costal margin and extends medially in a transverse direction (Fig. 10.1). The lateral half of the rectus muscle should be divided in young patients, however, in the elderly it is possible to split the muscle along its fibres and retract them to gain access to the abdomen. Exposure is facilitated by using a stabilized ring retractor such as a Bookwalter retractor (Codman and Shurleff Inc., New Bedford, MA, USA). In this circumstance one assistant is adequate. After dividing any adhesions around the gallbladder, dissection commences in the area of Calot's triangle. A single gauge pack suitably retracted is used to displace both hepatic flexure and duodenum from the operative field. A narrow Deaver retractor gently placed on the quadrate lobe of the liver improves the exposure of Calot's triangle. The cystic artery, cystic duct and the junction between the cystic duct and the common bile duct are identified as in conventional cholecystectomy. Cholangiography is performed in accordance with the policy of the operating surgeon. The cystic artery is traced up onto the gallbladder wall and then divided and ligated. Similarly, the cystic duct is also dissected proximally to identify its junction with the gallbladder before dividing and ligating it in a similar manner to the the cystic artery. Haemoclips may be used as an alternative to ligate cystic duct and artery. Good haemostasis can be achieved by use of electrocautery. Once the cystic duct has been divided the gallbladder can be removed in an antegrade or retrograde fashion taking care, at all times, to ensure that dissection takes place on the gallbladder wall. The gallbladder bed should be completely dry after the operation and no drains are required. Common bile duct exploration can also be performed without extending the incision. In the rare circumstance where Calot's triangle is obliterated by severe fibrosis and chronic inflammation it is wiser to open the gallbladder, empty its contents and perform a subtotal cholecystectomy or cholecystostomy. The wound is closed in a standard fashion. The fascial layers are closed with a suture such as No. 1 polydioxone, the

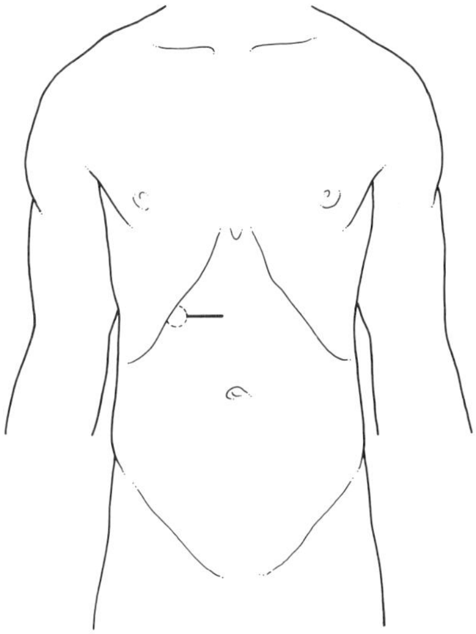

Fig. 10.1 Incision site for mini-cholecystectomy.

skin with subcuticular polyglycolic acid or paper tapes and the wound is infiltrated with 0.5% bupivacaine. Nasogastric tubes are not required and the patient can be allowed oral fluids on the morning after operation and a light diet by the evening. Young patients may be discharged on the second post-operative day and more elderly patients on the 4th post-operative day.

Results

Mini-cholecystectomy is associated with a shorter hospital stay and more rapid return to normal activiy than conventional cholecystectomy [1–11] (Table 10.1). In the only randomized trial comparing hospital stay for mini- and conventional cholecystectomy, median stay was significantly shorter for the mini-cholecystectomy group (3 days versus 5 days) [12]. Morbidity following mini-cholecystectomy varies between 0% and 15% and is similar in type to that following conventional cholecystectomy. In particular, there have been no reports of intestinal injury such as may have been anticipated by the reduced exposure for mini-cholecystectomy.

Bile duct injury

Mini-cholecystectomy has been criticized for limiting the exposure thought necessary for safe cholecystectomy. Many felt that this would result in an increased incidence of injury to the common bile duct. This, however, has not been borne out by the literature with only one major injury in over 2 700 cases reported [1–14]. This compares favourably with a 0.2% incidence of serious common bile duct injury following conventional cholecystectomy [15]. Although only one minor ductal injury has been reported after mini-cholecystectomy (2 mm injury to the common bile duct) it is likely that such injuries are under-reported presumably because they are recognized and repaired at the time of cholecystectomy and rarely go on to cause significant short- or long-term morbidity.

Comparison with laparoscopic cholecystectomy

The major advantage of mini-cholecystectomy

Table 10.1 Results of mini-cholecystectomy

Author	No. of patients	Incision size (cm)	Morbidity (%)	Mortality (%)	Hospital stay (days)	Return to work (days)
Dubois and Berthelot [1]	1500	3–6	–	–	–	–
Morton [2]	96	4–5	–	0	2.5	14
Russell and Shankar [3]	35	8	9	0.2	4.4	–
Goco and Chambers [4]	450	4	3.1	0.2	1.22	–
Merrill [5]	80	4–6	8.7	0	3.8–5.3	–
Reddick and Olsen [6]	25	–	0	0	2.8	34
O'Dwyer *et al.* [7]	55	5	9	0	3.9	–
Ledet [8]	200	5–10	–	0	Day case	21
Cheslyn-Curtis and Russell [9]	56	–	8	0	4	–
O'Kelly *et al.* [10]	32	5–10	9	0	3	–
Al-Tameem [11]	80	3–5	15	0	2	10

over laparoscopic cholecystectomy are reduced hospital costs. The extra time in hospital required for mini-cholecystectomy (Table 10.2) is offset by theatre costs and the use of disposable intruments (Table 10.3). Despite wound infiltration with bupivacaine, mini-cholecystectomy is more painful than laparoscopic cholecystectomy with significant differences in analgesia requirements, physical functioning, role limitation and pain for up to 1 week postoperatively. These differences result in increased respiratory depression following the open procedure [16] (Figs 10.2 and 10.3). Laparoscopic cholecystectomy also has a modest advantage in terms of return to normal activity (Table 10.4), however, education of patients and their primary care physicians is required before these differences translate into a more rapid return to paid employment. Patient satisfaction with the cosmetic result after mini-cholecystectomy is similar to that after laparoscopic cholecystectomy, with more than 95% of patients experiencing a good cosmetic result from these procedures. Wound-related and other minor complications are also similar to those observed with laparoscopic cholecystectomy (Table 10.5).

Table 10.2 Randomized trials comparing laparoscopic (LC) and mini-cholecystectomy (MC)

Author	No. of patients	Hospital stay LC	Hospital stay MC	Return to normal activity LC	Return to normal activity MC
Kunz *et al.* [13]	77	3.5	5.8	–	–
Barkun *et al.* [14]	62	3	4	8	13
O'Dwyer *et al.* [12]	299	2	4	10	15

Metabolic response

Despite significant differences in post-operative pain between laparoscopic and mini-cholecystec-

Table 10.3 Cost per patient for Mini-cholecystectomy and laparoscopic cholecystectomy

	Mini-cholecystectomy mean (SD)	Laparoscopic mean (SD)	*t* statistic	Significance level
Theatre	£577 (149)	£687 (126)	6.8	<0.001
Laparoscopic disposables	–	£303		
Laparoscopic equipment	–	£60		
Ward costs	£393 (190)	£299 (168)	4.5	<0.001
Pathology/Bacteriology	£87	£87		
ECG and Chest X-ray	£15 (8)	£15 (8)		
Additional (complications)	£17 (94)	£35 (176)	1.1	0.28
Total (excluding disposables)	£1 090 (296)	£1 183 (296)	2.7	0.008
Total (including disposables)	£1 090 (296)	£1 486 (296)	11.3	<0.001

Table 10.4 Time (days) to return to normal activities after mini-cholecystectomy and laparoscopic cholecystectomy

	Mini-cholecystectomy median (IQR)*	*n*	Laparoscopic median (IQR)*	*n*	Significance level (U test)
Hobbies	12 (7–21)	118	7 (4–14)	128	0.0014
Work in the home	15 (10–24)	114	10 (5–19)	122	<0.001
Social activities	21 (11–28)	111	14 (7–21)	125	<0.001
Sexual activity	21 (12–28)	64	21 (11–24)	60	0.33
Paid employment	41 (21–60)	37	36 (28–60)	31	0.86

* IQR = interquartile range.

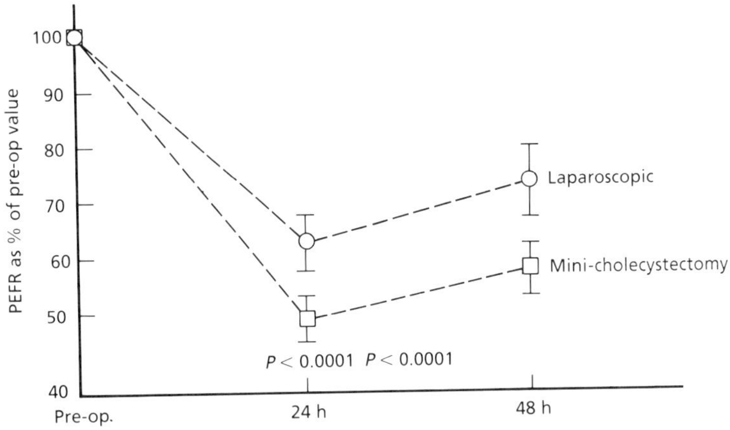

Fig. 10.2 Peak expiratory flow rate for laparoscopic and mini-cholecystectomy.

Table 10.5 Postoperative complications after mini-cholecystectomy and laparoscopic cholecystectomy

Complication	Mini-laparotomy (No.)	(*n* = 148) (%)	Laparoscopic (No.)	(*n* = 151) (%)
Wound infection	11	7.4	13	8.6
Wound haematoma	0	0	3	1.3
Urinary retention	6	4.1	2	1.3
Minor chest infection	5	3.4	1	0.7
Postoperative haemorrhage	3	3.0	3	2.0
Urinary tract infection	2	1.4	0	0
Septicaemic shock	1	0.7	0	0
Adhesive obstruction	1	0.7	0	0
Retained bile duct stone	0	0	1	0.7
Major bile duct injury*	0	0	1	0.7
Minor bile duct injury†	2	1.4	0	0
Cystic duct bile leak	0	0	1	0.7
Accessory bile duct leak	1	0.7	2	1.4
Readmission	3	2.0	5	3.3
Total number of patients with complications	30	20%	26	17%

* Complete transection and ligation of bile duct.
† 2 mm injuries of bile duct and junction of cystic and common bile duct.

tomy both exhibit a similar metabolic response to trauma [17] (Figs 10.4 and 10.5). This may be a result of the longer operating time required for laparoscopic cholecystectomy as the magnitude of the metabolic response has been shown to correlate with the duration of surgery [18]. In addition, diagnostic laparoscopy alone is associated with a substantial hormonal and glycaemic response which is thought to be evoked by the stimulus of peritoneal distension [19].

Conclusion

The relatively small number of cases of mini-laparotomy cholecystectomy published in the literature would suggest that this is an unpopular

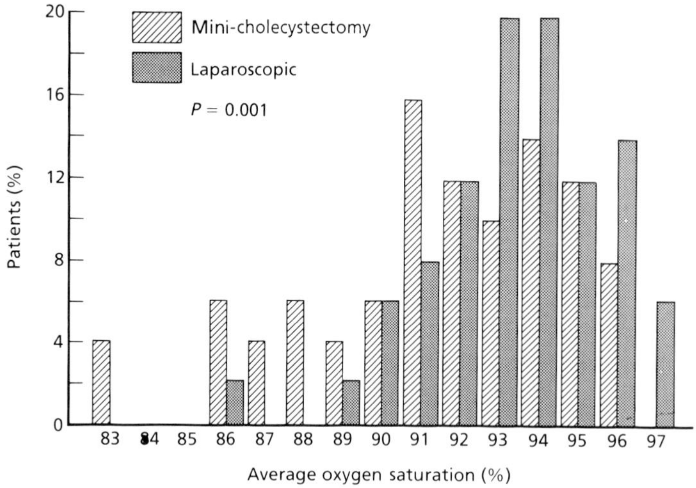

Fig. 10.3 Mean oxygen saturation following laparoscopic and mini-cholecystectomy.

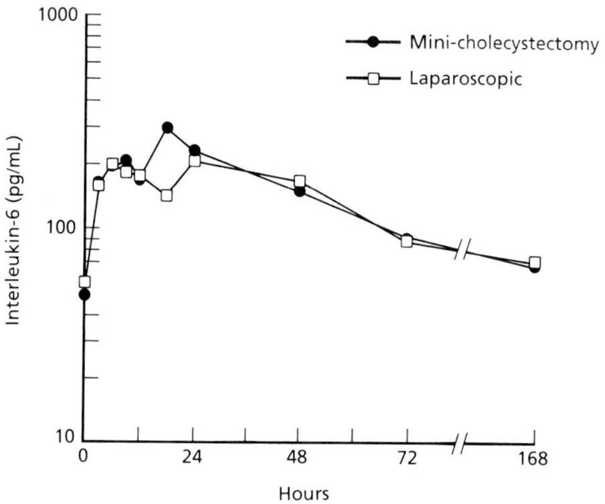

Fig. 10.4 Serum interleukin-6 following laparoscopic and mini-cholecystectomy.

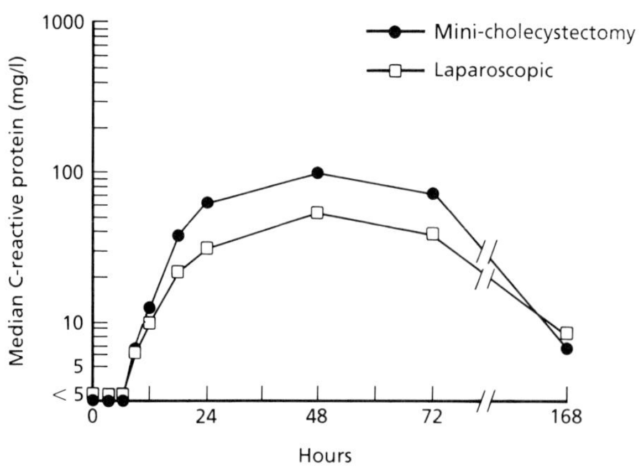

Fig. 10.5 C-reactive protein levels following laparoscopic and mini-cholecystectomy.

operation with surgeons. It is likely, however, that many surgeons practise small incision open cholecystectomy in selected cases without describing it as a mini-cholecystectomy. Mini-cholecystectomy is a satisfactory alternative to laparoscopic cholecystectomy particularly in situations where the modest differences in cost are important. As it requires similar skills to conventional cholecystectomy it is easier to adapt to than laparoscopic cholecystectomy and may, therefore, be a suitable alternative for surgeons who perform a small number of cholecystectomies annually.

References

1 Dubois F, Berthelot B. Cholecystectomie par mini-laparotomie. *Nouve Presse Med* 1982;**11**:1139–41.
2 Morton CE. Cost containment with the use of 'mini-cholecystectomy' and intraoperative cholangiography. *Am Surg* 1985;**51**:168–9.
3 Russell RC, Shankar S. The stabilised ring retractor: a technique for cholecystectomy. *Br J Surg* 1987;**74**:826.
4 Goco IR, Chambers LG. Dollars and cents: mini-cholecystectomy and early discharge. *South Med J* 1988;**81**:161–3.
5 Merrill JR. Minimal trauma cholecystectomy (a 'no-touch' procedure in a 'well'). *Am Surg* 1988;**54**:256–61.
6 Reddick EJ, Olsen DO. Laparoscopic laser cholecystectomy. A comparison with mini-lap cholecystectomy. *Surg Endosc* 1989;**3**:131–3.
7 O'Dwyer PJ, Murphy JJ, O'Higgins NJ. Cholecystectomy through a 5 cm subcostal incision. *Br J Surg* 1990;**77**:1189–90.
8 Ledet WP Jr. Ambulatory cholecystectomy without disability. *Arch Surg* 1990;**125**:1434–5.
9 Cheslyn-Curtis, Russell RCG. Laparoscopic cholecystectomy. *Br Med J* 1991;**302**:594.
10 O'Kelly TJ, Barr H, Malley WR, Kettlewell M. Cholecystectomy through a 5 cm subcostal incision. *Br J Surg* 1991;**78**:762.
11 Al-Tameem MM. Minilaparotomy cholecystectomy. *J R Coll Surg Edin* 1993;**38**:154–7.
12 O'Dwyer PJ, McGregor JR, McDermott EWM, Murphy JJ, O'Higgins NJ. Patients recovery following cholecystectomy through a 6 cm or 15 cm transverse subcostal incision: a prospective randomised clinical trial. *Postgrad Med J* 1992;**68**:817–19.
13 Kunz R, Orth K, Vogel J *et al.* Laparoskopische Cholecystektomie versus mini-lap-Cholecystektomie. *Chirug* 1992;**63**:291–5.
14 Barkun JS, Barkun AN, Sampalis JS *et al.* Randomised controlled trial of laparoscopic versus mini-cholecystectomy. *Lancet* 1992;**340**:116–19.
15 Roslyn JL, Gregory SB, Hughes EFX. Open cholecystectomy: a contemporary analysis of 42,474 patients. *Ann Surg* 1993;**218**:129–37.
16 McMahon AJ, Baxter JN, Russell IT *et al.* Laparoscopic and mini laparotomy cholecystectomy: a randomised trial comparing post-operative pain and pulmonary function. *Surgery* 1994;**115**:533–9.
17 McMahon AJ, O'Dwyer PJ, Cruikshank A *et al.* A comparison of the metabolic response to mini-laparotomy and laparoscopic cholecystectomy. *Br J Surg* 1993;**80**:1255–8.
18 Cooper GM, Scottins AM, Ward ID, Murphy D. Laparoscopy—a stressful procedure. *Anaesthesia* 1982; **37**:266–9.
19 Shenkin A, Fraser WD, Series J *et al.* The serum interleukin 6 response to elective surgery. *Lymphokine Res* 1989;**8**:123–7.

Chapter 11
Laparoscopic cholecystectomy

P.A. Grace & D. Bouchier-Hayes

In 1882, Langenbuch performed the first successful cholecystectomy [1] and for 100 years this procedure remained the standard surgical method for dealing with the diseased gallbladder. Alternative treatments for gallstone disease have been advocated in recent years. These include oral dissolution therapy, lithotripsy, percutaneous cholecystostomy and cholecystolithotomy, as well as contact dissolution therapy with methyl tert-butyl ether [2]. All of these approaches, however, leave the gallbladder *in situ* with the possibility of stone recurrence. The development of minimally invasive techniques in urology [3] and gastroenterology [4] stimulated general surgeons to explore the therapeutic potentials of such techniques in the management of gallbladder disease and the last 5 years has seen the development of both mini-cholecystectomy and laparoscopic cholecystectomy [2]. In many centres, laparoscopic cholecystectomy is now the treatment of choice for symptomatic gallbladder disease. The purpose of this chapter is to review the impact of laparoscopic cholecystectomy on the management of patients with gallstone disease.

Historical development

Developments in surgery and anaesthesia in the latter half of the 19th century revolutionized the management of many diseases for which there had previously been no safe or effective treatment. Thus, in 1882 Carl Langenbuch performed the first successful planned cholecystectomy [1] while in the same decade Fitz and McBurney reported their experiences with the diagnosis and treatment of appendicitis [5, 6]. The first laparoscopy was performed in 1902 in Dresden when Kelling inserted a cystoscope into the abdominal cavity of a dog [7]. Jacobeus had performed 100 laparoscopies by 1911 [8] and Kalk demonstrated the safety of the procedure when, in 1951, he reported 2 000 cases without a death [9]. Since then laparoscopy has been used extensively by gynaecologists and over 300 000 gynaecological laparoscopies were performed in the USA in 1984 [10].

More recently, general surgeons have adopted laparoscopy for diagnosis and treatment of intra-abdominal pathology [11]. The first laparoscopic cholecystectomy was performed in Lyons by Phillipe Mouret in 1987 and, following the pioneering work of Dubois *et al.* [12], Perissat *et al.* [13], Reddick and Olsen [14] and Cusheiri [15], several thousand of these procedures have been performed throughout the world [16–18].

Operative techniques

Laparoscopic cholecystectomy

Laparoscopic cholecystectomy requires general anaesthesia with endotracheal intubation. The patient is placed either in the lithotomy position with the feet down or simply supine on the table. In either case, the operating surgeon stands on the patient's left side facing a television monitor which is placed to the right of the patient's head. A second monitor placed to the left of the patient's head facilitates the assistants but it is not essential.

A nasogastric tube is passed to decompress the stomach and a urinary catheter is inserted to drain the bladder. Alternatively, the patient is asked to empty his or her bladder just prior to surgery. The patient is placed in the anti-Trendelenberg position and is rotated slightly to the left so that the abdominal vicera fall away from the gallbladder area. A Veres needle is inserted into the midline just below the umbilicus and approximately 5 000 mL of CO_2 is insufflated into the coelomic cavity to maintain a pressure of approximately 15 mmHg. The Veres needle is replaced by a 10 mm trocar and sheath, through which is passed a 25° laparoscope which is attached to a video camera. The rest of the procedure is performed by video dissection displayed on the television monitor(s).

If the patient has adhesions from previous abdominal surgery there is a risk of injuring the bowel when placing the Veres needle and the first trocar at the umbilicus. We have described a simple method to overcome this problem [19]. The Veres needle is inserted into the abdomen at some point away from the scarred area and a CO_2 pneumoperitoneum is created. The area over the liver is percussed and, if resonant, a small 5 mm trocar is inserted approximately 2 finger breadths below the costal margin in the mid-clavicular line, which is the site of insertion of the second grasping forceps for cholecystectomy by the Reddick technique [14]. Through this a 30° cystoscope or a 5 mm laparoscope is inserted and the posterior aspect of the anterior abdominal wall is inspected. The angulation of the 30° cystoscope makes visualization of the posterior abdominal wall easier than when a 0° 5 mm laparoscope is used. The 10 mm trocar for the standard laparoscope is now inserted under direct vision at the umbilicus. If adhesiolysis is needed prior to placement of the umbilical port, then one of the other accessory ports is placed under direct vision to allow placement of instruments for division of adhesions. The other trocars are placed under direct vision of the laparoscope and the cystoscope is removed.

Another alternative in the case of periumbilical scarring is the use of an 'open' technique for insertion of the umbilical cannula. A small incision is made into the fascia at the umbilicus and under direct vision a special cannula devised by Hasson is inserted.

Different port positions have been described [11–14] but the technique we favour is similar to that described by Reddick and Olsen [14, 20]. After a full laparoscopic examination of the abdomen trocars are placed under laparoscopic vision in the following positions.

1 A 5 mm trocar is placed in the right iliac fossa along the anterior axillary line halfway between the costal margin and the anterior superior iliac spine.

2 A 5 mm trocar is inserted approximately 2 finger breadths below the right costal margin in the mid-clavicular line.

3 A 10 mm operating trocar is placed a hand's breadth below the xiphisternum just to the left of the midline and the falciform ligament (Fig. 11.1).

Gallbladder grasping forceps are placed through the two 5 mm ports and the dissection is performed by instruments placed through the 10 mm port. Occasionally, it is possible to dispense with the upper grasping forceps (port No. 2) and perform the procedure through three ports.

The fundus of the gallbladder is grasped by a grasping forceps placed through the lower 5 mm trocar and pushed upwards and 'over' the liver. The area of Hartmann's pouch is grasped by a second grasping forceps placed through the upper

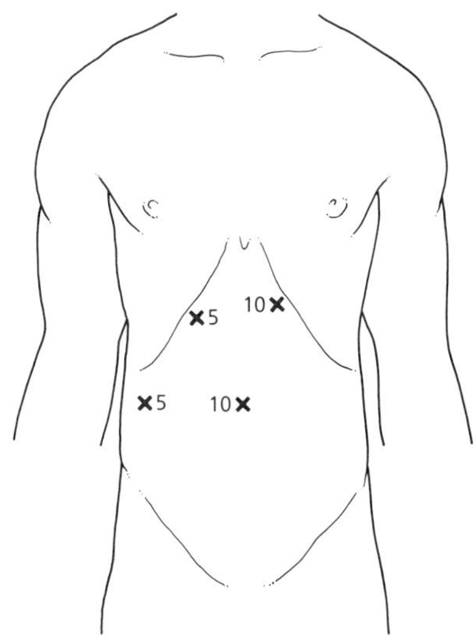

Fig. 11.1 Sites for insertion of ports for laparoscopic cholecystectomy.

5 mm trocar and is pulled gently upwards and laterally to the right. This manœuvre exposes Calot's triangle and by a combination of blunt and sharp dissection the cystic duct and artery are exposed. It is important that no electrocautery be used in the dissection of Calot's triangle as we believe that its use may predispose to duct injury. The dissection should start from the neck of the gallbladder sweeping the tissue from the gallbladder towards the common bile duct. An important technical point, emphasized by Ponsky [21], is that '. . . the cystic duct should be unequivocally traced up onto the gallbladder prior to any clipping or division'. The exposed cystic artery and duct are divided between clips. Using electocautery or laser the gallbladder is dissected from the gallbladder bed and removed via the 10 mm dissection port. Most surgeons now prefer to use electrocautery [22, 23] as laser technology is expensive and the use of laser may be associated with a higher rate of bile duct injury [24]. If a large stone is encountered, the gallbladder neck can be delivered onto the skin, opened and the stone crushed by an instrument placed inside the gallbladder. The gallbladder bed is inspected and irrigated with saline and if necessary a drain may be placed.

Peroperative cholangiography

Peroperative cholangiography is simple to perform and will be successful in 84–92% [25, 26] of patients. Following identification of the anatomy, a small incision is made with a microscissors in the cystic duct near its junction with the gallbladder. A flexible catheter is introduced into the cystic duct and held in position with one of a number of specially designed cholangiography clamps [27, 28] or a loosely applied clip or atraumatic grasping forceps [29]. While exposure of conventional films may be used with success, C-arm screening using image intensification with hard copy capability has several advantages: positioning is precise; radio-opaque instruments may easily be avoided; and the optimal volume of contrast material can be titrated accurately.

Exploration of the common bile duct

If common bile duct stones are identified the surgeon may:
1 opt to perform a laparoscopic cholecystectomy and deal with the stone by ERCP later;
2 convert to an open cholecystectomy and exploration of the common bile duct [30];
3 undertake laparoscopic exploration of the common bile duct by transcystic-duct flexible endoscopy or laparoscopic choledochotomy [31, 32];
4 place a small catheter via the cystic duct into the common bile duct through which the stones may subsequently be flushed or extracted using the Burhenne technique [33].

Flexible endoscopy is performed by passing a guidewire into the common duct and duodenum via the cystic duct. A 3 mm flexible ureteroscope is manipulated over the guidewire into the common duct and the stones can be pushed into the duodenum or retrieved with a wire stone basket passed through the working channel of the scope. Occasionally, contact lithotripsy is required if the stones are too large. Laparoscopic choledochotomy is performed via a longitudinal incision in the common bile duct. The stones are removed by a combination of irrigation, balloon catheter or wire basket extraction and choledochoscopy. After stone extraction the edges of the common duct incision should be sutured with 5–0 Vicryl over a T-tube [31, 32].

Laparoscopic cholecstectomy versus open cholecystectomy

Since the first laparoscopic cholecystectomy was performed by Mouret in 1987, thousands of surgeons have adopted this operation and the feasibility and safety of laparoscopic cholecystectomy has been attested to in several large series of patients [16–18, 25, 28, 34]. The ideal method for assessing any new drug or surgical technique is a randomized controlled trial. The difficulties of undertaking such a trial comparing laparoscopic with open cholecystectomy have been extensively reviewed by Neugebauer and colleagues from

Table 11.1 Results of laparoscopic cholecystectomy in 4 704 patients

Source	*n*	Conversion rate (%)	Mortality (%)	Major morbidity (%)	Bile duct injury (%)
Cushieri *et al.* [16]	1 236	3.6	0.0	1.6	0.2
Southern Surgeons [17]	1 518	4.7	0.07	1.5	0.5
Bailey *et al.* [28]	375	5.0	0.3	0.6	0.3
Spaw *et al.* [34]	500	1.8	0.0	1.0	0.0
Soper *et al.* [38]	618	2.9	0.0	1.6	0.2
Beaumont Group	457	8.5	0.0	3.5	0.4

Germany and they concluded that, '... the response of surgeons and patients to the new procedure now place ethical constraints on the planning of a randomized controlled trial' [35]. Similar concerns attended the introduction of extracorporeal shock-wave lithotripsy (ESWL) for renal calculi in the 1980s [36]. Paterson-Brown and colleagues recently commented editorially that in the absence of controlled studies 'meticulous audit of results will be of paramount importance' [37]. Several groups have examined in detail their experiences with laparoscopic cholecystectomy [16, 17, 28, 34, 38] and a number have compared their results with historical controls [39], concurrent non-randomized controls [14] or published reports of open cholecystectomy [18] (Table 11.1).

Our own experience reflects that of most series of laparoscopic cholecystectomy reported to date. Between February 1990 and August 1992 we attempted laparoscopic cholecystectomy in 457 consecutive patients with a conversion rate to open cholecystectomy of 8.5% (n = 39). The indications for laparoscopic cholecystectomy were biliary colic (n = 210), chronic cholecystitis (n = 136), acute cholecystitis (n = 81) and gallstone pancreatitis (n = 30). The reasons for conversion are given in Table 11.2. Thirty patients, of whom 19 had acute cholecystitis, were converted because of unclear anatomy where further dissection was deemed hazardous while five patients underwent laparotomy to control bleeding. Instrument failure resulted in conversion in three patients early in our experience and one patient had a laparotomy for suspected gallbladder carcinoma. We had no deaths and a major complication rate of 3.5%. The mean postoperative hospital stay was 3.6 days and the mean time to resumption of normal activities was 14 days.

Table 11.2 Reasons for conversion to open cholecystectomy in 457 patients undergoing laparoscopic cholecystectomy

Indication for laparoscopic cholecystectomy	*n*	Unsafe anatomy	Bleeding	Other	Total
Biliary colic	210	3	1	2	6
Chronic cholecystitis	136	8	3	0	11
Acute cholecystitis	81	19	1	2	22
Gallstone pancreatitis	30	0	0	0	0
Total	457	30	5	4	39

In our series most of the conversions to open cholecystectomy occurred in the group of patients with acute cholecystitis. Our success rate was only 63% in this group and uncertainty about the anatomy was the commonest cause for conversion. Recently, however, Wilson and colleagues from Edinburgh have reported a 94% success rate and minimal morbidity in a group of 31 patients with acute cholecystitis [40]. Thus, acute cholecystitis should not be considered a contraindication to laparoscopic cholecystectomy but we believe that in these patients the surgeon should have a very low threshold for conversion to open cholecystectomy.

From the published reviews of laparoscopic cholecystectomy a number of points emerge.

1 Laparoscopic cholecystectomy is a viable and safe alternative in the treatment of symptomatic gallstone disease.

2 Conversion to open cholecystectomy is required in about 5% of patients, usually due to the presence of severe inflammation.

3 Bile duct injury occurs in 0.5% of patients.

4 Overall morbidity and mortality rates are 3% and 0.08%, respectively.

More impressive, perhaps, is the fact that most patients (54–98%) are discharged from hospital within 24 hours of surgery and the majority (77–98%) have resumed full activity within 7–10 days of hospitalization [18]. While Ledet has reported a mean hospital stay of less than 1 day in 200 patients treated by open cholecystectomy [41], the average hospital stay for open cholecystectomy is 7–10 days and the time to full activity is more than 3 weeks [39, 42]. Finally, postoperative pain is reduced after laparoscopic cholecystectomy [43], there is improved pulmonary function compared to open cholecystectomy [44] and there are obvious cosmetic advantages.

Laparoscopic cholecystectomy versus mini-cholecystectomy

Mini-cholecystectomy is a technique for removing the gallbladder through a small (5–7 cm) subcostal incision [2, 45]. Proponents of this procedure cite reduced operation time, good cosmesis, less postoperative pain, diminished respiratory complications and shorter hospital stay as advantages for mini-cholecystectomy [2, 46]. Most patients are discharged on the 3rd postoperative day after mini-cholecystectomy [46] and are able to return to work after an average of 18.6 days [2]. Preliminary data from a randomized trial comparing laparoscopic cholecystectomy with mini-cholecystectomy indicate that laparoscopic cholecystectomy has advantages in terms of pain relief and better postoperative pulmonary function [47, 48], as well as hospital stay and return to normal activity (see Table 10.2).

Routine or selective cholangiography?

The advent of laparoscopic cholecystectomy has refocussed attention on the management of common bile duct stones and reopened the debate on the indications for cholangiography during cholecytectomy [49]. Symptomatic choledocholithiasis may be managed by pre-operative endoscopic retrograde cholangiopancreatography (ERCP) followed by laparoscopic cholecystectomy or by peroperative exploration of the common bile duct during laparoscopic (or open) cholecystectomy [32]. However, unsuspected common duct stones, which are detected in 1.2–14% of patients undergoing cholecystectomy [50], pose a more interesting problem. They may be detected by peroperative cholangiography or preoperative intravenous cholangiography [51]. The natural history of such stones is largely unknown. However, a number of reports have documented the spontaneous passage of common bile duct stones into the duodenum [33, 52, 53]. Moreover, it appears that only 0.5–0.8% of patients undergoing laparoscopic cholecystectomy will subsequently return with problems due to unsuspected common duct stones [54, 55]. In our own experience only 2 out of 240 patients (0.8%) undergoing laparoscopic cholecystectomy without cholangiography returned with symptomatic retained common bile duct stones, both of which were easily managed by ERCP [56].

Significant anatomical variation of the biliary tree may occur in 3–15% of patients [57, 58]. Advocates of routine peroperative cholangiography claim that demonstration of ductal anatomy will reduce iatrogenic injury to the common bile duct [26]. Open cholecystectomy is associated with a bile duct injury rate of 0.3–0.5% [56], although rates as low as 0.1% have been reported [59]. Similar rates of ductal injury have been reported in series of laparoscopic cholecystectomy in which routine (0.3%) [28] or selective (0.0%) [54] cholangiography was used. In our experience with selective cholangiography we have had two bile duct injuries in 418 laparoscopic cholecystectomies (0.5%). Subsequent cholangiography showed that there was no anatomical abnormality in either patient. In neither case was the common bile duct transected and repair was achieved easily in both.

Data collected by the Southern Surgeons Club indicate that most biliary injuries occur during a surgeon's initial experience with laparoscopic cholecystectomy. The rate of bile duct injury was 2.2% during a surgeon's first 13 laparoscopic cholecystectomies but only 0.1% for subsequent cases [17]. Thus, most biliary injuries are related to inexperience and are avoidable. The risk of iatrogenic injury can be minimized by adequate proctoring. This involves an experienced laparoscopic surgeon serving as an assistant for a surgeon's first cases [60]; assiduous attention to detail in the dissection of the cystic duct/gallbladder junction [21]; and a low threshold for conversion to open cholecystectomy when the dissection becomes difficult [60]. We concur with the view that cholangiography should be used selectively [61] and recommend the indications for cholangiography suggested by Corder and colleagues: abnormal liver function tests; a history of pancreatitis or jaundice; dilatation of the CBD demonstrated at operation or preoperatively on ultrasound and in the few patients in whom there is doubt about biliary ductal anatomy [62].

Training

The evolution of new techniques always brings in its wake implications for training. Minimally invasive approaches to surgical problems are now well established and laparoscopy is moving centre-stage in the management of a huge variety of intra-abdominal pathology. Thus, the time for confining laparoscopic techniques (especially cholecystectomy) to a few specialized centres is past [15] and it is incumbent upon all surgeons, who aspire to provide a modern state-of-the-art service to their patients and their communities to familiarize themselves with laparoscopic techniques.

The technical skills for laparoscopic surgery are video hand–eye coordination and remote dissection with novel endoscopic instruments. Continuing medical education programmes are the obvious method for teaching laparoscopic techniques to established surgeons. Initial instruction should be with bench models and all should subsequently attend an animal course. A surgeon's initial clinical experience should be supervised and, after a specified number of cases has been performed satisfactorily (probably about 12 cases) [60], certification in laparoscopic techniques should be awarded by an appropriate statutary body, for example the surgical colleges.

Surgeons in training also need to learn laparoscopic techniques as this will be the standard method of dealing with intra-abdominal (and possibly intrathoracic) pathology in the future. A system of supervision which advances the trainee from camera holding to operative assistance (e.g., creating the pneumoperitoneum or inserting ports) to chief operator is logical and works very well in practice [38]. There are real fears that 'old knowledge' will be lost and that trainees will have limited experience in conventional surgery. While this may be true for other minimally invasive therapies (e.g. ESWL) it is not true of laparoscopic surgery. Laparoscopic operations or laparoscopic-assisted operations are exactly the same as their open equivalents with the exception that exposure is far superior with the laparoscopic approach. Expertise in lararoscopic techniques can only enhance one's approach to the open operation on the rare occasion it will be required.

In conclusion, we agree with Soper and colleagues [38] that laparoscopic cholecystectomy is now the 'gold standard' for the management of symptomatic gallstones in the majority of patients. The management of symptomatic and asymptomatic choledocholithiasis remains controversial. Experience has shown that proctoring is an important aspect to ensure safety during a surgeon's initial experience with laparoscopic cholecystectomy. We believe that the fears that the laparoscopically trained surgical tyro will be unable to perform conventional surgery are unfounded.

References

1 Langenbuch C. Ein fall von extirpation der gallenblase wegen chronischer cholelithiasis. *Heilung*

Berl Klin Wochenschr 1882;**19**:725–7.
2 Cheslyn-Curtis S, Russell RCG. New trends in gallstone management. *Br J Surg* 1991;**78**:143–9.
3 Webb DR, Fitzpatrick JM. Percutaneous nephrolitotomy: a functional and morphological study. *J Urol* 1985;**134**:587–91.
4 Grace PA, Pitt HA. Biliary tract surgery: the role of percutaneous and endoscopic biliary drainage. In: ReMine WH, ed. *Problems in General Surgery*. Philadelphia: Lippincott, 1986;**3**:157–69.
5 Fitz RH. Perforating inflammation of the vermiform appendix with special reference to early diagnosis and treatment. *Am J Med Sci* 1886;**92**:321–5.
6 McBurney C. Experience with early operative interference in cases of diseases of the vermiform appendix. *N Y Med J* 1889;**50**:676–9.
7 Kelling G. Uber oesophagoskopie, gastroskopie und koelioskopie. *München Med Wochenschr* 1902;**49**:21.
8 Jacobeus HC. Uber die möglichkeit die zystoskopie bei untersuchung seroser hoblungen anzuweden. *München Med Wochenschr* 1911;**58**:2017–19.
9 Kalk H, Bruhl W. *Leitfaden der Laparoskopie und Gastroskopie*. Thieme: Stuttgart, 1951.
10 Rutkow M. Surgical operations in the United States: 1979–1984. *Surgery* 1987;**101**:192–200.
11 Fermelia D, Berci G. Diagnostic and therapeutic laparoscopy. *Surg Endosc* 1987;**1**:73–7.
12 Dubois F, Icard P, Berthelot G, Levard H. Coelioscopic cholecystectomy. *Ann Surg* 1990;**211**:60–3.
13 Perissat J, Colet D, Belliard R. Gallstones: laparoscopic treatment—cholecystectomy and lithotripsy. Our own technique. *Surg Endosc* 1990;**4**:15–17.
14 Reddick EJ, Olsen DO. Laparoscopic laser cholecystectomy. *Surg Endosc* 1989;**3**:131–3.
15 Cuschieri A. The laparoscopic revolution—walk carefully before we run. *J Roy Coll Surg Edin* 1989;**34**:295.
16 Cuschieri A, Dubois F, Mouiel J *et al.* The European experience with laparoscopic cholecystectomy. *Am J Surg* 1991;**161**:385–7.
17 Southern Surgeons Club. A prospective analysis of 1518 laparoscopic cholecystectomies. *N Engl J Med* 1991;**324**:1073–8.
18 Scott TR, Zucker MD, Bailey RW. Laparoscopic cholecystectomy: a review of 8016 patients. *Surg Endosc* 1992;**6**:107.
19 Grace PA, McEntee G, Bouchier-Hayes D. Laparoscopic cholecystectomy in the scarred abdomen. *Surg Endosc* 1991;**5**:118.
20 Olsen DO. Laparoscopic cholecystectomy. *Am J Surg* 1991;**161**:339–44.
21 Ponsky JL. Complications of laparoscopic cholecystectomy. *Am J Surg* 1919;**161**:393–5.
22 Voyles CR, Meena AL, Petro AB, Haick AJ, Koury AM. Electrocautery is superior to laser for laparoscopic cholecystectomy. *Am J Surg* 1990;**160**:457.
23 Hunter JG. Laser or electrocautery for laparoscopic cholecystectomy. *Am J Surg* 1991;**161**:345–9.
24 Moossa AR, Easter DW, VanSonnenberg E, Casola G, D'Agostino H. Laparoscopic injuries to the bile duct. A cause for concern. *Ann Surg* 1992;**215**:203–8.
25 Leahy AL, Bouchier-Hayes D, Hyland JM, Delaney PV, O'Sullivan G, Keane FB. Early experiences of laparoscopic cholecystectomy in five Irish Hospitals. *Ir J Med Sci* 1992;**161**:410–13.
26 Phillips EH, Berci G, Carroll B, Daykhovsky L, Sackier J, Paz-Pratlow M. The importance of intraoperative cholangiography during laparoscopic cholecystectomy. *Am Surg* 1990;**56**:792–5.
27 Nathanson LK, Shimi S, Cuschieri A. Laparoscopic cholecystectomy: the Dundee experience. *Br J Surg* 1991;**78**:155–9.
28 Bailey RW, Zucker KA, Flowers JL, Scovill WA, Graham SM, Imbembo AL. Laparoscopic cholecystectomy, experience with 375 consecutive patients. *Ann Surg* 1991;**214**:531–41.
29 Gompertz RHK, Rhodes M, Lennard TWJ. Laparoscopic cholangiography: an effective and inexpensive technique. *Br J Surg* 1992;**79**:233–4.
30 Berci G, Sackier JM. The Los Angeles experience with laparoscopic cholecystectomy. *Am J Surg* 1991;**161**: 382–4.
31 Reddick EJ, Olsen D, Spaw A *et al.* Safe performance of difficult laparoscopic cholecystectomy. *Am J Surg* 1991;**161**:377–81.
32 Petelin JB. Laparoscopic approach to common duct pathology. *Surg Laparosc Endosc* 1991;**1**:31–41.
33 Ireland A, Harte P, O'Sullivan G. Common bile duct calculi in patients selected for laparoscopic cholecystectomy—True incidence and management strategies. *Ir J Med Sci* 1992;**161** (Suppl. 11):36.
34 Spaw AT, Reddick EJ, Olsen DO. Laparoscopic laser cholecystectomy: analysis of 500 procedures. *Surg Laparosc Endosc* 1919;**1**:2–7.
35 Neugebauer E, Troidl H, Spangenberger W, Dietrich A, Lefering R. Conventional versus laparoscopic cholecystectomy and the randomized controlled trial. *Br J Surg* 1991;**78**:150–4.
36 Mays N, Challah S, Patel S *et al.* Clinical comparison of extracorporeal shock wave lithotripsy and percutaneous nephrolithotomy in treating renal calculi. *Br Med J* 1988;**297**:253–8.
37 Paterson Brown S, Garden OJ, Carter DC. Laparoscopic cholecystectomy. *Br J Surg* 1991;**78**:131–2.
38 Soper NJ, Stockmann PT, Dunnegan DL, Ashley SW. Laparoscopic cholecystectomy, the new 'Gold Standard'. *Arch Surg* 1992;**127**:917–23.
39 Grace PA, Quereshi A, Coleman J *et al.* Reduced postoperative hospitalization after laparoscopic cholecystectomy. *Br J Surg* 1991;**78**:160–2.
40 Wilson RG, Macintyre IMC, Nixon SJ, Saunders JH, Varma JS, King PM. Laparoscopic cholecystectomy as a safe and effective treatment for severe acute cholecystitis. *Br Med J* 1992;**305**:394–6.
41 Ledet WP. Ambulatory cholecystectomy without disability. *Arch Surg* 1990;**125**:1434–5.
42 Editorial. *Lancet* 1991;**338**:789–90.

43 Coleman J, Paul A, Spagenberger W, Klein J, Troidl H. Percutaneous cholecystolithotomy. *Br Med J* 1990;301:120.

44 Frazee R, Roberts JW, Okeson GC *et al.* Open versus laparoscopic cholecystectomy. A comparison of post-operative pulmonary function. *Ann Surg* 1991;213:651–4.

45 Dubois F, Berthelot G. Cholecystectomie par mini-laparotomie. *Nouv Presse Med* 1982;11:1139–41.

46 O'Dwyer PJ, Murphy JJ, O'Higgins NJ. Cholecystectomy through a 5 cm subcostal incision. *Br J Surg* 1990;77:1189–90.

47 McMahon AJ, Baxter JN, Anderson JR *et al.* Assessment of pain after laparoscopic cholecystectomy and minicholecystectomy. *Br J Surg* 1992;79:1224.

48 McMahon AJ, Baxter JN, Anderson JR *et al.* Pulmonary function after laparoscopic cholecystectomy. *Br J Surg* 1992;79:1226.

49 McEntee G, Grace PA, Bouchier-Hayes D. Laparoscopic cholecystectomy and the common bile duct. *Br J Surg* 1991;78:385–6.

50 Britton BJ. The management of stones in the common bile duct. In: Taylor I., ed. *Progress in Surgery*. Vol 2. Edinburgh: Churchill Livingstone, 1987:86–98.

51 Joyce WP, Keane R, Burke GJ *et al.* Identification of bile duct stones in patients undergoing laparoscopic cholecystectomy. *Br J Surg* 1991;78:1174–6.

52 Gardner AM, Holden WS, Monks PJW. Disappearing gallstones. *Br J Surg* 1966;53:114–20.

53 Johnson CD, Celestin LR. Large gallstones may pass spontaneously. *J Roy Soc Med* 1985;78:305–7.

54 Voyles CR, Petro AB, Meena AL, Haick A, Koury AM. A practical approach to laparoscopic cholecystectomy. *Am J Surg* 1991;77:368–72.

55 Grace PA, Qureshi A, Burke P *et al.* Selective cholangiography in laparoscopic cholecystectomy. *Br J Surg* 1993;80:244–6.

56 Smith EB. Iatrogenic injuries to extrahepatic bile ducts and associated vessels: a 25 year analysis. *J Natl Med Assoc* 1982;74:735–8.

57 Goor DA, Ebert PA. Anomalies of the biliary tree. *Arch Surg* 1972;304:102–9.

58 Issacs JP, Daves ML. Technique and evaluation of operative cholangiography. *Surg Gynecol Obstet* 1960;111:103–12.

59 Berci G, Sackier JM, Paz-Partlow M. Routine or selective intraoperative cholangiography during laparoscopic cholecystectomy. *Am J Surg* 1991;161:355–60.

60 Way LW. Bile duct injury during laparoscopic cholecystectomy. *Ann Surg* 1992;195.

61 Scott-Coombes D, Thompson JN. Bile duct stones and laparoscopic cholecystectomy. *Br Med J* 1991;303:1281–2.

62 Corder AP, Scott SD, Johnson CD. Place of routine operative cholangiography at cholecystectomy. *Br J Surg* 1992;79:945–7.

Chapter 12
Economic appraisal of alternative treatment options for gallstone disease

M.M. Wiley

Introduction

[cost effectiveness analysis] in health-care delivery is here to stay, and popular or not, it is becoming increasingly important in medical decision making. [1, p. 746]

Even a limited review of the literature suggests that this perspective currently represents a widely held view among practitioners and planners concerned with the provision of services for the treatment of gallstone disease. In this chapter, a cross-section of this literature is reviewed with the objective of identifying the relative cost-effectiveness of the different approaches to treating gallstone disease.

This chapter is not intended as a methodological lesson in the specifics of conducting an economic appraisal of health technology in general or treatment options for gallstone disease in particular. The main objectives include:

1 the identification of the predominant methods adopted by investigators concerned with assessing the relative merits of different approaches to treating gallstone disease;

2 the trends indicated by the findings of these studies.

This chapter is presented in three parts. Firstly, it is necessary to give a brief description of the type of approach which might be expected to be used from the more widely applied models of economic appraisal. The second section will be a review of selected studies undertaken with the objective of assessing the relative merits of different treatment options for gallstone disease. The final section will be concerned with the consolidation of the dominant trends emerging with respect to the cost-effectiveness of the treatment options considered by the studies reviewed.

Economic appraisal of health technology

As a framework for analysis and investigation, economics can help to clarify the issues involved in the distribution of medical services by providing a set of criteria for determining whether or not a person's welfare is improved by a specific policy or procedure. It is in facilitating the clarification of the cost of alternatives and by making values explicit that the application of economics may be useful in the arena of medical service provision. The application of economic appraisal to any health care programme would, therefore, be expected to take as its starting point the assumption that the scarcity of resources requires that the relative merits of different health service options should be assessed on the basis of their relative costs and benefits. From the economic perspective, it is the marginal costs and benefits of the service or programme under review which are most relevant in ensuring that choice between competing uses and scarce resources are made in an informed manner.

The main approaches to economic appraisal are usefully summarized by Drummond [2] and these are presented in diagrammatic form in Fig. 12.1. A fundamental tenet of any approach to economic appraisal is that the inputs used in the production of a particular health service may be compared with the outputs generated by the receipt of that service. It is in the enumeration, measurement and valuation of these inputs and outputs that the particular approaches available may be seen to differ. It is evident from Fig. 12.1 that inputs may

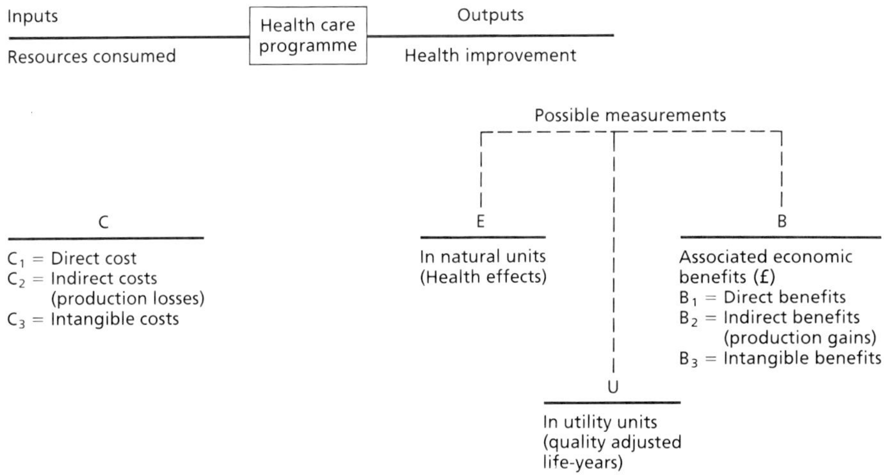

Common forms of analysis

1. Cost analysis: C_1, $C_1 + C_2$
2. Cost-effectiveness analysis (CEA): $(C_1 + C_2)/E$; $(C_1 - B_1)/E$; $(C_1 + C_2 - B_1 - B_2)/E$
3. Cost-utility analysis (CUA): $(C_1 + C_2)/U$; $(C_1 - B_1)/U$; $(C_1 + C_2 - B_1 - B_2)/U$
4. Cost-benefit analysis (CBA): $B_1 + B_2 - C_1 - C_2$; $(B_1 + B_2)/(C_1 + C_2)$

Also sometimes includes consideration of C_3 and B_3

Fig. 12.1 Components of economic appraisal. From [3].

be categorized as direct costs, indirect costs and the so-called intangible costs. The inputs may, therefore, be generally estimated in money terms, though this will not always be straightforward. One example of indirect costs is the estimation of the value of time lost from employment due to illness or treatment, while intangible costs could involve the attribution of a financial value to the experience of pain.

The assessment of the output side of the economic appraisal equation can be even more circuitous as there is rarely an output unit for health care programmes which parallels the function which money may serve in the estimation of costs. Drummond [3] suggests that such outputs may be considered in the following terms:

1 natural units like successful cases treated or years of life gained;

2 the application of a series of 'utility' weights to determine quality adjusted life-years or health year equivalents;

3 a money value like the increased value of production resulting from earlier return to work following medical treatment. Costs and benefits associated with the treatment/programme being evaluated which are expected to occur in the future should be taken into consideration in the analysis. This may be achieved by the application of the procedure of discounting expected costs/benefits to present values using an explicit discount rate.

Figure 12.1 indicates how the different approaches to economic appraisal involve different combinations of cost-types or output measures. Apart from a direct cumulation of costs, the remaining approaches all involve the assessment of some combination of costs relative to some valuation of outputs. Cost-benefit analysis is the most comprehensive approach, involving the assessment of all of the costs relative to all of the benefits. The availability of all the required information is, however, relatively rare which leads many researchers to pursue cost-effectiveness or cost-utility analysis. The distinguishing factor for cost-utility analysis is that costs are compared with health outcomes which are measured in terms of homogeneous life years [5]. This differs from the cost-effectiveness approach which is explained by Drummond as follows: 'If two alternative courses of action meet the objective equally well, then the less costly would be chosen on efficiency (or cost effectiveness) grounds' [2, p. 14].

In reviewing selected studies of different treatment options for gallstone disease in the next section, it will become clear that the majority of these studies applied the cost-effectiveness approach. In so doing, however, studies differ in the types of costs and benefits incorporated in the assessment undertaken. These will be identified as the studies are reviewed, together with the conclusions offered by the authors regarding the relative cost-effectiveness of the treatment options assessed.

Review of selected studies of alternative treatment options for gallstone disease

In reviewing the available literature for this study, the intention was not to attempt an exhaustive review of all published studies with any relevance to the area. Rather, the most feasible objective was considered to be a review of a number of critical studies which could be considered indicative of the approach adopted to the economic analysis of different treatment options for gallstone disease.

The studies reviewed for this exercise are listed in Table 12.1. Techniques covered by the studies reviewed include laparoscopic cholecystectomy (LC), open cholecystectomy (OC), extracorporeal shock wave lithotripsy (ESWL) and ursodiol treatment (UT). The studies are grouped by year of publication with the review being concentrated in the period during which the evaluations undertaken will be more likely to have included LC as one of the treatment options. The rationale for this is that while this approach has only come into general use since the late 1980s, its widespread use establishes an important alternative worthy of review in any subsequent assessment of treatment options for gallstone disease.

The sample size assessed for each treatment option in the studies reviewed is noted in Table 12.1. An initial review of this table, without any detailed knowledge of the individual studies, facilitates an understanding of the dominant approaches prevailing for the treatment of gallstone disease over the period. While the more recent

Table 12.1 Review of selected studies evaluating alternative treatment options for gallstone disease

		Treatment methods			
Studies		LC	OC	ESWL	UT
1992					
Kesteloot and Pennickx [4]	Sample size	21	26		
	Cost-effectiveness	*			
Cook, Richardson, Street [5]	Sample size	26	25	128	
	Cost-utility	*			
Schirmer and Dix [6]	Sample size	30	30		
	Cost-effectiveness	*			
Nicholl *et al.* [8]	Sample size		65	98	
	Cost-effectiveness				
	Small-bulk stone		*	*	
	Large-bulk stone		*		
1991					
Voyles *et al.* [7]	Sample size	453	47		
	Cost-effectiveness	*			
Bass *et al.* [11]	Decision analysis: ESWL/OC				
	Cost-effectiveness:				
	Single stone			*	
	Multiple stones		*		
Nealon *et al.* [10]	Sample size		100	52	
	Cost-effectiveness		*		
1990					
Rothschild, Holbrook, Reinhold [9]	Sample size		46	18	
	Cost-effectiveness			*	
Crain [12]	Decision analysis: OC/UT				
	Cost-effectiveness				*
Weinstein, Coley, Richter [13]	Decision analysis: OC/UT				
	Cost-effectiveness				*

* Treatment option which ranked best on the basis of the assessment criteria applied.
LC, laparoscopic cholecystectomy; OC, open cholecystectomy; ESWL, extracorporeal shock wave lithotripsy; UT, ursodiol treatment.

studies include an assessment of LC in the analysis of different treatment options, medical approaches feature frequently only in the earlier studies. Rather than dwelling in detail on the specifics of each study, this review will focus on issues concerned with the overall approach adopted including the sample, measures of cost and output, together with the final assessment of conclusions and recommendations.

When the studies undertaken by Kesteloot and Pennickx [4] and Cook *et al.* [5] are compared with studies by Schirmer and Dix [6] and Voyles *et al.* [7], it is clear that the first two studies are predominantly economic in their approach, while the second two are primarily clinical. The fact that all the studies include the relevant clinical factors together with an assessment of the costs of the different procedures does not alter the fundamental differences in approach. While Table 12.1 shows that these studies come to a similar conclusion, the differences in scope and methodology are worth considering in attempting to understand the approach adopted by the different studies.

An analysis of a consecutive series of 47 patients assigned on a non-random basis to LC or OC provide the basis for the Kesteloot and Pennickx study. The approach to costing adopted for this study was concerned with 'Only those components that are different for both procedures, and that hence may affect the decision to choose one or another procedure' [4, p. 4]. The cost-estimates derived from this study cannot, therefore, be taken as representing the full costs of each procedure but, rather, are intended to reflect the cost-differential between the procedures. It is important to recognize in interpreting the results from the study that no attempt was made to quantify such indirect patient costs as labour income loss, 'because of the controversies around the 'correct' financial translation of these indirect costs' [4, p. 11]. Notwithstanding the limitations in the approach adopted to costing the procedures, a number of interesting conclusions are presented by the study. These conclusions are specifically concerned with:

1 the relative cost-effectiveness of the different procedures;
2 the cost/volume implications of using laser or electrocautery and disposables/reusables;
3 the cost implications of learning effects.

With regard to cost-effectiveness, the authors conclude that, 'the laparoscopic procedure is more cost-effective for patients than the open cholecystectomy procedure, since the laparoscopy involves lower direct as well as indirect patient costs and superior effects' [4, p. 13]. They suggest that the use of electrocautery has advantages over the use of laser. With the electrocautery technique, total hospital costs will be lower if at least 140 cholecystectomies are performed laparoscopically whereas 300 would have to be performed to achieve the same cost reduction if the laser technique were used. With higher volumes, however, learning effects improve and there is a reduction in operating time which, in turn, results in a reduction in costs. The combined impact of learning effects, the use of electrocautery and the use of reusables/disposables is that total hospital costs will be lower if more than 70 laparoscopic procedures are performed with the electrocautery technique and the use of disposables, with this limit dropping to 50 if electrocautery is combined with the use of reusable equipment.

While the Kesteloot and Pennickx [4] study adopts a minimalist approach to cost-assessment, the study undertaken by Cook *et al.* [5] applies a classic cost-utility analysis approach to the assessment of the alternative options for the treatment of gallstone disease. This study differs from the others reviewed here in that three treatment options are reviewed (i.e., LC, OC and ESWL). This study is based on a trial which was undertaken at one hospital in Melbourne. While the trial was specifically concerned with the evaluation of biliary lithotripsy, information was also collected on the other two treatment methods. A random control trial could not be used. Patients in the ESWL arm of the trial received this procedure if they met selected predetermined criteria and were willing to accept this form of treatment. When LC became available, this option replaced ESWL and OC as the treatment of choice for patients meeting the selection criteria. The number of patients receiving each treatment option is specified in Table 12.1.

In recognition of the fact that quality of life is significantly affected by these procedures, cost-utility analysis was chosen by Cook *et al.* as the best option for the study. As this study constitutes a detailed assessment of costs relative to outcomes for the procedures reviewed, the approach adopted for each component of the analysis is worth considering briefly here. The costs involved in the analysis included hospital, patient and indirect costs. The hospital costs included medical, nursing, diagnostic, medications, overheads, capital and rental costs. Patient costs were based on travel time and indirect costs were based on estimations of lost production, both paid and unpaid. In addition, a provision was built in for conversion across treatments. It was estimated that 10% of patients undergoing LC would have to convert to OC and that 20% of lithotripsy patients would have to convert to LC, with the associated costs for these procedures.

The choice of outcome measure for this study was limited by the fact that the available data was retrospective. The approach adopted, therefore, involved the development of a number of standard scenarios from retrospective analysis of patient experience and the evaluation of these using an instrument for the measurement of patient utility. In this study, the authors adopted 'healthy year equivalents' (HYE-s) as the measure of final unit of outcome. The sequence involved in the estimation of HYE-s for each procedure included the following:

1 construction of an outcome tree for each intervention;
2 the construction of scenarios from patient interviews, questionnaires and expert judgement;
3 population interviews to evaluate scenarios using a rating scale and the 'time trade-off technique';
4 calculation of incremental benefits of the new technologies;
5 comparison with incremental costs;
6 sensitivity analysis.

While a number of interesting and important methodological issues are raised by this study, the conclusions advanced from the current stage of the analysis warrant serious attention given the sophistication of the approach to cost-utility analysis adopted. These conclusions may be usefully summarized here:

1 Laparoscopic cholecystectomy is the cheapest procedure both in terms of direct hospital costs and total costs; its outcome is also superior in terms of HYE-s.
2 Open cholecystectomy is inferior to LC and is a more expensive option than lithotripsy.
3 While lithotripsy has lower indirect costs, it has higher direct costs because of high capital costs, the cost of bile salts, and the number of repeat treatments required.

The authors comment that lithotripsy could be the procedure of first choice under the following circumstances:

1 the patient is suitable for lithotripsy treatment;
2 the use of ursodeoxycholic bile salts if these prove, in the event, to have no side-effects;
3 the use of the excess capacity of an independently justified lithotripter;
4 when patients exhibit a very strong preference for a non-invasive procedure [5].

The study by Schirmer and Dix [6] differs substantially from the previous two studies as it represents an assessment of performance within a single surgeon's practice. The general application of the findings are, therefore, open to question. It is presented here, however, as a potentially useful reference point for the two previous studies which were undertaken from a more classical economic perspective. The Schirmer and Dix study is based on an assessment of the first 30 consecutive patients undergoing LC successfully in a single surgeon's practice compared with the last 30 consecutive uncomplicated cases undergoing OC in the same surgeon's practice. While patients were followed up after surgery to determine the rate of return to normal activity, no other measures of outcome were attempted. In keeping with the findings of other studies, Schirmer and Dix found that LC is associated with a reduction in postoperative pain, length of hospitalization and a faster return to normal activity. The economic effect of these procedures was assessed on the basis of total hospital charges, including operative room charges. This analysis lead to the conclusion that total hospital charges for LC were less than those for OC, primarily due to the reduced length of hospital stay.

In attempting to explain the fact that operating room charges represented a higher proportion of hospital charges for LC compared with OC, learning effects and the use of the laser technique and disposables were identified as possible explanatory factors. The potential effects of these variables have already been shown to be substantial [3]. The fact that the LC group of patients assessed were the surgeon's first 30 LC patients provides some support for the contention that advancement along the 'learning curve' with greater experience could be expected to reduce operating room charges resulting in an even greater, cost differential favouring the LC option. While the findings of this study are consistent with the general trend of the previous studies reviewed, the results must be treated with caution as they are the experience of just one surgeon.

The study by Nicholl *et al.* [8] differs from the studies reviewed for 1992 in a number of respects, including the fact that LC is not included as a treatment option. This study is a randomized controlled trial of 163 patients, stratified by gallstone bulk, to ESWL or OC. The patients were originally recruited from nine surgeons in Sheffield, with the subsequent inclusion of patients from surgeons at two additional hospitals to accelerate recruitment. In evaluating the relative cost-effectiveness of the two procedures, the authors set out to assess health gain as well as costs for each procedure.

While this study, and the study of Cook *et al.* [5] both include an operational measure of outcome in their assessment, they differ in the particular approach adopted. The prospective basis of the Sheffield study opened up the range of options which could be applied. The outcome measures used were applied independently of those treating the patients and assessments were made at 4 weeks prior to intervention, and at 2 weeks, 5 weeks, 3 months, 6 months and 1 year after intervention. The measures of effectiveness assessed were health-related quality of life, biliary pain and gastrointestinal and other symptoms [8]. The Nottingham Health Profile was used to measure quality of life; a modified McGill pain questionnaire together with pain diaries were used to measure biliary pain; and visual analogue scales (VAS) were used in the assessment of the severity of gastrointestinal and other symptoms.

A detailed assessment of costs for both procedures was undertaken by the Sheffield study. The National Health Service (NHS) costs for each ESWL patient were estimated to include the suitability assessment, ESWL, ultrasound, hospital costs (including nursing, medical and hotel services), bile salts, the costs of any associated complication and patient time costs. In addition, the cost per ESWL session was calculated as the sum of the annual equivalent capital cost and the revenue costs divided by the expected total gallstone lithotripsy workload [8]. The NHS costs for OC were estimated to include the costs of the procedure, hospital stay, theatre costs, pre- and post-procedure investigations, outpatient follow-up, the costs of any associated complication and patient-time costs.

The findings presented for health status show that with the exception of sleep, after 1 year the health status of all patients with both procedures was similar to that of a similar age distribution in the general population. There were, however, differences recorded for both procedures under other criteria. An unexpectedly low clearance rate (24%) was found for patients undergoing ESWL. While the authors note that, 'It seems that patients with large-bulk stones tend to improve more if treated with cholecystectomy and those with small-bulk stones tend to do better with lithotripsy and bile salts', they acknowledge that patients' treatment preference may continue to influence treatment choice [8]. Notwithstanding these reservations, the authors conclude that after adjusting for stone bulk, the overall mean cost per patient of OC was significantly less than that for ESWL and bile salts. While this conclusion is different to that emerging from the Australian study [5], the authors of both studies make clear that differences in assumptions about the use of bile salts has a potentially substantial impact on the relative cost estimated for ESWL. In addition, the authors of the Sheffield study offer the opinion that, 'For small-bulk stone patients, conventional lithotripsy is at least as effective as cholecystectomy but relative cost will depend on length of stay' [8, p. 806].

The study reported by Voyles *et al.* [7] in 1991 was based on an analysis of 500 cholecystectomies carried out by five surgeons over a 9 month period. Data were collected on a prospective basis for the 47 patients which were initiated as OC and the 453 patients initiated as LC. Just 429 of the LC group were successful in having the procedure performed laparoscopically, with the remaining 24 patients requiring conversion to the open technique for clinical reasons. While the study deals in some detail with the process of undertaking LC and the complications arising, there is no attempt to apply a consistent outcome measure to the analysis.

The cost issues addressed by this study are specifically concerned with the use of the laser technique, disposable trocar/cannula charges and the use of routine operative cholangiography. The authors claim that, 'The laser appears to be completely unnecessary for laparoscopic cholecystectomy' and that their study has identified, 'a substantial subset of patients who do not require operative cholangiograms to exclude stones' [7]. In acknowledging that the potential cost savings of LC are substantial, the authors conclude that, 'The cost-effectiveness of laparoscopic cholecystectomy can be enhanced with no loss of patient benefit using the combination of electrosurgery, reusable trocars, and selective cholangiograms in low-risk patients' [7]. While the costing exercise attempted in this study is directed at a number of specific components rather than a comprehensive costing of the procedure, the findings regarding the use of electrosurgery and reusable trocars have clearly found further support in subsequent studies [4].

The studies by Rothschild and colleagues [9] and Nealon *et al.* [10] are worth considering together as they were both undertaken as part of a multi-centre Food and Drug Administration trial. In the Rothschild *et al.* [9] study, 18 patients received ESWL and 46 underwent OC, while in the Nealon *et al.* [10] study 52 patients received ESWL and 100 patients received OC. In their approach to costing each of these procedures, Rothschild *et al.* [9] took account of the treatment time, the length of stay and total hospital costs. Retreatment costs for ESWL were taken into consideration. In addition, the morbidity rate and the rate of return to work/normal activity were also estimated. Given the information available to the authors at the time of publication, they conclude that, 'extracorporeal shock wave lithotripsy is less costly, initially, with further reductions probable when performed on an outpatient basis' [9]. For this study, however, the costs of bile acid therapy were not included and the authors also noted that in their continuing assessment of the cost of lithotripsy they would have to take consideration of the cost of follow-up, serial testing, the need for retreatment and the rate of conversion to OC. This study, therefore, could not be considered to have taken account of all costs associated with ESWL.

In the Nealon *et al.* [10] study, the costs for individual ESWL patients were calculated on the basis of pre-operative evaluation, treatment, recovery room, follow up, and bile acid therapy. This costing procedure was further refined to enable the estimation of the cost per 'successful' ESWL procedure. The cost per OC procedure was estimated on the basis of length of hospital stay and total cost of treatment. Based on the results of this analysis, the cost of ESWL per 'successful' procedure was estimated to be more than four times that for OC, leading the authors to conclude that, 'Lithotripsy costs appear to be sufficiently high to render the procedure unlikely to emerge as the treatment of choice' [9, p. 645]. Notwithstanding limitations to the approach to costing in this study from an economic perspective, the fact that a more in-depth approach to costing ESWL services is used would suggest that estimates of resource intensity for this procedure relative to OC are more comprehensive.

The final group of studies reviewed falls within the research area known as decision analysis. Using available data sources, the authors of these studies estimate the probabilities of clinically important outcomes and service costs for the treatment options under consideration. These estimates are then incorporated into a computerized model which can be used to compare expected outcome and costs for different patient types receiving different treatment options. The predictive power and accuracy of the model will, therefore, be directly related to the specificity and comprehensiveness of the data originally used to estimate the model.

A model incorporating ESWL and OC is estimated by Bass *et al.* [11] and OC and UT are included in both the Crain [12] and Weinstein *et al.* [13] models. Bass *et al.* [11] report that the cost-effectiveness of the treatment options varies according to the age of patients and the number of stones. ESWL is projected to be more cost-effective for the elderly compared with the young, but less cost-effective for multiple stones. Crain [12] and Weinstein *et al.* [13] estimate that treatment with ursodiol is more cost-effective relative to the alternative. The findings offered by these studies offer some relevant reference points in assessing the relative potential of the different treatment options reviewed. Extreme caution is, however, urged by Diehl [14] in reviewing studies using the decision analysis methodology, 'Because decision analysis typically explores issues in which uncertainty is great, the probabilities assigned to chance nodes are difficult to set.' To illustrate this point, Diehl [14] notes that even if the findings of Weinstein *et al.* [13] were accepted uncritically, they would only apply to 10% of the US population with surgery being clinically indicated and/or more cost-effective for the remaining 90% [14].

In the final section which follows, the dominant trends indicated by the findings published from these studies will be reviewed.

Conclusion

With regard to cost-effectiveness of different treatment options assessed by the studies reviewed here, the main trends may be summarized as follows:

1 where the LC approach is compared with other options, this approach has been found to be the most cost-effective;

2 where OC and ESWL are compared, OC is generally found to be the more cost-effective, particularly for large-bulk stones and multiple stones;

3 the one study which concluded that ESWL was less costly than OC did not take account of the cost of bile acid therapy or the need for retreatment;

4 the conclusion offered by studies using decision analysis that UT was the most cost-effective option is heavily dependent on the specific set of assumptions adopted for these studies.

In terms of the approach adopted by the studies reviewed, it is interesting that the majority are presented as studies of the cost-effectivenes of the different treatment options, though the Australian study is the foremost example of the application of cost-utility analysis. Notwithstanding the declared common ground between the cost-effectiveness studies, there is considerable variation with regard to sample selection, the types of costs included in the analysis and the approach used for the assessment of treatment outcome. Given this variation in the application of the methodology by the different studies, it seems advisable to consider the cross-validation of those findings which may be used to inform decisions regarding service availability and delivery.

The approach adopted by studies for costing LC, in particular, resulted in the identification of a number of important cost factors which could be considered specific to this procedure. These factors include the impact of the learning curve on operating theatre costs, the relative costliness of laser versus the electrocautery technique and the use of reusables rather than disposables. All of the studies which took these factors into consideration concluded that as surgeons became more experienced with the LC procedure, operating time was reduced with an associated drop in costs; the electrocautery technique was found to be effective and cheaper than the laser alternative; and reusables were recommended as the cheaper option relative to disposables. It is clearly indicated by these studies that any future exercise concerned with costing the LC procedure would be stongly advised to take explicit account of these factors.

In addition to the mainstream costing issues arising for all treatment options, the studies concerned with costing the OC procedure reviewed here indicate that additional factors of critical importance are the length of hospital stay, complication rates associated with surgery and the cost-consequences of delayed return to work/normal activity. Failure to take account of any of these factors would warrant a critical analysis of the study under review. The costing for ESWL services was found to be particularly sensitive to assumptions made about the capital costs of the equipment, the clearance rate, retreatment, the conversion rate, site of service and the use of bile salts. It is reasonable to expect that these factors would be treated explicitly in any study currently undertaken to estimate the economic consequences of using ESWL for the treatment of gallstone disease.

In conclusion, therefore, it must be acknowledged that there is substantial variation in the application of the methodology of economic appraisal in the studies reviewed here relative to the theoretical framework outlined in Fig. 12.1. Despite this variation, however, the combined power of the published findings serve to advance our appreciation for the relative merits of the alternative approaches to the treatment of gallstone disease. In addition, these studies make an important positive contribution to our understanding of the specific cost and outcome factors which should be assessed in any future research involving the economic appraisal of these treatment options.

References

1 Fendrick AM. Cost-effectiveness of symptomatic gallstone management: what exactly are we measuring? *Gastroenterology* 1992;102:745–6.

2 Drummond MF. *Principles of Economic Appraisal in Health Care*. Oxford: Oxford University Press, 1987.

3 Drummond MF, ed. *Economic Appraisal of Health Technology in the European Community*. Commission of the European Communities Health Services Research Series No. 2. Oxford: Oxford Medical Publications, 1987.

4 Kesteloot K, Pennickx F. *The Costs and Effects of Open and Laparoscopic Cholecystectomies*. Colloque Europeen De L'Analyse Economique Aux Politiques de Sante, Paris, 16–18 December, 1992.

5 Cook J, Richardson J, Street A. Cost Utility Analysis of Treatment Options for Gallstone Disease: Preliminary Results and Methodological Issues. Paper presented to the Conference of Health Economists, Australian National University, 17–18 September 1992.

6 Schirmer BD, Dix J. Cost effectiveness of laparoscopic cholecystectomy. *J Laparosc Surg* 1992;2:145–9.

7 Voyles CR, Perto AB, Meena AL, Haick AJ, Koury AM. A practical approach to laparoscopic cholecystectomy. *Am J Surg* 1991; 161:365–70.

8 Nicholl JP, Brazier JE, Milner PC *et al.* Randomised controlled trial of cost-effectiveness of lithotripsy and open cholecystectomy as treatments for gallbladder stones. *Lancet* 1992;340:801–7.

9 Rothschild JG, Holbrook RF, Reinhold RB. Gallstone lithotripsy vs cholecystectomy. A preliminary cost-benefit analysis. *Arch Surg* 1990;125:710–14.

10 Nealon WH, Urrutia F, Fleming D, Thompson JC. The economic burden of gallstone lithotripsy. Will cost determine its fate? *Ann Surg* 1991;213:645–50.

11 Bass EB, Steinberg EP, Pitt HA *et al.* Cost-effectiveness of extracorporeal shock-wave lithotripsy versus cholecystectomy for symptomatic gallstones. *Gastroenterology* 1991;101:189–99.

12 Crain K. A computer model for evaluating the costs of cholecystectomy or ursodiol treatment in the management of cholelithiasis. *Clin Therap* 1990;12:250–62.

13 Weinstein MC, Coley CM, Richter MD. Medical management of gallstones. A cost-effectiveness analysis. *J Gen Int Med* 1990;5:277–84.

14 Diehl AK. Cost-effectiveness of ursodiol: the creature from the black box. *J Gen Int Med* 1990;5:374–5.

Chapter 13
Acute calculous and acalculous cholecystitis

R.M. Howerton & R.C.N. Williamson

Incidence and spectrum of disease

Acute cholecystitis is characterized by acute biliary pain with evidence of constitutional upset: pyrexia greater than 37.5 °C, right hypochondrial tenderness with guarding, and persistence of symptoms beyond 24 hours [1]. Patients with acute cholecystitis form a subset of a larger group of patients with acute biliary pain or 'biliary colic'; however, the pain is typically not colicky in nature as it is with ureteric or intestinal obstruction. Patients with biliary colic have episodic attacks of right hypochondrial pain and tenderness thought to result from temporary impaction of a calculus in the cystic duct or neck of the gallbladder. Acute biliary pain is reported to be the third most common cause of admission to a general surgical ward in the UK [2].

Distinguishing those patients with acute cholecystitis is imperative as they are more seriously ill and at greater risk of complications.

Acute cholecystitis is associated with gallstones in 90% of cases and predominantly affects the middle-aged and elderly. It generally shows a female preponderance [3–6] though some report a more even distribution between the sexes [7, 8]. The disease is widely accepted to be increasing in frequency and afflicting a more elderly population. This increase in elderly patients was substantiated in a recent review of patients with acute cholecystitis over two different time periods in an Israeli hospital [9].

Acute cholecystitis is not associated with gallstones in 10% of cases. This condition is termed acute acalculous cholecystitis. A historical survey indicates that the first case was reported by J. Duncan in 1844, although wide appreciation of this dangerous condition did not come until much later [10–13]. The incidence of acalculous cholecystitis has been reported to be between 6% and 17% of all episodes of cholecystitis [14], and this proportion may be increasing [15]. Frequently, acalculous cholecystitis develops in the setting of other serious conditions such as trauma, sepsis or major surgical procedures, but sometimes it complicates specific infections (e.g. typhoid fever, leptospirosis, candida and hepatitis A) or auto-immune diseases (e.g. Sjögren's disease, poly-arteritis nodosa and rheumatoid arthritis) [14, 16–19] and it can develop spontaneously. It has been reported in a child with Crohn's disease [20]. Acute acalculous cholecystitis is increasingly seen in patients in an intensive therapy unit [21], and it is an accepted complication of total parenteral nutrition [22, 23]. In seriously ill patients the condition may be difficult to recognize and may cause death [14].

Acute acalculous cholecystitis has been reported in a variety of iatrogenic settings including interleukin 2-lymphokine activated killer cell therapy [24], intra-arterial lipiodol therapy [25], following percutaneous transhepatic cholangiography [26] and following stenting of the common bile duct for pancreatic carcinoma [27]. In a series of 364 patients undergoing insertion of a biliary endoprosthesis at the Middlesex Hospital, London in 1989, six patients (1.6%) developed gallbladder sepsis [28]. Despite this multiplicity of potential causes up to one-half of the cases of acalculous cholecystitis appear to be idiopathic [29]. A recent report found that 77% of cases of acalculous cholecystitis developed in outpatients, although these patients were generally older [30–31]. One unusual variant is acute emphysematous cholecystitis, in which the gallbladder is infected with gas-forming organisms, usually in the absence of gallstones. This is typically a condition of elderly male diabetics, and it causes quite a high mortality rate.

Aetiology and pathogenesis

Acute calculous cholecystitis

Acute calculous cholecystitis is thought to begin with impaction of a gallstone in the gallbladder neck or cystic duct, resulting in the formation of abnormal bile (see below). However, in the experimental setting ligation of the cystic duct seldom results in acute mucosal inflammation, but rather causes simple dilatation of the gallbladder (hydrops) or shrinkage of the organ [32, 33]. In the clinical setting mucosal damage appears to follow obstruction, and predispose to bacterial infection. Bacteria have been cultured from the bile in up to 65% of patients with acute calculous cholecystitis, but the exact proportion depends upon the timing of operation following the onset of symptoms [34]. If operation is undertaken within 48 hours of the onset of symptoms, 81% of bile cultures are positive, a finding contrary to the prevailing opinion that bacterial infection is a secondary phenomenon [35]. Intestinal organisms predominate, 20% being anaerobic bacteria [34]. The same organism can often be cultured simultaneously from blood and bile, supporting the hypothesis that infection may be bloodborne [13, 36].

Several clues suggest that bacteria in the bile are not the only culprits. Components of normal bile can be injurious to biliary mucosa. Bile acids have been shown to damage mucosa experimentally, and the effect can be countered by lecithin [37]. Furthermore, patients with acute cholecystitis have less lecithin and more deoxycholic acid in their bile than normal [37]. Lysolecithin has been shown to induce chemical cholecystitis in experimental animals [38]. Though lysolecithin is present in small amounts in normal bile, the lysolecithin:lecithin ratio has been found to be increased 25-fold in acute cholecystitis [39]. β-glucuronidase from luminal bacteria might convert lecithin to lysolecithin [35]. Phospholipase-A can perform the same function and may be released in response to epithelial trauma [35]. Since phospholipase also interacts with lecithin to release arachadonic acid, this prostaglandin precursor could mediate the inflammatory response [38, 40]. In summary, it is probable that gallstone impaction and the accompanying mucosal trauma stimulate the formation of abnormal bile, which may lead to further mucosal damage with or without the assistance of enteric bacteria.

Acute acalculous cholecystitis

Many factors contribute to the pathogenesis of acute acalculous cholecystitis, the final common pathway probably being tissue hypoxia in the gallbladder mucosa. The mucosa is then injured by the irritants present in abnormally concentrated bile and/or by circulating organisms [41]. One-third of patients with acute acalculous cholecystitis have sterile bile upon culture, and many with positive bile cultures have other aetiological factors to explain the attack [13, 36, 42, 43]. One classification of acute acalculous cholecystitis separates the population into three groups (Table 13.1): those with primary (i.e., idiopathic disease); those with disease secondary to some other serious illness or stress; and those with certain rare variants.

The sex distribution is reversed in acute acalculous cholecystitis in comparison to calculous cholecystitis, the disease being commoner in men (3:2). In certain subgroups the ratio is even higher. One postoperative series had a M:F ratio of 7:1, and a series of post-traumatic cases

Table 13.1 Types of acute acalculous cholecystitis [150]

Primary	Secondary	Rare causes
Idiopathic	Surgical operations	Torsion of the gallbladder
	Multiple trauma	Abdominal trauma
	Burns	Intra-arterial chemotherapy
	Severe sepsis	Radiological embolization therapy
	Recent childbirth	Biliary endoprosthesis
		Collagen diseases

(a condition disproportionately affecting young men) had a ratio of 21:1 [44].

Several aetiological factors may lead to the development of acute acalculous cholecystitis. These include biliary stasis, ischaemia and infection.

Biliary stasis

Among wounded American soldiers in Vietnam acalculous cholecystitis was attributed to large volumes of transfused blood. It was suggested that increased pigment loads resulted in increased biliary viscosity and chemical irritation of the gallbladder mucosa [13]. Postoperative or post-traumatic patients who become dehydrated could be at similar risk [11]. Reduction in circulating cholecystokinin during prolonged parenteral nutrition can result in decreased gallbladder contraction and bile stasis [11, 45–47]. Subsequent forceful attempts to empty the gallbladder might trigger acute inflammation. Other factors impeding the egress of bile could include sphincter spasm secondary to the regular administration of opioid analgesics [48], as well as mechanical narrowing of the cystic duct by congenital stenosis, local inflammation or enlarged lymph nodes [49, 50]. Congenital stenosis could explain why acute cholecystitis is frequently acalculous in children. In at least one study of primary papillitis, 'tortuosity of the cystic duct' and recent vagotomy were common in an adult population with acute acalculous cholecystitis, supporting the theory of mechanical obstruction and biliary stasis [51]. Acute cholecystitis is a well recognized complication in post-gastrectomy patients, who are prone to biliary stasis with sludge and subsequent stone formation [52].

Ischaemia

Decreased blood supply to the gallbladder is also thought to play a part in the pathogenesis of cholecystitis [36]. Since many patients with acute acalculous cholecystitis are elderly, atherosclerotic narrowing of the cystic artery could be a factor [53, 54]. A recent study of standardized specimen radiographs revealed 'multiple arterial occlusions, with minimal or absent venous filling' in patients with acute acalculous cholecystitis. This is in comparison to normal specimens or those of patients with acute calculous cholecystitis, where there was arterial dilatation and extensive venous filling [55]. Increased sympathetic tone is a probable factor in post-traumatic and postoperative patients. Exaggeration of the sympathetic effect may occur in shocked patients receiving inotropes [56]. Similarly occlusion to blood flow may be a factor in patients with polyarteritis nodosa [57]. Two patients have been reported whose only apparent risk factor was severe visceral atherosclerosis [58]. A recent Japanese paper stresses the importance of reperfusion in addition to ischaemia in an experimental model of acalculous cholecystitis [59]. Increased phospholipase activity was also noted in this model, and oxygen-derived free radicals might conceivably have been important. The role of prostanoids in the production of acute acalculous cholecystitis is receiving increasing attention [60].

Infection

This could be either a primary or a secondary phenomenon. Patients with immune deficiencies such as AIDS may not require mucosal hypoxia as a precipitating factor in gallbladder injury. A variety of infectious agents including cytomegalovirus [61, 62] and fungi [63] have been implicated in causing acalculous cholecystitis in these patients [64].

Clinical assessment

Symptoms and signs

Up to 25% of patients develop acute cholecystitis as the first manifestation of gallstone disease, but most have had previous episodes of 'biliary colic' or flatulent dyspepsia [35]. A rich or heavy meal frequently precipitates the attack, bringing on pain in the right hypochondrium which may or may not radiate to the epigastrium or back. Nausea and/or vomiting are commonly present. As inflammation proceeds, the pain becomes localized to the region of the gallbladder.

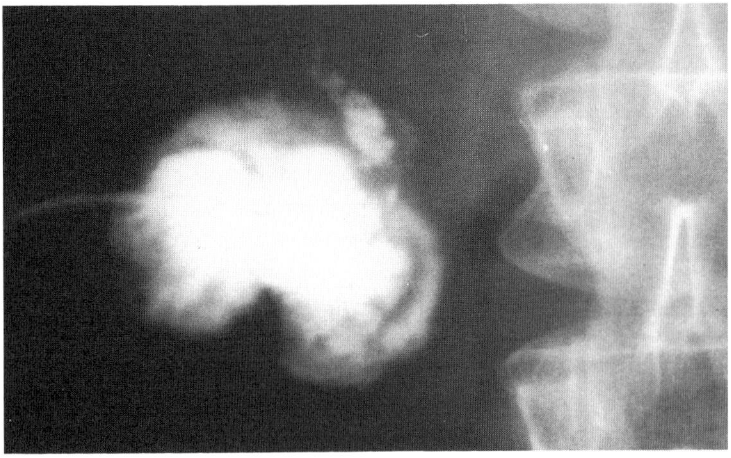

(a)

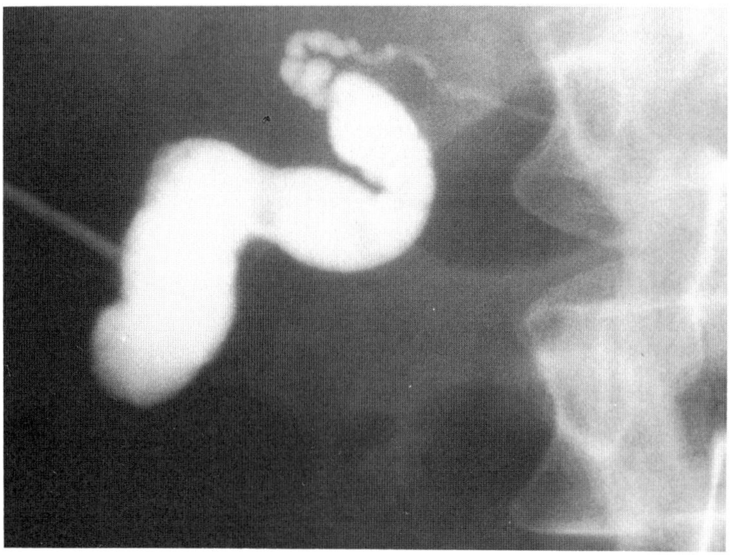

(b)

Fig. 13.1 Percutaneous cholecystostomy in a case of acute acalculous cholecystitis. The gallbladder is outlined (Fig. 13.1(a)) following initial transhepatic puncture and insertion of a catheter. Subsequent catheter cholecystograms (Figs 13.1(b) and 13.1(c)) show a patent cystic duct and a normal common bile duct.

Tenderness, rebound tenderness and a positive Murphy's sign are the physical signs of acute cholecystitis. If guarding is not too severe, the distended gallbladder may be appreciated as a mass. A self-portrait was given by Zachary Cope:

> I felt a dull, severe, deep pain in the middle of the epigastrium. My attention was then directed to the abdomen. I palpated the left side and right iliac region without finding anything abnormal. In the right hypochondrium however, a surprise awaited me, for in the normal position of the gallbladder was a rounded, tense and firm swelling, about the size of a small golf ball. [65]

Mild jaundice is present in 10–15% of patients [3, 35]. Possible causes include concurrent stones in the common duct, coexisting acute cholangitis or partial obstruction of the common duct by inflammatory oedema surrounding an impacted stone in Hartmann's pouch (Mirrizzi's syndrome) [5, 66]. Pyrexia is frequently mild, although ascending cholangitis or Gram-negative septicaemia give rise to high swinging fevers.

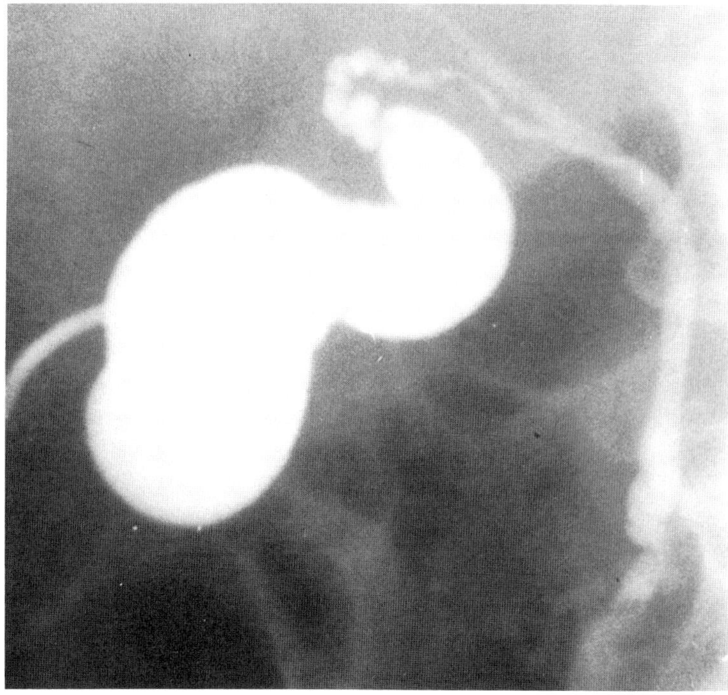

Fig. 13.1 (*Continued*)

(c)

Laboratory tests

Laboratory analysis usually reveals a leucocytosis (WBC (white blood cell) count greater than $10 \times 10^9/L$), and liver function tests are frequently abnormal. Even without clinical jaundice, modest increases in serum bilirubin and one or more aminotransferase enzymes are often encountered [5]. Bile in the urine suggests biliary disease and may be useful in refining the differential diagnosis, which includes peptic ulcer, retrocaecal appendicitis, renal colic, pyelitis, angina and the Fitz–Hugh–Curtis syndrome (gonococcal or chlamydial perihepatitis) [35]. Marked elevation of serum alkaline phosphatase and bilirubin suggest concomitant common bile duct obstruction. It is common for serum amylase to be mildly elevated in uncomplicated cholecystitis, but a substantial increase is consistent with coexisting acute pancreatitis. Fever and toxicity are indicative of Gram-negative septicaemia and mandate blood cultures; this is particularly true in elderly patients. Such seriously ill patients are at risk of renal failure, necessitating careful measurement of urea, creatinine and urine output.

Radiological diagnosis

Ultrasonograpy will suffice in the radiological diagnosis of most cases of acute cholecystitis. Cholescintigraphy should confirm virtually all the remaining cases [67]. The many advantages of ultrasonography include its ready availability, non-invasive nature, and ability to be used in a real-time mode at the bedside of critically ill patients in an intensive therapy unit. Findings in acute cholecystitis include gallstones, mural thickening, pericholecystic fluid, a distended gallbladder and a positive 'ultrasonographic Murphy's sign': pain when pressure is applied to the transducer while it is positioned directly over the gallbladder, although the latter may be absent in gangrenous cholecystitis (Fig. 13.1) [68]. In acute acalculous cholecystitis, the oedema of malnutrition and serious illness can be difficult to distinguish from a thickened, diseased gallbladder wall, though mural striations suggest cholecystitis. Serial ultrasonographic scans will show progressive changes in those with true cholecystitis.

Cholescintigraphy is used to diagnose cystic duct obstruction. An iminodiacetic acid (IDA) derivative, such as ethylhydroxy IDA (HIDA) or paraisopropyl IDA (PIPIDA), is labelled with radioactive technetium and injected intravenously. In the presence of liver uptake and excretion of isotope into the duodenum without filling of the gallbladder, acute cholecystitis can be diagnosed with confidence in the correct clinical setting [69]. While its specificity is lower than that of ultrasound in acalculous cholecystitis, the sensitivity of cholescintigraphy is higher [70]. The false-positive rate of cholescintigraphy can be reduced by injection of morphine, which increases common duct pressure and aids in the visualization of the gallbladder [71]. The presence of gangrene may be revealed on cholescintigraphy by the 'rim' sign of increased pericholecystic activity [72]. Rarely, the isotope may be seen to spill freely into the peritoneal cavity, indicating perforation of the gallbladder [73, 74]. Hyperperfusion of the gallbladder fossa on radionucleotide angiography combined with the 'rim' sign on hepatobiliary imaging have been shown to have a positive predictive value of 90%, although this combination is not in wide use [75]. Another infrequently used test is the indium-labelled leucocyte scan, which may detect an acutely inflamed gallbladder [76, 77].

Other investigations are seldom needed. Calcified gallstones are seen on plain abdominal radiographs in only 10–20% of patients [35, 78]. However, the plain film appearance of acute emphysematous cholecystitis is pathognomonic, with gas bubbles in the wall of the gallbladder, in the lumen and occasionally in the biliary tree. Oral cholecystography is of no use in acute cholecystitis. Endoscopic retrograde cholangiography is similarly unhelpful in the acute setting unless there is concomitant acute cholangitis (an exception to this predominant view is mentioned below where endoscopic therapy is used to treat acute cholecystitis). Computed tomography and magnetic resonance imaging have been used but are seldom necessary [79, 80].

In a very small subset of seriously ill patients with uncertain disease, the percutaneous aspiration of gallbladder contents may play a role in the diagnosis of acute cholecystitis [81]. In these same patients percutaneous drainage of the gallbladder may also have a therapeutic role (see below) [81, 82]. One group has suggested that for the occasional patient who is seriously ill with undiagnosed sepsis and a distended gallbladder on ultrasound, routine percutaneous drainage of the gallbladder may be the optimum management [83]. The use of imaging techniques in the diagnosis and therapy of acute cholecystitis has recently been reviewed in detail [84].

Management

Pre-operative treatment

The treatment of choice for most patients with acute cholecystitis is cholecystectomy, despite the fact that most episodes will settle quickly with appropriate medical therapy. Operation is indicated because of the risk of complications and the likelihood of recurrence. The timing of operative intervention has been the subject of much dispute.

Generally accepted principles of conservative treatment and pre-operative management include intravenous fluid replacement, nasogastric suction if vomiting continues, opiate analgesia, antibiotic therapy and diligent clinical monitoring for signs of disease progression. Proof of the benefit of antibiotic treatment over no antibiotic treatment is difficult to find in a controlled trial, but the risks of ascending cholangitis, septicaemia and empyema of the gallbladder justify its routine use in acute cholecystitis [35]. Traditionally, a single broad-spectrum antibiotic such as a cephalosporin has been used in most cases, with combination therapy reserved for seriously ill patients. The specific antibiotic regimen has been the source of many trials, and there is no clear-cut consensus at present [85–89]. Some preliminary data on the possible beneficial effect of the prostacyclin inhibitor indomethacin on the course of acute cholecystitis are of particular interest in view of the proposed role for prostaglandins in the pathogenesis of the disease [90–92]. During the phase of conservative management the opportunity should be taken to confirm the diagnosis (as discussed above).

Timing of operation

In a small percentage of patients the initial presentation of acute cholecystitis is so severe as to necessitate immediate operation. In one series from Oxford, only 7% of 304 patients were deemed to require immediate operation [1]. In this same series 5% of patients were considered unfit for any surgical treatment on presentation, mandating initial medical therapy only. In the remaining 88% of patients a choice was possible between early and late cholecystectomy.

Conservative management of the initial attack with subsequent confirmation of the diagnosis and interval cholecystectomy has been the traditional approach to acute cholecystitis. Two factors have guided this rationale: the perceived difficulty and risk of operating in the inflamed field around the gallbladder during the acute attack; and the observation that delay is not associated with serious complications in many cases [93]. Concern about spreading infection at the time of operation is also a consideration.

In the Oxford study three-quarters of the 267 patients for whom choice was possible received initial conservative management [1]. The mortality rate in this group was only 1.4% and the subsequent operations were largely uneventful, suggesting the relative safety of interval cholecystectomy. However, in 23% of patients, failure to respond to initial management led to operation during the first admission. No less than half the group (54%) developed symptoms while awaiting cholecystectomy; one-third of these required emergency re-admission. Among those patients receiving early operation, the mortality rate (1.5%) was similar to the constructively managed group. The only significant difference between the two groups was a shorter hospital stay in those having an early operation. Such a treatment plan also eliminated the possibility of a patient being lost to follow-up or declining the interval operation and presenting later with severe or complicated cholecystitis.

This issue has been similarly addressed in at least four prospective controlled trials, and the data have been summarized by Pellegrini and Way (Table 13.2) [94–97, 35]. The benefits of early operation were several: shorter hospital stay (11 versus 20 days), lower mortality rate (0/214 patients versus 5/192 patients), fewer treatment failures (defined as cholecystectomy not being performed as planned) and the occasional detection of a missed diagnosis. The operations were not found to be risky in the early period; in particular, no bile duct injuries were recorded. This policy was considered especially justified in those at apparently greater risk of complications (e.g. the elderly and diabetics [8, 35]). Indeed, Jenkinson [8] recommended that elderly men who developed symptoms of gallstones should have early cholecystectomy to prevent the development of a bout of acute cholecystitis with its attendant danger. This view is supported by data from Sweden, in which a series of elderly patients receiving early cholecystectomy for acute cholecystitis were compared with historical controls; again early operation emerged superior [98]. Further support for the safety of early cholecystectomy in acute cholecystitis in the elderly comes from a recent Spanish study [99]. Another analysis of previous series found lower failure rates (defined above) and shorter hospital stays in the early groups, with no deaths or ductal injuries in either the early or late groups [100].

The policy at Hammersmith Hospital is to admit patients with suspected acute cholecystitis and treat them expectantly unless generalized peritonitis is pre-sent necessitating emergency laparotomy. Failure of constitutional symptoms to settle, marked tenderness and/or a mass result in opera-

Table 13.2 Meta-analysis of four controlled trials comparing early and delayed cholecystectomy for acute cholecystitis [35]

No. of patients	Deaths	Ductal injuries	Total mean hospital stay (days)	Failure of regimen (%)
Early (214)	0	0	10.9	9
Delayed (192)	5	0	20.1	19

Original data from [94–97].

tion within the first 48 hours to alleviate the risk of gangrene or perforation. Those responding to initial conservative treatment have the diagnosis confirmed by appropriate imaging studies in hospital, and cholecystectomy is performed on the next convenient operating list. It is to be expected that one-third of patients presenting with cholecystitis will already be known to have gallstones and only require clinical confirmation of the diagnosis before proceeding to cholecystectomy [1].

The choice of operation

Cholecystectomy

The goal of this definitive treatment is complete excision of the gallbladder, and this can usually be accomplished without undue difficulty [96]. In urgent operations for severe cholecystitis with incipient or established gangrene, however, cholecystectomy may be a formidable and bloody technical exercise [1]. Sometimes the surgeon is fortunate to find that the oedema simplifies the separation of the gallbladder from its bed, but this same oedema may obscure the crucial anatomical details in Calot's triangle. Of course, fibrosis can also obscure the operative field at interval cholecystectomy performed 1–2 months after the acute episode. Variations in technique sometimes useful in the acute setting include early decompression of a distended gallbladder with an Ochsner suction trocar, blunt dissection from the liver bed after incising the gallbladder peritoneum, and the fundus-first technique [101, 35]. This last technique facilitates the safe identification of the common duct by following the cystic duct from the gallbladder to the cystic duct–common duct junction. Common duct injury is rare during early cholecystectomy, with no bile duct injuries in five series cited above [1, 94–97]. However, this serious complication is always a threat unless the surgeon is continually aware of the frequent anatomical anomalies affecting the biliary tree and its arterial supply.

An operative cholangiogram is indicated unless the patient is too ill or the periductal inflammation is too severe. Stones in the common duct will be found in 12–20% of patients with acute cholecystitis [2, 5]. It is sometimes necessary to suture-ligate the extremely friable cystic duct stump in the acutely inflamed state. Bile cultures and adequate drainage to the subhepatic space are also important in acute cholecystitis. A 5% incidence of wound infection and a 2% incidence of subhepatic abscess following cholecystectomy in the setting of acute cholecystitis mean that peri-operative antibiotic cover should be given routinely. Postoperative antibiotics are required in toxic patients, the particular agents sometimes requiring modification according to bile culture results. Analysis of several predictive factors may allow prediction of bactobilia, according to a recent report, and may provide a useful guide to the duration of antibiotic treatment [88].

Subtotal cholecystectomy

This procedure is sometimes more appropriate than complete cholecystectomy or cholecystostomy when the cystic duct–common duct junction is extremely difficult to identify owing to severe inflammation and fibrosis [35]. Stones are removed under direct vision after opening the neck of the gallbladder. The neck, frequently adherent to the common duct, is not removed. It is oversewn after obtaining a cholangiogram through the stump (whenever possible). The body and fundus are then removed, sometimes without the back wall if it is too densely adherent to the liver for safe removal. In this case diathermy is used to destroy the remaining mucosa. A running suture controls any bleeding from the residual cut edge of the gallbladder [102]. Excepting the case of residual bile duct stones, further biliary surgery should not be required following this procedure. A recent prospective review of partial cholecystectomy in 16 high-risk patients found it a 'fast and safe procedure [to] . . . be considered as an option in the emergency situation in the high-risk patient' [103].

Choledochotomy

Ductal stones identified pre-operatively or intraoperatively should be removed, thereby relieving or preventing cholangitis and obstructive jaundice. Clearance is confirmed with choledochoscopy and/or a post-exploration cholangiogram, and T-tube drainage is instituted [101]. The extent of ductal exploration is a matter of surgical judgement in the setting of suppurative cholangitis and/or severe periductal sepsis such as that found in association with a perforated gallbladder. Ascending cholangitis, septicaemia and liver abscess formation are usually arrested by incising the duct, removing as many calculi as possible, irrigating and then draining the duct to provide decompression. Meticulous searching for small stones may be inappropriate in the presence of gross sepsis. Many options exist for dealing with small retained calculi after recovery from the life-threatening situation. These include T-tube extraction or dissolution, extracorporeal lithotripsy and endoscopic extraction. The risk of anastomotic breakdown argues against the use of choledochoduodenostomy or transduodenal sphincteroplasty in the presence of suppurative cholangitis, though these procedures are useful in the absence of gross sepsis for patients with multiple ductal stones.

Cholecystostomy

This procedure, involving opening of the gallbladder under local or light general anaesthesia, removal of as many stones as possible and the placement of a drain, has a long history. Used as an alternative in patients deemed too ill for cholecystectomy, its role has fluctuated greatly. Reportedly performed by W.S. Halsted upon his mother in 1881, it later fell out of favour [2, 104]. Several major series have assessed its place [4, 105–107]. Having been used in up to 35% of patients presenting with acute cholecystitis it carried a high mortality rate of 8–25%, probably reflecting the desperately ill nature of the patients in whom it was applied. Retained stones, recurrent cholecystitis, extrusion of the drain and persistent biliary fistula were frequently encountered problems. Subsequent cholecystectomy is often needed, especially if follow-up tube cholangiography does not reveal a patent cystic duct. It is not an effective technique for treating gangrene of the gallbladder, and it does not address the possibility of gallbladder cancer as the cause of acute cholecystitis, a situation we have recently reported [108]. If this technique is used we recommend biopsy of the gallbladder during chole-cystostomy and early interval cholecystectomy.

In two more recent series cholecystostomy was used less frequently. It was performed in 10% of the urgent operations undertaken in the Oxford study [1] but in only 1 of 163 patients in a series from Florida [109]. Although still an option, particularly in a seriously ill, elderly patient, with a palpable gallbladder mass, the open operation as described above is being superseded in many cases by percutaneous and laparoscopic methods for achieving the same goal.

Percutaneous cholecystostomy

While this procedure has enjoyed increasing usage to treat both calculous and acalculous cholecystitis in the last decade, percutaneous puncture of the gallbladder is not a new technique. It was used for diagnostic opacification of the gallbladder in 1921 [110]. In a patient with malignant biliary obstruction and cholangitis in 1976, ultrasound was used to percutaneously catheterize and drain the gallbladder [111]. In 1980, a similar procedure was undertaken on a patient with empyema of the gallbladder [112]. This patient recovered to undergo an interval cholecystectomy at 9 months. Detailed description of the technique is beyond the scope of this chapter, but it is especially useful in decompressing the gallbladder and relieving toxicity in patients too ill for an anaesthetic [113]. Some have suggested that it may be the treatment of choice for critically ill patients in the intensive therapy unit with acalculous cholecystitis [114]. Subsequent tube cholangiography and the patient's general condition after recovery from the acute event determine the need for interval cholecystectomy.

We have some reservations about this technique because of the relatively high incidence of gangrene in the gallbladder wall, particularly in acalculous disease. Delayed gallbladder rupture following 'technically successful percutaneous drainage has been reported [115]. The open technique for cholecystostomy at least allows limited inspection of the gallbladder. A compromise may be the 'mini-cholecystostomy' involving ultrasonographic localization of the gallbladder followed by surgical drainage through a small skin incision under local anaesthesia [116]. Use of percutaneous drainage requires close clinical attention until recovery to detect a possible need for further surgical intervention. Hypotension secondary to profound vasovagal reaction has been reported [117]. There is also a theoretical risk of biliary peritonitis. Nevertheless, most reported complications of the technique have been minor and easily correctable [81]. Most survivors should probably be advised to undergo interval cholecystectomy.

Laparoscopic techniques

A laparoscopically assisted technique for percutaneous cholecystostomy has recently been developed [118]. This method employs a direct fundal puncture in contrast to the transhepatic approach preferred by radiologists. The laparoscopic removal of the gallbladder for symptoms of cholelithiasis and chronic cholecystitis has achieved rapid and widespread usage as discussed extensively in another chapter. While initially considered inappropriate for use in acute cholecystitis, this technique has been applied with success for the treatment of this condition by several major laparoscopic centres [18, 119–121]. It has also been used to treat empyema of the gallbladder [122]. Some experts have attempted the technique in all patients presenting with acute cholecystitis [120], although the rate of conversion to open cholecystectomy has been reported to be higher in acute rather than elective cases (33% versus 5%) [119]. This careful approach has resulted in complication rates no higher than in elective laparoscopic cholecystectomy [119, 120]. Though feasible, laparoscopic cholecystectomy is certainly more difficult in the acute setting. The laparoscopic surgeon should possess expertise in elective operations before treating a patient with acute cholecystitis. Familiarization with the experience and suggestions of experts as mentioned above is also essential.

Management in special circumstances

Gangrene of the gallbladder

Gangrene is thought to result from increased luminal pressure in the gallbladder following cystic duct obstruction rather than from cystic artery occlusion [35]. However, the development of cholecystitis following hepatic artery ligation and the frequency of gangrene and perforation in diabetics with cholecystitis suggests that vascular occlusion may also be a cofactor.

The incidence of gangrenous cholecystitis is uncertain. Careful inspection of the specimen in patients undergoing early cholecystectomy for acute cholecystitis frequently shows patchy necrosis. At presentation, 10% of patients with acute cholecystitis have peritonitis, and emergency laparotomy reveals a gangrenous gallbladder with or without perforation [2]. Acalculous cholecystitis is associated with gangrene more often than calculous disease. In patients with postoperative or post-traumatic acalculous cholecystitis the incidence of gangrene may be as high as 60% [14]. It is important to be aware of the frequency of this complication. Its presence or impending arrival requires resectional therapy (total or subtotal) in contrast to the various drainage techniques.

Empyema of the gallbladder

This uncommon but serious complication, consisting of an inflamed gallbladder containing pus, has a predilection for elderly patients. Usually occurring in the setting of a cystic duct obstructed by stones, it has also been reported in cases of acalculous cholecystitis [42, 43]. One large series (1 372) of patients with gallbladder disease seen at Bristol Royal Infirmary between 1976 and 1981 reported a 2.4% incidence of empyema of the gallbladder [123]. These 32 patients had a mean age of 71 years and a mortality rate of 25%. While right hypochondrial tenderness, leucocytosis and abnormal liver function tests were nearly always present, only half of the patients had fever or a gallbladder mass. Almost 20% of the patients had no history of cholecystitis. In these infection of a pre-existing mucocoele is a possible explanation for the development of empyema. The prevalence of this serious problem, particularly in the elderly, and its sometimes subtle presentation argue for an aggressive policy of early operation in acute cholecystitis. As already mentioned, peroral endoscopic transpapillary stenting has been used to treat this condition [124]. This technique can be used successfully to treat other forms of acute cholecystitis as well, but at present the total reported experience is very small and the eventual place of the technique is unclear [125].

Perforation of the gallbladder

The diagnosis of perforation is often not made until laparotomy or even autopsy [126]. The diagnostic imaging modalities mentioned previously may detect fluid collections around the gallbladder, though a pericholecystic abscess may be mistaken for empyema of the gallbladder. Acute calculous cholecystitis is complicated by perforation in 3–15% of cases [96, 97, 127, 128]. An even higher rate of perforation is reported in acalculous cholecystitis, ranging from 11% to 28% [36, 42, 43, 54, 56]. The insidious onset in patients with concomitant illness and the lack of a gallbladder wall thickened by chronic cholecystitis may explain the higher incidence of perforation in acute acalculous disease. Elderly patients, diabetics, and those with acute typhoid cholecystitis have higher rates of perforation [126].

Infected bile is a severe irritant in the peritoneal cavity, and the profound toxicity accompanying perforation requires energetic resuscitation with intravenous fluids and antibiotics followed by urgent laparotomy. A collected review of six series revealed the following statistics for patients with perforated gallbladders: a 31% mortality rate overall in free perforation, falling to 22% with surgical treatment, and an 18% mortality rate overall with localized perforation, falling to 6% with surgical treatment [128]. The need for aggressive removal of gangrenous gallbladders before perforation is clear. Expeditious cholecystectomy once perforation does occur is imperative to prevent further dissemination of bile.

Acute acalculous cholecystitis

The diagnosis of this entity remains problematic requiring a high index of suspicion. While the signs and symptoms can mimic those of calculous disease, the lack of a history of gallstones and the frequent presence of serious coexistent illness may confound the clinician. Laboratory evidence of increased serum bilirubin, amylase, liver enzymes and leucocytes is common [21]. Helpful findings on diagnostic imaging include a distended gall bladder, mural thickening, intraluminal sludge and a halo of subserosal edema during ultra-sound examination [129]. The diagnosis may be confirmed or perforation can occasionally be detected with HIDA scanning [73, 130]. Nevertheless, diagnosis is frequently delayed until gangrene and even perforation are present [14].

The high incidence of complications and the higher mortality rate of acalculous cholecystitis demand early intervention [41]. The frequency of gangrene makes cholecystectomy the preferred treatment [70] with subtotal cholecystectomy as an acceptable alternative [102]. Children may be an exception to this policy for they have a lower incidence of gangrene and may best be served by percutaneous cholecystostomy [49]. Conservative measures alone have been reported to be successful in a few cases, although we cannot commend this course [131, 132]. Cholecystectomy has a higher reported survival rate than cholecystostomy, although selection bias may be partly responsible for this discrepancy [29, 46, 48]. Percutaneous cholecystostomy (see above) has enjoyed wider usage in this setting recently [113, 114] and not all survivors have undergone subsequent cholecystectomy [46, 133]. We remain concerned about the application of this treatment modality given the high incidence of gangrene and further experience is awaited. As already noted the difficulty in diagnosing acute acalculous cholecystitis in critically ill patients has led one group of investigators to treat all patients with a distended gallbladder on ultrasound by means of percutaneous cholecystostomy [83]. Though the numbers are small, half the patients are said to improve dramatically. Again further data are awaited.

Acute emphysematous cholecystitis

Gas-forming anaerobes, particularly clostridia, coliforms and streptococci, are primarily responsible for this rare variant of acute cholecystitis [134]. Gas bubbles are seen in the wall and lumen of the gallbladder on plain radiography, although gallstones are seldom observed on these films. Bright echoes without calculi are found on ultrasonographic examination. The imaging signs are unlikely to be mistaken for the similar picture of biliary–enteric fistula, as emphysematous cholecystitis presents far more acutely. Pneumoperitoneum is the extremely rare result of perforation in this condition [135].

Males are three times more likely to develop this condition, particularly the elderly. Vascular occlusion may be important as 20–30% of these patients are diabetic [134] and endarteritis obliterans can be seen in the cystic artery [136]. The cycle of cystic duct occlusion increased gallbladder wall tension, ischemia, and secondary infection is an alternative explanation.

Severe toxicity associated with sudden onset of pain and a palpable gallbladder mass are the clinical features. Urgent resuscitation is imperative with appropriate antibiotics such as penicillin and metronidazole. Cholecystectomy follows soon in the patient who responds or is performed urgently in the patient who does not respond. Gangrene is a frequent operative finding, and mortality rates are probably highest in this type of acute cholecystitis [35].

Torsion of the gallbladder

This rare variant of acute necrotizing cholecystitis can occur when the gallbladder has a long cystic duct and is excessively mobile. Two anatomical configurations have been described:

1 a gallbladder unattached to the liver and connected only to a cystic duct and artery;
2 a gallbladder suspended on a very long mesentery from the liver [137].

Torsion of the entire organ is most common, but the process may occasionally be confined to the fundus. The condition is almost never diagnosed preoperatively as the presentation mimics commoner varieties of cholecystitis and imaging studies are non-specific. The treatment is prompt laparotomy. Reduction of the torsion prior to excision of the gallbladder is useful in preventing injury to the common duct [138]. Recurrent pain and swelling may occasionally result from subacute torsion with spontaneous resolution [139].

Iatrogenic cholecystitis

The increasing variety of iatrogenic causes of acute cholecystitis has been previously mentioned. Acute cholecystitis with gangrene and perforation can follow hepatic artery chemotherapy, usually given for colorectal liver metastases. Chronic cholecystitis with recurrent painful attacks can also follow this treatment [140, 141]. A sensible policy would be to perform cholecystectomy at the time of hepatic artery cannulation for infusional therapy. Transcatheter embolization of liver tumours has also caused gallbladder infarction [142]. Haemodialysis for renal failure is another reported cause of gangrenous cholecystitis [143]. We have seen patchy mucosal necrosis in a patient with an indwelling biliary endoprosthesis stenting a stricture secondary to chronic pancreatitis [41].

Cholecystitis in pregnancy

A recent review of 26 patients with biliary disease in pregnancy included five patients who were operated upon for acute cholecystitis during pregnancy [144]. The fetus was lost in five patients, two of these by intent. Two of the cholecystectomies were successfully undertaken in the last trimester. The optimum diagnostic modality is ultrasound, and if operative cholangiography is performed lead shielding of the lower abdomen is required.

Cholecystitis in children

This long-recognized condition [145] is uncommon and is rarely complicated by gangrene. Thus a more conservative approach to management may be adopted. Acalculous disease is relatively common, occurring in up to 30% of cases. Mechanical narrowing in the cystic duct region is one possible cause [49, 50], and torsion of the gallbladder (see above) is another [146].

The percutaneous approach is particularly applicable when emergency drainage is needed. Cholecystostomy of some variety usually allows the gallbladder inflammation to subside [49], and it is a safe and quick procedure in these often critically ill patients. If there is radiological evidence of an obstructed gallbladder or inability to empty the gallbladder contents by direct pressure at laparotomy, cholecystectomy is indicated. The rarity of this condition in children often leads to delay in diagnosis, a contributing factor to increased mortality in acalculous cholecystitis.

Prognosis

Overall risk of death

An overall mortality rate of 5% has been given for acute cholecystitis [35], but better mortality figures can be obtained with an aggressive approach to management [41]. Two separate experiences from the same institution over different time intervals are instructive [1, 3]. Acute cholecystitis treated between 1953 and 1962 had a 7.7% mortality rate. Between 1974 and 1978 the same condition was treated with a 1.6% mortality rate. The increasing percentage of patients operated upon in the first hospitalization (45% versus 27%) was thought to contribute to the improvement observed in the later period. A 1.9% mortality rate reported in 1969 was achieved with a policy of early operation and lends further support to this approach [147]. No deaths occurred in the 133 patients actually operated upon in the 1969 series. A 1986 series of 120 patients with acute cholecystitis had only 2 deaths (1.7%) [148].

Prognostic factors

Age

In Glenn's comprehensive series of 2 087 patients treated surgically for acute cholecystitis between 1932 and 1975 the overall mortality rate was 3.5% [4]. Patients over 65 years of age had a mortality rate of 9.3%, compared with a rate of 1.4% for patients under 65 years. Similar results have been published in more recent reports [1, 7, 149]. Older patients are prone to complications such as empyema and perforation of the gallbladder, and they are also more likely to develop fatal cardiorespiratory complications.

Diabetes mellitus

Whether diabetics with acute cholecystitis fare worse than non-diabetics with this condition is unclear. Recent authors have both supported [35] and refuted this postulate [148]. The postoperative recovery in diabetics might be expected to be complicated by concomitant cardiovascular and renal disease. A policy of recommending prophylactic cholecystectomy for diabetics with asymptomatic gallstones has been challenged recently after no increase in deaths among diabetics with acute cholecystitis was found [149].

Acalculous cholecystitis

This condition carries a higher mortality rate than that of calculous disease, 9.6% versus 4.3%. The subset of patients with postoperative or post-traumatic acalculous cholecystitis has a particularly grave prognosis, with mortality rates ranging from 32 to 47% being reported [42, 43, 56]. Patients with acalculous disease are often elderly and systemically ill, and are especially likely to develop gangrene and perforation. In critically ill patients in the intensive therapy unit, acute necrotizing acalculous cholecystitis is often a terminal event.

Conclusions

The surgical treatment of acute cholecystitis is

more than 100 years old. This experience has led to many advances in diagnosis, preoperative care, surgical technique and postoperative care. Better antibiotics and a clearer understanding of the pathophysiology of acute cholecystitis have been important improvements. Ultrasound has established itself as the diagnostic modality of choice, supplemented as needed by cholescintigraphy. A particular advance in caring for critically ill patients with suspected cholecystitis has been the availability of portable real-time ultrasound scanners allowing bedside examination in the intensive therapy unit.

An aggressive policy of early or urgent cholecystectomy has replaced the more traditional approach of initial medical management and interval cholecystectomy. Four prospective studies have substantiated this policy and we have adopted this approach, generally operating on the next available list and almost always during the initial hospital admission. Suspicion of perforation, gangrene or failure to respond to medical therapy results in prompt operation. Operation is postponed only for the profoundly unfit and those reluctant for operation. The use of laparoscopic techniques to remove the gallbladder in acute cholecystitis will probably continue to increase.

The place of cholecystostomy merits reappraisal. Desperately ill patients benefit from its speed and safety. It may be all that is required in children with acalculous disease. Formal or open cholecystostomy is often unsatisfactory, for it has a substantial complication rate and leaves the gallbladder *in situ*. The newer laparoscopic or percutaneous methods may allow a simpler method of improving the patient's condition. Subsequent cholecystectomy may then be undertaken in a healthier patient. All drainage procedures suffer from the possible drawback of leaving gangrenous tissue *in situ* as a focus of continuing sepsis. If operation has been embarked upon and difficulties are encountered, then subtotal cholecystectomy may be a better option than cholecystostomy.

Death from calculous cholecystitis is mostly confined to the elderly. Acalculous cholecystitis remains a highly lethal disease for all, with a mortality rate approaching 10%. This rate will be reduced only with prompt diagnosis and early treatment of this serious condition.

References

1 Mitchell A, Morris PJ. Trends in management of acute cholecystitis. *Br Med J* 1982;**284**:27–30.

2 Jones PF. Acute cholecystitis: a case for early surgery? *Br Med J* 1982;**285**:1376–7.

3 Essenhigh DM. Management of acute cholecystitis. *Br J Surg* 1966;**53**:1032–8.

4 Glenn F. Cholecystectomy in the high risk patient with biliary tract disease. *Ann Surg* 1977;**185**:185–91.

5 Stryker SJ, Beal JM. Acute cholecystitis and common duct calculi. *Arch Surg* 1983;**118**:1063–4.

6 Addison NV, Finan PJ. Urgent and early cholecystectomy for acute gallbladder disease. *Br J Surg* 1988;**75**:141–3.

7 Huber DF, Martin EW Jr. Cooperman M. Cholecystectomy in elderly patients. *Am J Surg* 1983;**146**: 719–22.

8 Jenkinson LR, Crumplin MKH, Kassab JY, Whitaker CJ. Early elective cholecystectomy—an alternative to early cholecystectomy in acute cholecystitis? *Ann R Coll Surg Eng* 1985;**67**:162–3.

9 Reiss R, Nudelman I, Gutman C, Deutsch AA. Changing trends in surgery for acute cholecystitis. *World J Surg* 1990;**14**:567–70.

10 Glenn F. Acute cholecystitis following the surgical treatment of unrelated disease. *Ann Surg* 1947;**126**: 411–20.

11 Genn F, Wantz GE. Acute cholecystitis following the surgical treatment of unrelated disease. *Surg Gynecol Obstet* 1956;**102**:145–53.

12 Howard RJ, Delaney JP. Postoperative cholecystitis. *Amer J Digest Dis* 1972;**17**:213–18.

13 Lindberg EF, Grinnan GLB, Smith L. Acalculous cholecystitis in Vietnam casualties. *Ann Surg* 1970; **171**:152–7.

14 Williamson RCN. Acalculous disease of the gallbladder. *Gut* 1988;**29**:860–72.

15 Glenn F, Becker CG. Acute acalculous cholecystitis. *Ann Surg* 1982;**195**:131–6.

16 Fernandez-Nebro A, Valdivielso P, Sanchez-Carrillo JJ, Domenech I, DeRamon E, Gonzalez-Santos P. Localized rheumatoid vasculitis presenting as acute alithiasic cholecystitis. *Am J Med* 1991;**91**:90–2.

17 Parangi S, Oz MC, Blume RS *et al.* Hepatobiliary complications of polyarteritis nodosa. *Arch Surg* 1991;**126**:909–12.

18 Jacobs M, Verdeja JC, Goldstein HS. Laparoscopic cholecystectomy in acute cholecystitis. *J Laparoendosc Surg* 1991;**1**:175–7.

19 Black MM, Mann NP. Gangrenous cholecystitis due to hepatitis A infection. *J Trop Med Hyg* 1992;**95**:73–4.

20 Hyams JS, Baker E, Schwartz AN, Ricci A Jr,

McGowan G. Acalculous cholecystitis in Crohn's disease. *J Adoles Health Care* 1989;10:151–4.
21 Fabian TC, Hickerson WL, Mangiante EC. Post-traumatic and postoperative acute cholecystitis. *Am Surg* 1986;**52**:188–92.
22 Hwang TL, Chen MF. Percutaneous gallbladder drainage for acute acalculous cholecystitis during total parenteral nutrition. *Br J Surg* 1992;**79**:237–8.
23 Bower R, Mrdeza MA, Block GE. Association of cholecystitis and parenteral nutrition. *Nutrition* 1990; **6**:125–30.
24 Chung-Park M, Kim B, Marmolya G, Karlins N, Wojcik E. Acalculous lymphoeosinophilic cholecystitis associated with interleukin-2 and lymphokine-activated killer cell therapy. *Arch Pathol Lab Med* 1990;**114**:1073–5.
25 Yeung E, Jackson J, Finn JP, Thomas MG, Benjamin IS, Adam A. Acalculous cholecystitis complicating hepatic intraarterial lipiodol: case report. *Cardiovasc Intervent Radiol* 1989;**12**:80–2.
26 Lillemoe KD, Pitt HA, Kaufman SL, Cameron JL. Acute cholecystitis occurring as a complication of percutaneous transhepatic drainage. *Surg Gynecol Obstet* 1989;**168**:348–52.
27 Gardner AMN. Acalculous cholecystitis. *J Roy Soc Med* 1989;**82**:242.
28 Ainley CC, Williams SJ, Smith AC, Hatfield ARW, Russell RCG, Lees WR. Gallbladder sepsis after stent insertion for bile duct obstruction: management by percutaneous cholecystostomy. *Br J Surg* 1991;**78**: 961–3.
29 Glenn F. Acute acalculous cholecystitis. *Ann Surg* 1979;**189**:458–65.
30 Malet PF. Acalculous cholecystitis: a new perspective. *Gastroenterology* 1990;**99**:1529–30.
31 Savoca PE, Longo WE, Zucker KA, McMillen MM, Modlin IM. The increasing prevalence of acalculous cholecystitis in outpatients. Results of a 7-year study. *Ann Surg* 1990;**211**:433–7.
32 Morris CR, Hohf RP, Ivy AC. An experimental study of the role of stasis in the etiology of cholecystitis. *Surgery* 1952;**32**:673–85.
33 Salomonowitz E, Frick MP, Simmons RL *et al.* Obliteration of the gallbladder without formal cholecystectomy. *Arch Surg* 1984;**119**:725–9.
34 Claesson BEB, Holmlund DEW, Matzsch TW. Microflora of the gallbladder related to duration of acute cholecystitis. *Surg Gynecol Obstet* 1986;**162**: 531–5.
35 Pellegrini CA, Way LW. Acute cholecystitis. In: Way LW, Pellegrini CA, eds. *Surgery of the Gallbladder and Bile Ducts*. Philadelphia: Saunders, 1987:251–64.
36 Orlando R III, Gleason E, Drezner AD. Acute acalculous cholecystitis in the critically ill patient. *Am J Surg* 1983;**145**:472–6.
37 Heuman R, Norrby S, Sjodahl R, Tiselius HG, Tagesson C. Altered gallbladder bile composition in gallstone disease: Relation to gallbladder wall permeability. *Scand J Gastroent* 1980;**15**:581–6.
38 Sjodahl R, Tagesson C. On the development of primary acute cholecystits. *Scand J Gastroent* 1983; **18**:577–9.
39 Sjodahl R, Wettefors J. Lysolecithin and lecithin in the gallbladder wall and bile; their possible roles in the pathogenesis of acute cholecystitis. *Scand J Gastroent* 1974;**9**:519–25.
40 Jivegard L, Thornell E, Svanvik J. Pathophysiology of acute obstructive cholecystitis: implications for non-operative management. *Br J Surg* 1987;**74**:1084–6.
41 Williamson RCN. Acute cholecystitis, calculous and acalculous. In: Williamson RCN, Cooper MJ, eds. *Clinical Surgery International Vol. 17: Emergency Abdominal Surgery*. Edinburgh: Churchill Livingstone, 1990:1110–27.
42 Ottinger LW. Acute cholecystitis as a postoperative complication. *Ann Surg* 1976;**184**:162–5.
43 Devine RM, Farnell MB, Mucha P Jr. Acute cholecystitis as a complication in surgical patients. *Arch Surg* 1984;**119**:1389–93.
44 Jonsson PE, Andersson A. Postoperative acute acalculous cholecystitis. *Arch Surg* 1976;**111**:1097–101.
45 Gullick HD. A roentgenologic study of gallbladder evacuation following nonbiliary tract surgery. *Ann Surg* 1960;**151**:403–8.
46 Long TN, Heimbach DM, Carrico CJ. Acalculous cholecystitis in critically ill patients. *Am J Surg* 1978;**136**:31–6.
47 Petersen SR, Sheldon GF. Acute acalculous cholecystitis: a complication of hyperalimentation. *Am J Surg* 1979;**138**:814–17.
48 Flancbaum L, Majerus TC, Cox EF. Acute post-traumatic acalculous cholecystitis. *Amer J Surg* 1985; **150**:252–32.
49 Ternberg JL, Keating JP. Acute acalculous cholecystitis. Complication of other illness in childhood. *Arch Surg* 1975;**110**:543–7.
50 Traynelis VC, Hrabovsky EE. Acalculous cholecystitis in the neonate. *Amer J Dis Child* 1985;**139**:893–5.
51 Lygidakis NJ. Surgery for acalculous cholecystitis. An organic and not a functional disease. *Am J Gastroenterol* 1981;**76**:27–31.
52 Takahashi T, Yamamura T, Utsunomiya J. Pathogenesis of acute cholecystitis after gastrectomy. *Br J Surg* 1990;**77**:536–9.
53 Fox MS, Wilk PJ, Weissmann HS, Freeman LM, Gliedman ML. Acute acalculous cholecystitis. *Surg Gynecol Obstet* 1984;**159**:13–16.
54 Johnson LB. The importance of early diagnosis of acute acalculous cholecystitis. *Surg Gynecol Obstet* 1987;**164**:197–203.
55 Warren BL. Small vessel occlusion in acute acalculous cholecystitis. *Surgery* 1992;**111**:163–8.
56 DuPriest RW Jr, Khaneja SC, Cowley RA. Acute cholecystitis complicating trauma. *Ann Surg* 1979; **189**:84–9.
57 LiVolsi VA, Perzin KH, Porter M. Polyarteritis nodosa

of the gallbladder, presenting as acute cholecystitis. *Gastroenterology* 1973;**65**:115–23.
58 Savoca PE, Longo WE, Pasternak B, Gusberg RJ. Does visceral ischemia play a role in the pathogenesis of acute acalculous cholecystitis? *J Clin Gastroenterol* 1990;**12**:33–6.
59 Taoka H. Experimental study on the pathogenesis of acute acalculous cholecystitis, with special reference to the role of microcirculatory disturbances, free radicals and membrane-bound phospholipase A2. *Gastroenterol Japon* 1991;**26**:633–44.
60 Kaminski DL, Andrus CH, German D, Deshpande YG. The role of prostanoids in the production of acute acalculous cholecystitis by platelet-activating factor. *Ann Surg* 1990;**212**:455–61.
61 Ong ELC, Ellis ME, Tweedle DEF, Ferguson G, Haboubi NY, Know WF. Cytomegalovirus cholecystitis and colitis associated with the acquired immunodeficiency syndrome. *J Infect* 1989;**18**:73–5.
62 Aaron JS, Wynter CD, Kirton OC, Simko V. Cytomegalovirus associated with acalculous cholecystitis in a patient with acquired immune deficiency syndrome. *Am J Gastroenterol* 1988;**83**:879–81.
63 Cervia JS, Murray HW. Fungal cholecystitis and AIDS. *J Infect Dis* 1990;**161**:358.
64 Vao L, Scialdone C. Empyema of the gallbladder in a patient with AIDS-related complex. *Clin Imag* 1990;**14**:157–8.
65 Silen W. *Cope's early diagnosis of the acute abdomen.* New York: Oxford University Press, 1979;129–130.
66 Witte CL. Choledochal obstruction by cystic duct stone: Mirrizzi's Syndrome. *Am Surg* 1984;**50**:241–3.
67 Gill PT, Dillon E, Leahy AL, Reeder A, Peel ALG. Ultrasonography, HIDA scintigraphy or both in the diagnosis of acute cholecystitis? *Br J Surg* 1985;**72**: 267–8.
68 Simeone JF, Brink JA, Mueller PR *et al.* The sonographic diagnosis of acute gangrenous cholecystitis: importance of the Murphy sign. *Am J Roentgenol* 1989;**152**:289–90.
69 Cabellon S, Brown JM, Cavanaugh DG. Accuracy of the hepatobiliary scan in acute cholecystitis. *Am J Surg* 1984;**148**:607–8.
70 Kang JY, Williamson RCN. Review article: Cholecystitis without gallstones. *HPB Surg* 1990;**2**:83–103.
71 Flancbaum L, Alden SM. Morphine cholescintigraphy. *Surg Gynecol Obstet* 1990;**171**:227–32.
72 Bushnell DL, Perkman SB, Wilson MA, Polcyn RE. The rim sign: association with acute cholecystitis. *J Nuc Med* 1986;**27**:353–6.
73 Swayne LC. Acute acalculous cholecystitis: sensitivity in detection using technitium-99m iminodiacetic acid cholescintigraphy. *Radiology* 1986;**160**:33–8.
74 Siskind BN, Hawkins HB, Cinti DC, Zeman RK, Burrell MI. Gallbladder perforation. An imaging analysis. *J Clin Gastroenterol* 1987;**9**:670–8.
75 Aburano T, Yokoyama K, Taniguchi M. Diagnostic values of gallbladder hyperperfusion and the rim sign in radionuclide angiography and hepatobiliary imaging. *Gastrointest Radiol* 1990;**15**:229–32.
76 Datz FL. Utility of Indium-111-labelled leukocyte imaging in acute acalculous cholecystitis. *Am J Roentgenol* 1986;**147**:813–14.
77 Fink-Bennett D, Clarke K, Tsai D, Nuechterlein P, Gora G. Indium-111-leukocyte imaging in acute cholecystits. *J Nuc Med* 1991;**32**:803–4.
78 Watts J McK, Toouli J. Cholecystitis and choledocholithiasis. In: Bouchier IAD, Allan RN, Hodgson HJF, Keighley MRB, eds. *Textbook of Gastroenterology.* London: Baillière Tindall, 1984:1416.
79 Varma DG, Faust JM. Computed tomography of gangrenous acute postoperative acalculous cholecystitis. *J Comput Tomog* 1988;**12**:29–31.
80 Weissleder R, Stark DD, Compton CC, Simeone JF, Ferrucci JT: Cholecystitis: diagnosis by MR imaging. *Magnet Reson Imag* 1988;**6**:345–8.
81 Werbel GB, Nahrwold DL, Joehl RJ, Vogelzang RL, Rege RV. Percutaneous cholecystostomy in the diagnosis and treatment of acute cholecystitis in the high-risk patient. *Arch Surg* 1989;**124**:782–6.
82 Blankenberg F, Wirth R, Jeffrey RB Jr, Mindelzun R, Francis I. Computed tomography as an adjunct to ultrasound in the diagnosis of acute acalculous cholecystitis. *Gastrointest Radiol* 1991;**16**:149–53.
83 Lee MJ, Saini S, Brink JA *et al.* Treatment of critically ill patients with sepsis of unknown cause: value of percutaneous cholecystostomy. *Amer J Roentgenol* 1991;**156**:1163–6.
84 Adam A, Roddie ME. Acute cholecystitis: radiological management. *Baillière's Clin Gastroenterol* 1991;**5**: 787–816.
85 Muller EL, Pitt HA, Thompson JE Jr, Doty JE, Mann LL, Manchester B. Antibiotics in infections of the biliary tract. *Surg Gynecol Obstet* 1987;**165**:285–92.
86 Chacon JP, Criscuolo PD, Kobata CM, Ferraro JR, Saad SS, Reis C. Prospective randomized comparison of pefloxacin and ampicillin plus gentamicin in the treatment of bacteriologically proven biliary tract infections. *J Antimicrob Chemother* 1990;**26**(Suppl. B):167–72.
87 Friedlender J, Meyer P, Marti MC, Rohner A. Comparative study of ceftriaxone and cefoperazone in the treatment of acute cholecystitis. *Chemotherapy* 1988;**34**(Suppl. 1):30–3.
88 Thompson JE Jr, Bennion RS, Doty JE, Muller EL, Pitt HA. Predictive factors for bactibilia in acute cholecystitis. *Arch Surg* 1990;**125**:261–4.
89 Hjortrup A, Moesgaard F, Jensen F, Johansen C, Nielsen R. Antibiotic prophylaxis in high risk biliary surgery: one dose of ceftriaxone compared with two doses of cefuroxime. *Europ J Surg* 1991;**157**:403–5.
90 Thornell E, Nilsson B, Jansson R, Svanvik J. Effect of short-term indomethacin treatment on the clinical course of acute obstructive cholecystitis. *Europ J Surg* 1991;**157**:127–30.
91 Goldman G, Kahn PJ, Alon R, Wiznitzer T. Biliary

colic treatment and acute cholecystitis prevention by prostaglandin inhibitor. *Digest Dis Sci* 1990;**34**:809–11.
92 Kaminski DL, Andrus CH, German D, Deshpande YG. The role of prostanoids in the production of acute acalculous cholecystitis by platelet-activating factor. *Ann Surg* 1990;**212**:455–61.
93 Paterson-Brown S, Chan STF. Early versus delayed cholecystectomy for acute cholecystitis. *Br J Hos Med* 1987;**37**:546–8.
94 Van der Linden W, Sunzel H. Early versus delayed operation for acute cholecystitis: A controlled clinical trial. *Am J Surg* 1970;**120**:7–13.
95 McArthur P, Cuschieri A, Sells RA, Shields R. Controlled clinical trial comparing early with interval cholecystectomy for acute cholecystitis. *Br J Surg* 1975;**62**:850–2.
96 Lahtinen J, Alhava EM, Aukee S. Acute cholecystitis treated by early and delayed surgery. A controlled clinical trial. *Scand J Gastroenterol* 1978;**13**:673–8.
97 Jarvinen HJ, Hastbacka J. Early cholecystectomy for acute cholecystitis: A prospective randomized study. *Ann Surg* 1980;**191**:501–5.
98 Edlund G, Ljungdahl M. Acute cholecystitis in the elderly. *Am J Surg* 1990;**159**:414–16.
99 Hidalgo LA, Capella G, Pi Figueras J *et al.* The influence of age on early surgical treatment of acute cholecystitis. *Surg Gynecol Obstet* 1989;**169**:393–6.
100 Motson RW, Way LW. Cholecystitis. In: Blumgart LH, ed. *Clinical Surgery International Vol. 5: The Biliary Tract.* Edinburgh: Churchill Livingstone, 1982:121.
101 Williamson RCN. Surgery of the biliary tract and pancreas. In: Kirk RM, Williamson RCN, eds. *General Surgical Operations.* Edinburgh: Churchill Livingstone, 1987:171–95.
102 Bornman PC, Terblanche J. Subtotal cholecystectomy: For the difficult gallbladder in portal hypertension and cholecystitis. *Surgery* 1985;**98**:1–6.
103 Schein M. Partial cholecystectomy in the emergency treatment of acute cholecystitis in the compromised patient. *J Roy Coll Surg Edin* 1991;**36**:295–7.
104 Ross FP, Dunphy JE. Studies in acute cholecystitis. *New Eng J Med* 1950;**242**:359–64.
105 Gingrich RA, Awe WC, Boyden AM, Peterson CG. Cholecystostomy in acute cholecystitis. Factors influencing morbidity and mortality. *Am J Surg* 1968; **116**:310–15.
106 Pheils MT, Duraiappah B. Cholecystostomy for acute cholecystitis. *Med J Aust* 1975;**1**:418–19.
107 Welch JP, Malt RA. Outcome of cholecystostomy. *Surg Gynecol Obstet* 1972;**135**:717–20.
108 Thomas MG, Grace PA, Benjamin IS, Williamson RCN. Carcinoma of the gallbladder, acute cholecystitis and cholecystostomy. *Europ J Gastroenterol Hepatol* 1991;**3**:277–9.
109 Ganey JB, Johnson PA Jr, Prillaman PE, McSwain GR. Cholecystectomy: clinical experience with a large series. *Am J Surg* 1986;**151**:352–7.
110 Burkhardt H, Mueller W. Versuche uber die Punktion der Gallblase und ihre Roentgendarstellung. *Deutsche Zeitsch Chirurg* 1932;**161**:632–5.
111 Elyanderani MK, McDowell DE, Gabriele OF. A preliminary report of percutaneous cholecystostomy under ultrasonography and fluoroscopy guidance *J Clin Gastroenter* 1983;**5**:277–81.
112 Radder RW. Ultrasonically guided percutaneous catheter drainage for gallbladder empyema. *Diag Imag Clin Med* 1980;**49**:330–3.
113 Klimberg S, Hawkins I, Vogel SB. Percutaneous cholecystostomy for acute cholecystitis in high-risk patients. *Am J Surg* 1987;**153**:125–9.
114 Eggermont AM, Lameris JS, Jeekel J. Ultrasound guided percutaneous transhepatic cholecystostomy for acute acalculous cholecystitis. *Arch Surg* 1985;**120**: 1354–6.
115 LaBerge JM, Gordon RL, Kerlan RK Jr, Ring EJ. Delayed gallbladder rupture following percutaneous cholecystostomy. *J Vasc Intervent Radiol* 1991;**2**: 539–41.
116 Burhenne HJ, Stoller JL. Minicholecystostomy and radiologic stone extraction in high risk cholelithiasis patients. *Am J Surg* 1985;**149**:632–5.
117 van Sonnenberg E, Wittich GR, Casola G *et al.* Diagnostic and therapeutic percutaneous gallbladder procedures. *Radiology* 1986;**160**:23–6.
118 Cuschieri A, Berci G. *Laparoscopic Biliary Surgery.* Oxford: Blackwell Scientific Publications, 1990.
119 Flowers JL, Bailey RW, Scovill WA, Zucker KA. The Baltimore experience with laparoscopic management of acute cholecystitis. *Am J Surg* 1991;**161**:388–92.
120 Reddick EJ, Olsen D, Spaw A *et al.* Safe performance of difficult laparoscopic cholecystectomies. *Am J Surg* 1991;**161**:377–81.
121 Baird DR, Wilson JP, Mason EM *et al.* An early review of 800 laparoscopic cholecystectomies at a university-affiliated community teaching hospital. *Am Surg* 1992;**58**:206–10.
122 Hugh TB, Chen FC, Li B. Empyema of the gallbladder treated by laparoscopic cholecystectomy. *Med J Aust* 1991;**154**:417–18.
123 Thornton JR, Heaton KW, Espiner HJ, Eltringham WK. Empyema of the gallbladder–reappraisal of a neglected disease. *Gut* 1983;**24**:1183–5.
124 Feretis CB, Manouras AJ, Apostolidis NS, Golematis BC. Endoscopic transpapillary drainage of gallbladder empyema. *Gastrointest Endosc* 1990;**36**: 523–5.
125 Tamada K, Seki H, Sato K *et al.* Efficacy of endoscopic retrograde cholecystoendoprosthesis (ERCCE) for cholecystitis. *Endoscopy* 1991;**23**:2–3.
126 Roslyn JJ, Thompson JE Jr, Darvin H, DenBesten L. Risk Factors for gallbladder perforation. *Am J Gastroenterol* 1987;**82**:636–40.
127 Essenhigh DM. Perforation of the gall-bladder. *Br J Surg* 1968;**55**:175–8.
128 Ranson JHC. Perforation of the gallbladder. In: Way

LW, Pellegrini CA, eds. *Surgery of the Gallbladder and Bile Ducts*. Philadelphia: Saunders, 1987:265–73.
129 Beckman I, Dash N, Sefczek RJ *et al*. Ultrasonographic findings in acute acalculous cholecystitis. *Gastrointest Radiol* 1985;10:387–9.
130 Fox MS, Wilk PJ, Weissmann HS, Freeman LM, Gliedman ML. Acute acalculous cholecystitis. *Surg Gynecol Obstet* 1984;**159**:13–16.
131 Gately JF, Thomas EJ. Acute cholecystitis occurring as a complication of other diseases. *Arch Surg* 1983;**118**:1137–41.
132 Bauer T, Steven K. Acute acalculous cholecystitis after radical cystectomy. *J Urol* 1988;**139**:128–9.
133 McDermott MW, Scudamore CH, Boileau LO, Snelling CFT, Kramer TA. Acalculous cholecystitis: its role as a complication of major burn injury. *Canad J Surg* 1985;**28**:529–33.
134 Rosoff L, Meyers H. Acute emphysematous cholecystitis. An analysis of ten cases. *Am J Surg* 1966;**111**: 410–23.
135 Radin DR, Halls JM. Emphysematous cholecystitis presenting with pneumoperitoneum. *Am J Roentgenol* 1987;**149**:1175–6.
136 May RE, Strong R. Acute emphysematous cholecystitis. *Br J Surg* 1971;58:453–8.
137 Schlinkert RT, Mucha P Jr, Farnell MB. Torsion of the gallbladder. *Mayo Clinic Proceed* 1984;59:490–2.
138 Butsch JL, Luchette F. Torsion of the gallbladder. *Arch Surg* 1985;**120**:1323.
139 Ashby BS. Acute and recurrent torsion of the gallbladder. *Br J Surg* 1965;**52**:182–4.
140 Carrasco CH, Freeny PC, Chuang VP, Wallace S. Chemical cholecystitis associated with hepatic artery infusion chemotherapy. *Am J Roentgenol* 1983;**141**: 703–6.
141 Pietrafitta JJ, Anderson BG, O'Brien MJ, Deckers PJ. Cholecystitis secondary to infusion chemotherapy. *J Surg Oncol* 1986;**31**:287–93.
142 Simons RK, Sinanan MN, Coldwell DM. Gangrenous cholecystitis as a complication of hepatic artery embolization: Case report. *Surgery* 1992;**112**:106–10.
143 McFadden DW, Smith GW. Hemodialysis-associated hemorrhagic cholecystitis. *Am J Gastroenterol* 1987; **82**:1081–3.
144 Hiatt JR, Hiatt JCG, Williams RA, Klein SR. Biliary disease in pregnancy: strategy for surgical management. *Am J Surg* 1986;**151**:263–5.
145 Lowenburg H Jr, Mitchell AG. Cholecystitis in childhood. *J Pediat* 1938;**12**:203–8.
146 Greenwood RK. Torsion of the gall bladder. *Gut* 1963;**4**:27–9.
147 Payne RA. Evaluation of the management of acute cholecystitis. *Br J Surg* 1969;**56**:200–2.
148 Pickleman J, Gonzalez RP. The improving results of cholecystectomy. *Arch Surg* 1986;**121**:930–4.
149 Ransohoff DF, Miller GL, Forsythe SB, Hermann RE. Outcome of acute cholecystitis in patients with diabetes mellitus. *Ann Int Med* 1987;**106**:829–32.
150 Sen M, Williamson RCN. Acute cholecystitis: surgical management. *Baillière's Clin Gastroenterol* 1991;**5**: 817–40.

Chapter 14
Acute cholangitis

P.A. Lipsett & H.A. Pitt

Introduction

Acute cholangitis is a life-threatening infection of the biliary tree. First described in 1877, Charcot recognized the triad of jaundice, fever, and right-upper quadrant pain [1]. Charcot postulated that 'stagnant bile' caused cholangitis and that gallstones and benign and malignant strictures were most often the underlying causes of biliary obstruction. However, obstruction without infection is insufficient to cause cholangitis and vice versa. The biliary tree is normally sterile but biliary pathology is often associated with secondary bacterial colonization.

The spectrum of clinical presentation of patients with acute cholangitis is widely variable. Some patients are mildly ill and others present with hypotension and mental obtundation. This group of patients with septic shock are best described as having 'toxic' rather than suppurative cholangitis. Purulent bile does not define the degree of a patient's illness. Some patients without purulent bile are gravely ill while other patients with grossly purulent bile are only mildly ill.

Currently, the treatment of acute cholangitis is primarily supportive with intravenous hydration and antibiotics being the mainstay of therapy. A high-risk group of patients warranting early biliary decompression have been identified in recent studies. However, standard indications that warrant biliary decompression include septic shock, clinical deterioration or failure to improve. This chapter will discuss the pathophysiology, aetiology, clinical presentation, laboratory and radiological evaluation of the spectrum of patients with acute cholangitis. Treatment options will be presented along with outcome data in patients with and without the 'toxic' form of cholangitis.

Pathophysiology

Acute cholangitis results from the combination of biliary tract obstruction and infection (Fig. 14.1). In the early stages of biliary obstruction normal hepatic bile secretion continues; and thus, an increase in intraductal pressure ensues. Furthermore, obstruction results in stagnation of bile which allows any microbe present the potential for rapid proliferation. As obstruction continues, biliary pressures approach the secretory pressure of bile, 25–30 as H_2O. Systemic bacteremia can result from increased intraductal pressure when biliary bacteria reflux into hepatic veins and perihepatic lymphatics [2]. Moreover, the systemic release of inflammatory mediators can produce profound hemodynamic effects in the 'toxic' form of cholangitis. Gallstones, parasites, and other foreign bodies can all cause obstruction and also act as a nidus for increased bacterial overgrowth [3].

Obstruction

With normal biliary physiology, biliary ductal pressures usually range from 7–14 cm H_2O [4]. Intraductal pressure can rapidly rise to 20–30 cm H_2O with either partial or complete obstruction [4]. At biliary pressures greater than 15 cm H_2O Jacobson *et al.* have demonstrated systemic reflux of radiolabelled biliary bacteria [2]. Normally, however, even when biliary pressures are elevated, most bacteria are killed within the liver and only an estimated 10% enter the blood stream. Huang

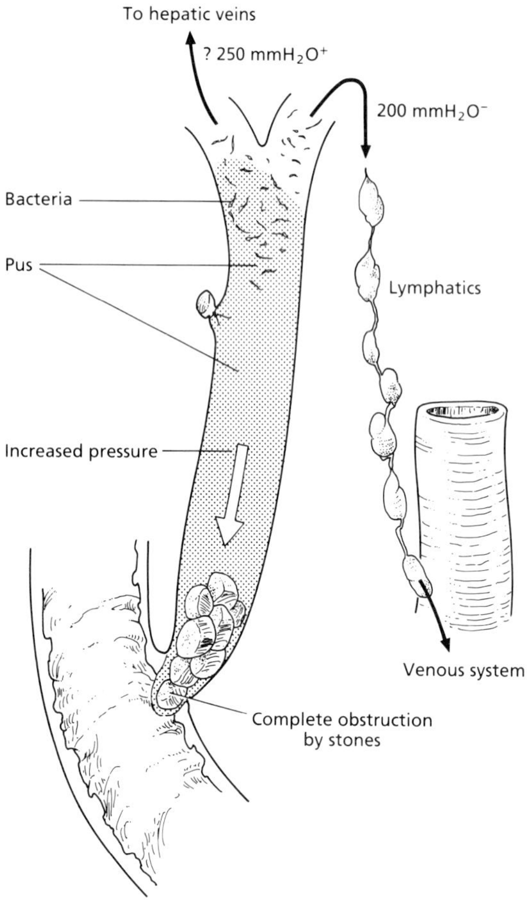

Fig. 14.1 Cholangitis is caused by the combination of biliary obstruction, often related to distally impacted stones and bactibilia. Bacteria then reflux into the hepatic veins and perihepatic lymphatics, resulting in systemic bacteremia. (From Pitt and Longmire [44].)

et al. [5] and Flemma and colleagues [6] have in separate models confirmed the importance of biliary obstruction in illness. In the canine model Huang *et al.* demonstrated that cultures were sterile when the biliary pressure was less than 20 cm H_2O but became positive when intraductal pressure exceeded 25 cm H_2O [5]. In Flemma's work infected bile (10^5 organisms) did not produce bacteremia and illness unless biliary obstruction was present [6]. These and other studies form the basis of our knowledge that clinical cholangitis is not produced by infected bile without obstruction, or by obstruction without infected bile. Furthermore, the degree of obstruction is directly related to the intraductal pressure. Even though patients with malignant obstruction tend to have more complete biliary obstruction, their bile is often initially sterile. However, in patients with gallstones or other foreign bodies, infection is often present in combination with partial or total biliary obstruction.

The systemic signs of clinical cholangitis, fever, chills, and occasionally mental confusion, and hypotension are caused by bacterial, toxin and inflammatory mediator release via cholangiolymphatics or cholangiovenous pathways. Patients with 'toxic' cholangitis usually have systemic endotoxemia as well as high serum levels of tumor necrosis factor even in the absence of documental bacteremia.

Bacteria

In normal patients the gallbladder and biliary tree are sterile [7]. However, in the presence of gallstones either within the gallbladder or biliary tree, positive cultures are seen in 15–50% and 70–90%, respectively [8, 9, 10]. Moreover, in patients with complete ductal obstruction secondary to malignancy 25–40% of patients have positive cultures. Thus, the aetiology of the bile duct obstruction, gallstones versus malignancy influences the likelihood of a positive bile culture. Advancing age also increases the likelihood of a positive bile culture. The organisms most often isolated are the Gram-negative aerobes, *Escherichia coli* and *Klebsiella pneumonia*, the Gram-positive enterococci and the Gram-negative anaerobe, *Bacteroides fragiles* [11, 12, 13, 14]. In 30–50% of patients multiple organisms are present [15–19]. In some series anaerobes are present in 25–30% of patients, but rarely as an isolated pathogen [15, 16, 19].

The origin of biliary bacteria is not precisely known and several possible anatomic explanations exist [20]. Possibilities include ascending infection from the duodenum, lymphatic spread, vascular spread from portal venous or hepatic arterial flow, or seeding from a chronically infected gallbladder. Because the bacteriology of the duodenum and infected bile are similar, the ascending infection theory is quite plausible. However, the sphincter of Oddi normally prevents bacterial reflux into bile. Dineen [21] has demonstrated that lymphatic flow is caudal from the liver to the duodenum; thus, this mechanism of infection is somewhat unlikely. Furthermore, hepatic arterial infection and resulting hepatic abscesses do occur but in only a small percentage of patients with cholangitis.

In 1964 Dineen demonstrated that portal venous bacteremia resulted in bacterial infection and that the concentration of bacteria was related to the degree of biliary obstruction [21]. Portal venous bacteremia has been demonstrated in patients with cholangiohepatitis. However, not all patients with portal venous bacteremia were ill. One possible explanation for this observation is that the bacteria, and/or its by-products and inflammatory mediators are destroyed in the liver by an efficient hepatic reticuloendothelial system which eliminates bacteria by excretion into the biliary tree and subsequent elimination in stool. However, in the presence of a foreign body or partial obstruction bacteria will stagnate and multiply. One objection to the portal venous theory for the origin of cholangitis is the relatively low proportion of anaerobic infecting organisms. One might expect a similar spectrum and proportion of ileal or colonic organisms as biliary tract pathogens in acute cholangitis. However, Gram-negative and Gram-positive anaerobes are disproportionately few in number when compared with typical gastrointestinal tract contents. Two factors may explain this discrepancy, the difficulty in handling and processing anaerobic organisms, and the fact that bile salts inhibit the growth of most anaerobic organisms.

In the rat model used by Rapier *et al.* [22], constant infusion of bacteria retrograde into the biliary tree resulted in an increase in intraductal pressure and a proportional increase in bacteremia. In this model bacterial reflux into the blood stream occurred via intracellular pathways, and pre-existing biliary obstruction was not a major determinant of bacteremia. Though this model provides important information about obstruction and bacteremia, the rat does not have a gallbladder and, thus, is not equivalent to the human situation. The gallbladder is enormously efficient at absorption of water and may function to relieve some biliary pressure when a distal ductal obstruction is present. Obviously, an infected gallbladder itself can serve as a source of biliary infection.

Aetiology

Biliary obstruction is most commonly caused by choledocholithiasis, benign strictures, postoperative anastomotic strictures and malignant processes. In older series, up to 80% of all cases of biliary obstruction and cholangitis were caused by choledocholithiasis [9]. However, more recently in a series reported by Thompson *et al.* [23], malignancy and congenital problems accounted for the majority of problems at a tertiary referral centre. In addition, the use of biliary stents, both endoscopic and percutaneous, have increased the incidence of bacterial infection.

Over the last 4 decades at The Johns Hopkins Hospital and the University of California at Los Angeles we have noticed a marked change in the aetiology of biliary obstruction (Fig. 14.2). As expected, in the earliest time period from 1952–78, choledocholithiasis was by far the most common aetiology of cholangitis. However, in the last 2 decades malignant obstruction and sclerosing cholangitis have been seen with increasing frequency. Undoubtedly, these changes are multifactorial and can be explained, in part, by the tertiary referral nature of these institutions and by the increased use of endoscopic and percutaneous stents for the treatment and palliation of biliary obstruction [7, 8].

Clinical presentation

Patients with cholangitis can present with a wide spectrum of disease. Some patients may be mildly ill and may not seek medical attention. On the other end of the spectrum is the patient who presents in septic shock with hypotension and confusion or mental obtundation, as first described by Reynolds and Dargan [24], in addition to Charchot's triad of fever, jaundice, and right-upper quadrant pain. Much as the aetiology of

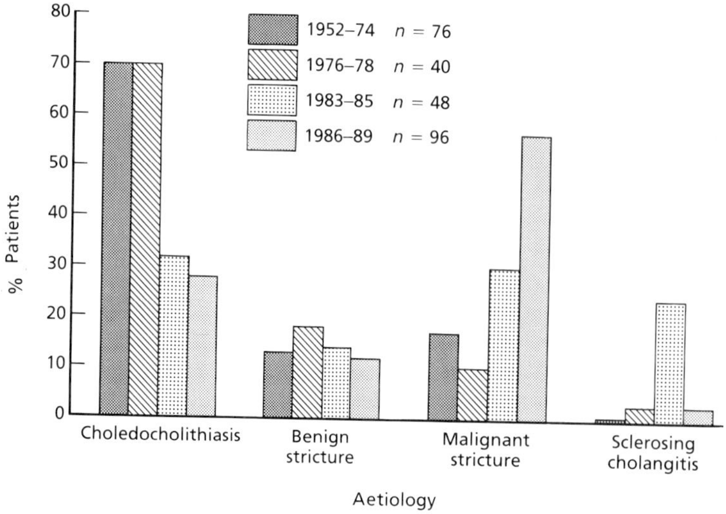

Fig. 14.2 The changing aetiology of acute cholangitis at The Johns Hopkins Hospital.

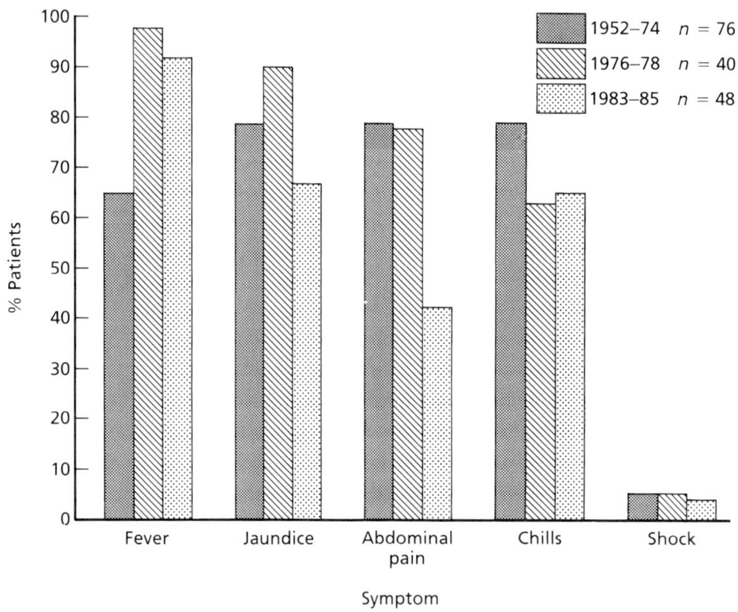

Fig. 14.3 Clinical presentation of cholangitis at The Johns Hopkins Hospital.

cholangitis has changed over the last 40 years, so too has the clinical presentation.

In a recent series from Johns Hopkins and the Olive View Medical Center in Los Angeles, the mean age of patients presenting with cholangitis was 51 years and did not vary with the aetiology of the biliary obstruction [23]. Fever is the most common presenting symptom, but jaundice, a previous hallmark of the disease is now present in only two-thirds of our patients at Johns Hopkins (Fig. 14.3) [7, 23]. Again this change may be due, in part, to the increased number of patients with malignancy and indwelling biliary catheters.

Abdominal pain if present is usually mild. Since both jaundice and abdominal pain are seen less commonly in patients with acute cholangitis, the classic Charcot's triad of fever, jaundice, and right-upper quadrant pain is now seen even less commonly than previously [23]. However, the severe form of 'toxic' cholangitis has remained constant at approximately 5% of all cases of cholangitis.

The physical examination of a patient, much like the clinical presentation, is somewhat variable. The combination of jaundice and mild right-upper quadrant tenderness is seen in as many as two-thirds of patients. The presence of severe tenderness on physical examination should prompt consideration of an alternative diagnosis such as acute cholecystitis.

Diagnosis

The diagnosis of cholangitis should be considered in any patient who presents with jaundice, fever, or right-upper quadrant pain. In patients who are known to have gallstones, previous biliary reconstruction, or indwelling biliary catheters, this possibility should be high on the differential diagnosis. Virtually all patients with cholangitis will have some abnormality in laboratory information. In the series by Saharia and Cameron an elevated white blood cell count greater than 10 000/mm^3 was seen in 79% of all patients with cholangitis [25]. Thompson *et al.* have found the mean white blood cell count to be 13 600/mm^3 [23] while others have reported a higher mean white blood cell count of greater than 19 000/mm^3 [26, 27]. In a small minority of patients with overwhelming Gram-negative sepsis, leukopenia may be seen.

Abnormalities of liver function tests are common in patients with cholangitis. The pattern and degree of liver function abnormalities has been correlated to the aetiology of the biliary obstruction as noted by Thompson *et al.* [23]. In patients with a malignant obstruction a higher elevation of alkaline phosphatase was observed (531 versus 278 iu, $P < 0.05$) when compared with patients who had a benign biliary obstruction. Patients with benign disease more often have elevations of transaminase values, likely secondary to an acute common duct obstruction. Although liver function abnormalities are usually seen in patients with acute cholangitis, many other disease processes can have these non-specific elevations in liver function values. Specifically, sepsis of any origin and hepatitis must be considered. However, the presence of entirely normal liver function tests is unusual in patients with cholangitis.

In addition to liver function tests, serum amylase may be elevated in some patients [8]. In this subgroup, the aetiology of the cholangitis is often choledocholithiasis. The serum tumour marker CA19-9 has been evaluated in patients with cholangitis by Albert *et al.* [28]. They noted that the CA19-9 could be markedly elevated in patients with benign biliary obstruction and acute cholangitis, but with therapy the elevated values returned to normal.

Radiographs of the abdomen, though often obtained, are rarely helpful in establishing this diagnosis. Occasionally, radiopaque gallstones may be seen or, even more rarely, pneumobilia may be detected [25]. Nucleotide scans are helpful in establishing the diagnosis of acute cholecystitis but not cholangitis. Ultrasonography and computed tomography (CT) scans can visualize dilated biliary ducts, or may find a potential aetiology for cholangitis such as common duct stones or a pancreatic mass, but these studies do not establish a diagnosis of acute cholangitis (Fig. 14.4).

At some time point, either in acute treatment or in defining ultimate management, cholangiography will be required. Direct cholangiography via the endoscopic (ERC) or percutaneous (PTC) route are equally informative. If common duct stones or a periampullary tumour is suspected, in general, the endoscopic route is preferred. On the other hand, if a perihilar tumour is expected, the percutaneous route has some advantages. Cholangitis can be a complication of either procedure, but with appropriate attention to biliary pressures, a generally low incidence of 3–7% can be expected [29–31].

The timing of cholangiography can be important. With the exception of patients who have 'toxic' cholangitis, cholangiography should be delayed until fever has resolved [32]. Lai and colleagues have suggested that ERC should be delayed for 72 hours after the patient has

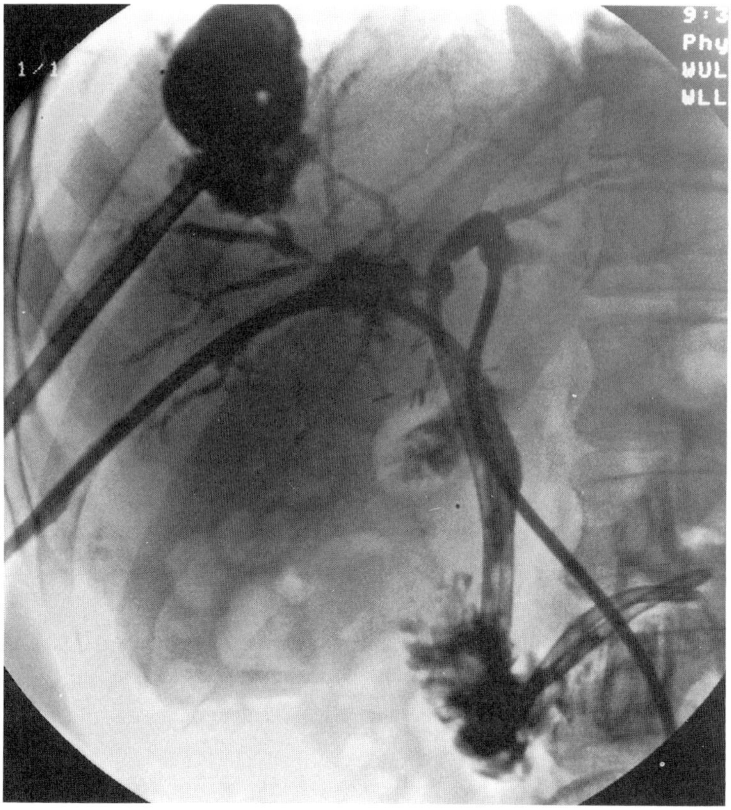

Fig. 14.4 Percutaneous transhepatic cholangiogram and liver abscess drainage. Note right hepatic abscess drainage catheter in a patient with biliary obstruction secondary to a proximal cholangiocarcinoma.

defervesced when performed for diagnostic reasons alone. In patients who have a malignant obstruction or recent cholangitis the incidence of ERC associated cholangitis is higher; and thus, these patients warrant early elective biliary decompression [33].

Microbiology

The combination of biliary obstruction and infection cause bacteremia. Systemic signs such as high fever, rigors, and particularly hypotension signify that Gram-negative bacteremia is likely in patients with acute cholangitis. In the Saharia series, 50 of 78 patients with acute cholangitis had blood cultures drawn shortly after admission, and 20 patients (26%) had bacteremia [25]. *E. coli* and *Klebsiella* species accounted for 17 of these 20 cases. In the most recent series from Johns Hopkins, 21% of patients with cholangitis had bacteremia, but *E. coli* and *Klebsiella* species represented a much smaller proportion of the total number of isolated organisms [23].

In most of the current series more than one organism is typically cultured from the biliary tree [19, 23, 26, 27, 34]. As the aetiology of biliary obstruction has changed, so too has the bacteria isolated from the biliary tree (Table 14.1). The enteric Gram-negative aerobes *E. coli* and *Klebsiella* and the Gram-positive aerobe, enterococci, formerly were the most common isolates. However, the more resistant Gram-negative organisms *Enterobacter* and *Pseudomonas* are being seen with increasing frequency [23]. These changes may again be due to a new patient population with indwelling biliary stents, and in many patients, multiple previous episodes of cholangitis and antibiotic therapy. Anaerobes, such as the *Bacteroides* species, continue to play a small, but significant, role in biliary infection [11, 19].

Table 14.1 Biliary bacteriology at The Johns Hopkins Hospital

	Patients (%)		
Bile culture	1976–8 (*n* = 40)	1983–5 (*n* = 48)	1986–9 (*n* = 96)
Escherichia coli	55	55	39
Klebsiella species	41	32	54
Enterococcus	41	55	34
Bacteroids species	28	9	15
Enterobacter species	0	33	34
Pseudomonas species	0	23	24

Treatment

Patients with acute cholangitis represent a wide spectrum of illness. Those patients with a minor degree of illness may not require hospitalization and may be treated with oral antibiotics. An equally small minority of patients with the 'toxic' form of cholangitis may require intensive care admission, invasive monitoring, and the use of vasoactive agents to support blood pressure. Maintenance of euvolemia is important to preserve organ function, and hydration is usually required. If vasopressors are necessary or renal impairment is present, low dose dopamine may be helpful in maintaining renal blood flow.

Antibiotic therapy

Antibiotics are required for the treatment of all patients with acute cholangitis. However, the specific agent selected for use is a matter of choice. In part, the antibiotics chosen should be based on an institutional experience with cholangitis. For example, at Johns Hopkins, an increased incidence of the Gram-negatives typically associated with nosocomial disease, *Pseudomonas* and *Enterobacter* have been seen in patients with acute cholangitis. In part, this experience is related to the underlying changing etiology of the disease and the use of indwelling catheters. Nonetheless, the antibiotics chosen empirically must include the Gram-negative aerobes and, possibly, enterococci.

The aminoglycosides offer excellent spectrum of activity against the Gram-negatives [35, 36]. However, the use of aminoglycosides in patients with jaundice and renal compromise must be cautious. In patients who are critically ill the volume of distribution is often markedly underestimated and aminoglycosides are frequently underdosed with initial low peak levels [35, 36]. The mortality from Gram-negative sepsis when treated with aminoglycosides is directly related to:

1 the time until a therapeutic peak level is reached;

2 low initial drug trough levels [37].

The renal toxicity of aminoglycosides is also related to the trough level, and prolonged dosing intervals, with trough levels falling to at least below 2 mg/dL, is recommended [35]. To account for a larger volume of distribution, the initial loading dose for gentamicin and tobramycin in the critically ill patient is 4–6 mg/kg. A peak serum level can be obtained to insure initial adequate doses. If aminoglycosides are administered on a once daily dosing schedule, then a trough level is recommended at the second dose. This regimen insures that the kidneys have cleared adequate drug in order to prevent renal toxicity. This method of administering aminoglycosides also insures high initial serum levels and also allows for the post-antibiotic effect of aminoglycosides to be utilized.

Aside from the aminoglycosides, Gram-negative aerobes are well covered by the third generation cephalosporins, ureidopenicillins, monobactams, and the fluroquinolones. Ureidopenicillins, such as pipercillin, offer the advantage of Gram-positive coverage, including the enterococci and of anaerobic coverage [23]. The monobactam, imipenem, also covers the Gram-negatives, the Gram-positives, and the anaerobes. However, the fluroquinolones do not cover the anaerobes, but they provide excellent Gram-negative and reasonable Gram-positive coverage.

Several randomized prospective trials for the antibiotic treatment of acute cholangitis have been performed [11, 23, 34]. In a study done at the Mayo Clinic, mezlocillin, a ureidopenicillin, favourably compared with the combination of ampicillin/gentamicin [34]. Twenty of 24 patients (83%) treated with mezlocillin were cured, compared with only nine of 24 (41%) patients treated with ampicillin/gentamicin. In addition, fewer toxic effects were seen in the mezlocillin arm. However, aminoglycosides were administered in the traditional every 8 hour dosing schedule.

In a recent study from, Johns Hopkins, UCLA, and the Olive View Medical Center, 90 patients were randomized to either pipercillin or ampicillin and tobramycin [23]. The cure rates of both treatment groups were similar, but the outcome was noted to be related to the aetiology of the obstruction (benign versus malignant) (Fig. 14.5). In this study population, the single agent pipercillin was as effective as the penicillin/aminoglycoside combination in the treatment of cholangitis.

Biliary decompression

Most patients who present with acute cholangitis will respond to initial therapeutic measures of intravenous hydration and antibiotics. However, up to 15% of patients with acute cholangitis will require urgent biliary decompression for the treatment of ongoing sepsis. Several investigators have proposed risk factors that predict the need for urgent biliary decompression. Gigot *et al.* have found seven independent risk factors which predicted mortality [38]. These factors were:

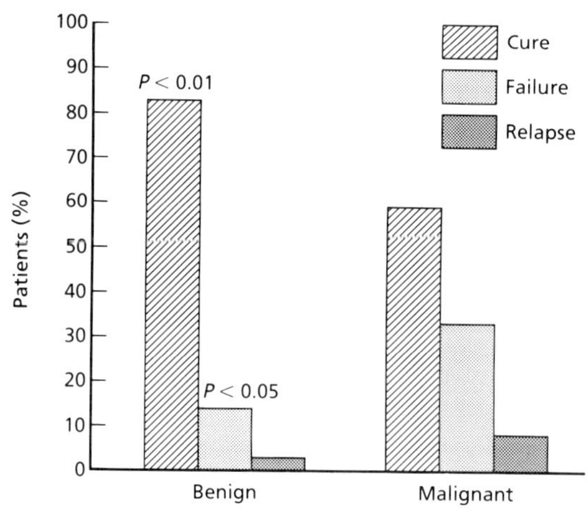

Fig. 14.5 Cure, failure and relapse rates among 96 patients with cholangitis caused by either benign or malignant obstruction. Outcome was significantly worse with malignant obstruction. (From Thompson *et al.* [45].)

1 acute renal failure;
2 liver abscess;
3 cirrhosis;
4 high malignant strictures;
5 percutaneous transhepatic cholangiography;
6 female gender;
7 age.

In a multiple regression formula with proportional weight given to the individual factors, a score from 0–27 could be obtained. If the score was less than seven the predicted mortality was 1.8%; while if the score was greater than seven, the predicted mortality was 49%. These data were obtained from a retrospective study and have not been used in a prospective fashion to predict mortality or to guide management decisions. Nonetheless, it seems reasonable that high-risk patients identified by a score greater than seven be considered for urgent biliary decompression. Identification of patients with a high predicted mortality would target a group of patients who might benefit most from an intensive and aggressive approach to the treatment of biliary tract sepsis. Aside from this group of patients, biliary decompression is warranted in patients who fail to improve with supportive care alone.

Non-operative means for establishing biliary decompression are now available in many hospitals. Percutaneous transhepatic decompression (PTD) is a well established technique for biliary drainage in patients with obstructive jaundice [29–31]. In patients who are already ill, this technique alleviates the need for general anesthesia and an operative intervention. In most series urgent percutaneous decompression in patients can be done with a morbidity less than 10% and a mortality of 5% [30, 39]. If a patient is known to have a previous biliary-enteric anastomosis or a proximal perihilar obstruction, then percutaneous transhepatic drainage is the preferred route.

The treatment of patients with 'toxic' cholangitis secondary to choledocholithiasis who require urgent biliary decompression has been prospectively studied by Lai *et al.* [27]. In this study, 82 patients with 'toxic' cholangitis were randomized to receive either urgent endoscopic treatment or surgical decompression. In the patients who underwent operative treatment respiratory failure, ventilatory support and mortality were all more common than in the endoscopically managed group (Table 14.2). Thus, this study suggests that if the expertise is available for urgent endoscopic decompression, then this treatment is preferable for patients with 'toxic' cholangitis secondary to choledocholithiasis.

In institutions where endoscopic or percutaneous biliary decompression is not available, operative drainage is still a useful and life-saving intervention for seriously ill patients with acute cholangitis. These patients can survive when managed in a timely fashion. Lai *et al.* demonstrated that even patients with persistent shock can be successfully managed by operative decompression. He demonstrated that the outcome of 30 patients who were managed with operative decompression was not different from a similar group of patients who were successfully resuscitated prior to surgery [26].

The haemodynamic status of the patient in the operating room should guide the extent of the surgical procedure. Cholangiography and choledochoscopy should not be performed in an unstable patient. Operative drainage alone may be life saving. Biliary drainage alone was performed in 24 of the 44 patients in the Lai series [27]. In this series choledocholithiasis was the most common aetiology for acute cholangitis and choledochotomy and placement of a T-tube was required. Since the common bile duct is the sight of the biliary obstruction in most series, cholecystostomy is not adequate treatment and biliary decompression of some type is required. Additional, and often definitive, therapy should not be performed at the same operative procedure, when the indication for intervention has been 'toxic' cholangitis and the patient remains haemodynamically unstable during surgery.

Table 14.2 Outcome of endoscopic versus surgical decompression for toxic cholangitis

	Endoscopic papillotomy nasobiliary drainage	Surgical decompression
No. of patients	41	41
Ventilatory support	29%	63*%
Morbidity	34%	66 %
Mortality	10%	32*%

* $P < 0.03$ versus papillotomy. After Lai *et al.* [27].

Outcome

In high-risk patients with 'toxic' cholangitis, considerable morbidity and mortality may be expected. These high-risk patients are at particular risk for the development of end organ dysfunction or organ failure, and careful management is necessary to alleviate the development of these complications. The development of renal dysfunction and renal failure is common in this group of patients and undoubtedly is related to inflammatory mediators released by the severe infection which in turn cause a low systemic vascular resistance, altered permeability and relative hypovolaemia. Direct and indirect effects of hormonal and sympathetic control on renal blood flow can cause acute or relative renal ischemia. The maintenance of adequate intravascular volume is essential and, in the very ill, renal dose dopamine (1–3 μg/kg/min) can help preserve renal blood flow. In some cases where hepatic and renal failure is present, circulating endotoxin has been documented and may contribute to continued or additional morbidity and mortality. Therapies directed at decreasing absorption of endotoxin through the small bowel mucosa and thus decreasing the amount in the portal bloodstream have been proposed. These methods include oral bile acids, lactulose, and internal bile drainage [40–42].

The development of one or more liver abscesses considerably increases morbidity and mortality (91%). A liver abscess should be considered in any patient with cholangitis who is either seriously ill or fails to improve after initial therapy. If multiple small abscesses are present, biliary drainage and systemic antibiotics may be all that is required. However, if a large hepatic abscess is present, usually separate drainage will be required. Often, this drainage can be accomplished percutaneously, but occasionally surgical drainage and debridment is required for persistant sepsis.

In most series the overall mortality of patients with acute cholangitis is 5%. The highest mortality occurs in the small subgroup of patients who present with 'toxic' cholangitis. Several authors have suggested additional risk factors for patients who present with acute cholangitis. As might be expected, concomitant medical disease, acute renal failure, and low serum albumin are additional risk factors [26, 38, 43]. These findings have been noted specifically in patients with acute cholangitis, but are also described in more general and more widely applicable prognostic scoring systems such as the Acute Physiology and Chronic Health Score (APACHE). This score is a measure of illness and prognosis on admission to the intensive care unit, and recent modifications (APACHE III) apply to all patients irrespective of the specific underlying disease process.

In patients with acute cholangitis the underlying cause of the biliary obstruction does have prognostic importance as demonstrated by Thompson *et al.* [23]. In this study designed to evaluate antibiotic therapy, the benign or malignant nature of the biliary obstruction was an independent and important predictor of outcome. The initial cure rate of the patients with a benign obstruction was 83% which compared with only 59% of patients with a malignant obstruction. In this study there was a 5% mortality, but all of these patients had end-stage malignancy, and many also had liver failure and/or renal failure. Thus, identification of patients at a high risk of mortality by history, clinical presentation, and laboratory investigation may lessen the expected morbidity and mortality by targeting a high-risk patient group for urgent biliary decompression. In future years, these high-risk patients may also benefit from biologic response modifying drugs designed for patients with severe sepsis.

References

1 Charcot JM. Leçons sur les maladies du fore des voices biliares et des veins. Recueillies et Publices Par. Bourneville et Sevestre, 1877. Paris: Faculté de Médicine de Paris 1–102.

2 Jacobson K, Ellander J, Rosengren B. Cholangiovenous reflux. *Acta Chir Scan* 1962;**123**:316–21.

3 Kaufman HW, Magnuson TH, Lillemoe KD, Pitt HA. The role of bacteria in gallbladder and common duct stone formation. *Ann Surg* 1989;**209**:584–92.

4 Mallet-Guy P. Value of preoperative manometric and roentgenographic examination in the diagnosis of pathologic changes and functional disturbances of the biliary tract. *Surg Gynecol Obstet* 1952;**94**:385–91.

5 Huang T, Bass JA, Williams RD. The significance of biliary pressure in cholangitis. *Arch Surg* 1969;**98**: 629–32.

6 Flemma RJ, Flint LM, Osterhout S, Shingleton WW. Bacteriologic studies of biliary infection. *Ann Surg* 1967;**166**:563–70.

7 Csendes A, Fernandez M, Uribe P. Bacteriology of the gallbladder bile in normal subjects. *Am J Surg* 1975;**129**:629–31.

8 Lipsett PA, Pitt HA. Acute cholangitis. *Surg Clin N Amer* 1990;**70**:1297–1312.

9 Pitt HA, Couse NF. Biliary sepsis and toxic cholangitis. In: Moody FG, ed. *Surgical Treatment of Digestive Disease*, 2nd edn. Chicago: Year Book Medical Publishers, 1990:332–50.

10 Pitt HA, Longmire WP Jr. Suppurative cholangitis. In: Hardy JM, ed. *Critical Surgical Illness*, 2nd edn. Philadelphia: Saunders, 1980:380–408.

11 Muller EL, Pitt HA, Thompson JE Jr, Doty JE, Mann LL, Manchester B. Antibiotics in infections of the biliary tract. *Surg Gynecol Obstet* 1987;**165**:285–292.

12 Stewart L, Pellegrini CA, Way LW. Cholangiovenous reflux pathways as defined by corrosion casting and scanning electron microscopy. *Am J Surg* 1988;**155**: 23–8.

13 Edlund YA, Mollstedt BO. Ouchterlong Bacteriologic investigation of the biliary system and liver in biliary tract disease correlated to clinical data and microstructure of the gallbladder and liver. *Acta Chir Scand* 1959;**116**:461–76.

14 Pitt HA, Postier RG, Cameron JL. Consequences of preoperative cholangitis and its treatment on the outcome of surgery for choledocholithiasis. *Surgery* 1983;**94**:447–52.

15 Keighley MR, Flinn R, Alexander-Williams J. Multivariate analysis of clinical and operative findings associated with biliary sepsis. *Br J Surg* 1976;**63**:528–31.

16 Pitt HA, Postier RG, Cameron JL. Biliary bacteria: significance and alterations after antibiotic therapy. *Arch Surg* 1982;**117**:445–59.

17 O'Connor MJ, Schwartz ML, McQuarrie DG, Sumner HW. Cholangitis due to malignant obstruction to biliary outflow. *Ann Surg* 1981;**193**:341–5.

18 Keighley MR, Drysdale BB, Quorashi AH. Antibiotic treatment of biliary sepsis. *Surg Clin N Am* 1975;**55**: 1379–90.

19 Lee W, Chang KJ, Lee CS, Chen KM. Surgery in cholangitis: Bacteriology and choice of antibiotic. *Hepatogastroenterology* 1992;**39**:347–9.

20 Scott AJ, Kahn GA. Origin of bacteria in the bile duct. *Lancet* 1967;**2**:790–3.

21 Dineen P. The importance of the route of infection in experimental biliary obstruction. *Surg Gynecol Obstet* 1964;**119**:1001–1008.

22 Raper SE, Barker ME, Jones AL *et al.* Anatomic cor-

relates of bacterial cholangiovenous reflux. *Surgery* 1989;105:352–9.
23 Thompson JE Jr, Pitt HA, Doty JE, Coleman JA, Irving C. Broad spectrum penicillin as adequate therapy for acute cholangitis. *Surg Gynecol Obstet* 1990;171: 275–82.
24 Reynolds BM, Dargan EL. Acute obstructive cholangitis: a distinct clinical syndrome. *Ann Surg* 1959; 150:299–303.
25 Saharia PC, Cameron JL. Clinical management of cholangitis. *Surg Gynecol Obstet* 1976;**142**:369–72.
26 Lai ECS, Tam PC, Paterson IA *et al.* Emergency surgery for severe acute cholangitis: the high risk patients. *Ann Surg* 1990;**211**:55–9.
27 Lai ECS, Mok FPT, Tan ESY *et al.* Endoscopic biliary drainage for severe acute cholangitis. *N Eng J Med* 1992;**326**:1582–6.
28 Albert MA, Steinberg WM, Henry JP. Elevated serum levels of tumor marker CA19-9 in acute cholangitis. *Dig Dis Sci* 1988;**33**:1223–5.
29 Gould RJ, Vogelzang RL, Neiman HL *et al.* Percutaneous biliary drainage as an initial therapy in sepsis of the biliary tract. *Surg Gynecol Obstet* 1985; **160**:523–7.
30 Kadir S, Baassiri A, Barth RH *et al.* Percutaneous biliary drainage in the management of biliary sepsis. *Am J Radiol* 1982;**138**:25–9.
31 Lois JF, Gomes AS, Grace PA *et al.* Risks of percutaneous transhepatic drainage in patients with cholangitis. *Am J Radiol* 1987;**148**:367–71.
32 Lai ECS, Lo CM, Choi TK *et al.* Urgent biliary decompression after endoscopic retrograde cholangiopancreatography. *Am J Surg* 1989;**157**:121–5.
33 Davis JL, Milligan FD, Cameron JL. Septic complication following endoscopic retrograde cholangiopancreatography. *Surg Gynecol Obstet* 1975;**140**:365–7.
34 Gerecht WB, Henry NK, Hoffman WW *et al.* Prospective randomized comparison of mezlocillin therapy alone with combined ampicillin and gentamicin therapy for patients with cholangitis. *Arch Internal Med* 1989;**149**:1279–84.
35 Parker Se, Davey PG. Practicalities of once daily aminoglycoside dosing. *J Antimicrob Chemother* 1993; 31:4–7.
36 Miyagawa CI. Aminoglycosides in the intensive care units: An old drug in a dynamic environment. *New Horizons* 1993;1:172–80.
37 Moore RD, Smith CR, Lietman PS. Association of aminoglycoside plasma levels with therapeutic outcome in gram-negative pneumonia. *Am J Med* 1984;77: 657–62.
38 Gigot JF, Leese T, Dereme T *et al.* Acute cholangitis: multivariate analysis of risk factors. *Ann Sur* 1989; **209**:435–8.
39 Pessa ME, Hawkins IF, Vogell SB. The treatment of acute cholangitis: percutaneous transhepatic biliary drainage before definitive therapy. *Ann Surg* 1987; 205:389–92.
40 Dawson JL. Acute postoperative renal failure in obstructive jaundice. *Ann Roy Col Surg Eng* 1968; **42**:163–72.
41 Dawson JL. Acute postoperative renal function in obstructive jaundice: effect of mannitol diuresis. *Br Med J* 1965;1:82–6.
42 Pain ME, Cahill CJ, Bailey ME. Perioperative complications in obstructive jaundice: therapeutic considerations. *Br J Surg* 1985;73:775–8.
43 Little JM. A prospective evaluation of computerized estimates of risk in the management of obstructive jaundice. *Surgery* 1987;**102**:47–76.
44 Pitt HA, Longmire WP. Suppurative cholangitis. In: Hardy JM, ed. *Critical Surgical Illness*, 2nd edn. Philadelphia: Saunders, 1980;380–408.
45 Thompson JE Jr, Pitt HA, Doty JE *et al.* Broad spectrum penicillin as adequate therapy for cholangitis. *Surg Gynecol Obstet* 1990;171:275–82.

Chapter 15
Gallstone pancreatitis

P.J. Broe & K. Mealy

Gallstones remain a frequent cause of acute pancreatitis. In the UK gallstones are the most frequent cause of pancreatitis, unlike the USA where alcohol-induced pancreatitis is more common [1, 2]. Epidemiological studies indicate that the relative proportion of aetiological factors in acute pancreatitis may be changing as in Scandinavia the proportion of alcohol-induced pancreatitis appears to be on the increase [3, 4]. The importance of gallstone-induced pancreatitis, however, should not be underestimated as not infrequently the diagnosis is still missed and considerable numbers of patients with gallstone-induced pancreatitis are still diagnosed at autopsy [5]. While the majority of patients with acute pancreatitis have a self-limiting disease and recover, there is a mortality of up to 10% in unselected series [6, 7]. This figure may be higher if autopsy figures are included.

While little progress has been made in our understanding of pathophysiological events underlying gallstone pancreatitis in recent years, two developments have altered our approach to the management of this condition. These have been the rapid availability of endoscopic retrograde cholangiopancreatography (ERCP) and the introduction of laparoscopic biliary surgery. Both of these minimally invasive techniques have altered management of patients with gallstone disease, however, as yet there is little evidence that outlook is altered. The purpose of this chapter will be to briefly review our understanding of gallstone pancreatitis and discuss management strategies in dealing with biliary calculi in the light of these recent developments.

Pathophysiology

The association of pancreatitis and gallstones stems from an observation by Opie in 1901 of a gallstone impacted in the ampulla of Vater in a patient who died of acute pancreatitis [8]. Since then this association has been firmly established, however, the mechanism of gallstone induced pancreatitis remains contentious. The reasons for this are that only a small proportion of patients with gallstones develop pancreatitis [9], ductal or ampullary calculi are present in only a small proportion of patients operated on for pancreatitis [10] and patients with ampullary impaction do not necessarily develop pancreatitis [11]. These issues, however, have been clarified to a certain extent by increased understanding of extrahepatic biliary anatomy and the temporal sequence of gallstone migration in the induction of pancreatitis.

Acosta and colleagues were among the first to highlight the importance of gallstone passage in patients who develop pancreatitis [12, 13]. Biliary calculi are found in the faeces in the majority of patients with pancreatitis. Furthermore, the incidence of biliary calculi is greater in patients operated on promptly for gallstone pancreatitis in comparison to those undergoing delayed surgery. Kelly demonstrated stones in the stools of 84% of patients with gallstone pancreatitis whereas this only occurred in 11% of patients with uncomplicated gallstones [14]. Stone and colleagues examined the location of gallstones in patients undergoing immediate and delayed surgery for gallstone pancreatitis. The locations of gallstones in patients undergoing early versus delayed surgery were, respectively: 97% and 100% in the gallbladder; 75% and 28% in the biliary tree; and 31% and 0% in the duodenum [15]. Of interest sphincteroplasty in this early group led to a 'gush' of pancreatic juice from the pancreatic duct in contrast to those in the delayed group, implying pancreatic duct obstruction [15].

Patients with gallstone pancreatitis are also more likely to have smaller stones, in greater number in a gallbladder with a larger calibre cystic duct [16, 17]. In addition the 'common channel' between common bile and pancreatic ducts is longer in those with a history of gallstone pancreatitis. Armstrong and coworkers found a common channel of 5 mm or longer in 73% of patients with pancreatitis but in only 19% of patients with gallstones but no pancreatitis [16]. These features support the concept that patients with gallstone pancreatitis have anatomical differences in their biliary tree which facilitate gallstone migration. Another important variable appears to be sex. Males, despite having a lower incidence of cholelithiasis than females, are more prone to gallstone-associated pancreatitis. Taylor and colleagues have examined an exhaustive data base on 664 patients with symptomatic cholelithiasis and shown that gallstone associated pancreatitis occurs in 19.7% of men with gallstones in comparison to 5.5% of women [18]. Furthermore, males have on average a fewer number of gallstones than females, however, the male cystic duct is larger in diameter which may predispose to pancreatitis at an earlier age [18].

Other features which may be important are the greater frequency of pancreatic reflux in patients with gallstone pancreatitis and possible associated biliary motility disorders. Pancreatic reflux occurs in approximately 60% of patients undergoing operative cholangiograpy in comparison to 15% of controls [14, 16, 19]. Guelrud and colleagues demonstrated that basal sphincter of Oddi pressures and the amplitude of pressure waves in the ampullary region are higher in patients with a history of recurrent gallstone pancreatitits than in those with choledocholithiasis alone indicating that intrinsic biliary motility disorders may be a contributing factor in gallstone induced pancreatitis [20] (Table 15.1).

Table 15.1 Features which predispose to gallstone pancreatitis

Male sex
Larger number of gallstones
Smaller diameter stones
Larger diameter cystic duct
Longer 'common channel'
More frequent pancreatic reflux
Sphincter of Oddi and biliary motility disorders

Despite the strong association between migrating gallstones and pancreatitis the actual mechanism leading to the induction of pancreatic inflammation and necrosis are unknown. However, a consensus of opinion suggests that pancreatic 'autodigestion' is the mechanism which leads to the process of pancreatitic inflammation and eventual tissue destruction. This concept was in fact first suggested by Chiari in 1896 and while generally accepted has remained difficult to prove [21]. It is clear that the biliary anatomy described above does lead to an increased incidence of bile and duodenal content reflux up the pancreatic duct [22], which in turn may predispose to pancreatic duct epithelium damage, enzyme activation and pancreatic tissue destruction. Increased pancreatic duct pressure can lead to epithelial cell damage, increased pancreatic capillary permeability to macromolecules, extravasation of pancreatic juice and premature activation of pancreatic enzymes [23–27]. Experimental studies of pancreatitis by duodenal or pancreatic duct ligation, intravenous injection of caerulein and retrograde infusion of taurocholate up the pancreatic duct all support this concept.

The multiple systemic aetiological factors associated with clinical pancreatitis such as alcohol, hypercalcaemia, hyperlipidemia and drug induced pancreatitis all suggest that local mechanical factors alone are not responsible for all the pathophysiological events leading to pancreatitis. More recent studies have concentrated on cellular events leading to pancreatic destruction. Oxygen-derived free radical activity leading to increased capillary permeability and subsequent pancreatic tissue destruction has been proposed as one of the final local mechanisms in the process of pancreatitis [28], although this has been discounted by other studies [29]. Gough and colleagues have demonstrated that oxygen-free radical generation as measured by chemiluminescence, an indicator of energy release by activated neutrophils, is increased in both caerulein and taurocholate induced experimental pancreatitis [30]. Increased free radical release corresponded to the degree of pancreatitis. In an attempt to reverse this process, superoxide dismutase a free radical scavanger, was administered which limited chemiluminescence and the degree of hyperamylasemia. Unfortunately, the clinical usefulness of superoxide dismutase may be limited as pretreatment is required [30]. Other vasoactive agents such as prostaglandin E_2 either primarily or in conjunction with oxygen free radicles may be involved in this process [31].

Diagnosis

The diagnosis of gallstone pancreatitis rests on the clinical evidence of gallstone disease in addition to specific plasma enzyme changes and radiological confirmation of both the gallstones and pancreatic involvement.

The clinical picture will vary depending on the associated biliary tract disease. Acute cholecystitis or biliary colic may present as right-upper quadrant pain, radiating into the back with a variable systemic upset such as nausea, vomiting, pyrexia and rigors. Duct calculi may in addition lead to jaundice. The presence of pus in the biliary tree, usually associated with ductal calculi is referred to as ascending cholangitis and exhibits the triad of pain, jaundice and rigors (Charcot's triad) and may lead to septic shock, collapse and death if not dealt with by appropriate antibiotic therapy and urgent biliary decompression. Pancreatitis frequently presents with epigastric pain which because of the retroperitoneal nature of the organ radiates through to the back. The patient may sit forward in the knee-chest position for relief. Symptoms and abdominal signs again may be variable from a mild abdominal upset to an acute abdomen, cardiovascular collapse and shock.

Because of the variability of the presentation emphasis has been placed on plasma enzyme levels for diagnosis. Likewise, because of the unpredictability of outcome attention has been placed on diagnostic criteria for establishing severity of disease which may allow more invasive monitoring and possible remedial action at an earlier stage.

Laboratory tests in the diagnosis of pancreatitis

Amylase

The usefulness of serum amylase in the diagnosis of pancreatitis was first demonstrated by Elman *et al.* in 1929 [32]. Since then it has become the cornerstone of diagnosis in this condition. Unfortunately, many different assays are available, making comparisons between different centres impossible [33]. With gallstone pancreatitis serum amylase levels rapidly rise and are maximal within 24–48 hours [34, 35]. If patients present late serum amylase levels may be normal. The peak level also appears to be higher than in alcohol induced pancreatitis.

In an attempt to increase the diagnostic accuracy of amylase levels, measurement of the isoenzyme amylase p-type or isoamylase, has been proposed [36]. This is specific for pancreatic amylase and not for that derived from the salivary gland (amylase s-type). Isoamylase allows differentiation between pancreatic and extrapancreatic amylase elevations. Some evidence indicates that up to a third of patients with abdominal pain and hyperamylasaemia do not in fact have pancreatitis and the elevated amylase is derived from extrapancreatic tissue [36–38]. Difficulties arise, however, in that clinical conditions which may mimic pancreatitis with elevated isoamylase levels such as mesenteric ischaemia and perforated peptic ulceration will not be distinguished with this test.

Other enzymes

Abnormalities in liver enzymes can be useful in delineating gallstone pancreatitis from other forms of pancreatitis. McMahon and Pickford demonstrated elevations in serum aspartate aminotransferase (AST) (originally referred to as serum glutamate oxaloacetate transaminase (SGOT)) greater than 60 iu/L in 88% of patients with gallstone pancreatitis whereas in all patients with non-gallstone pancreatitis AST levels were less than this [39]. Other serum enzymes may also be of use in the diagnosis of acute pancreatitis. However, the time duration of the assay limits the usefulness of many of these tests in the clinical setting. Lipase, although not completely specific for the pancreas is increased with acute pancreatitis, with a specificity of about 90% [40]. Its degree of rise is greater than amylase in alcoholic pancreatitis and persists longer [41]. Elastase is also elevated in acute pancreatitis, however difficulties in measurement give it no advantage over amylase or lipase [42]. Phospholipase A_2 levels have also been examined in acute pancreatitis as early increased phospholipase A_2 levels may be a guide to severity of disease. Bird and coworkers found a good correlation between early phospholipase A_2 levels with multiple prognostic criteria and clinical outcome [43]. Gronroos and colleagues have also demonstrated a good correlation between phospholipase A_2 levels and impaired renal function in acute pancreatitis [44].

Acute phase reactants

The measurement of acute phase reactants offers potential in that they are non-specific indicators of inflammation and may aid in the prediction of severity of acute pancreatitis. The specific function of acute phase proteins is unclear. It is thought that they act as antiproteases which limit tissue damage and also act as non-specific opsonins. Thus they augment phagocytosis of bacteria and other foreign particles by polymorphonuclear cells and macrophages. C-reactive protein is the major acute phase protein in humans [45].

Wilson and colleagues have demonstrated that C-reactive protein, in contrast to other acute phase reactants such as complement components, α_2-macroglobulin and α_1-antiprotease, is a reliable indicator of severity in acute pancreatitis [46]. C-reactive protein levels were found to provide the best discrimination between mild and complicated acute pancreatitis and was similar in accuracy to either Ranson or Glasgow multiple scoring systems, particularly for gallstone pancreatitis [46] (Table 15.2).

Table 15.2 Serum markers useful in the diagnosis of gallstone pancreatitis

Enzymes	*Acute phase reactants*
Amylase	C-reactive protein
Amylase isoenzyme p-type	α_2-Macroglobulin
Liver enzymes–AST	Fibrinogen
Elastase-1	
Lipase	
Phospholipase A_2	
Ribonuclease	
Carboxypeptidase	

α_2-macroglobulin is one of the more important antiproteases in man. Along with other antiproteases (α_1-proteinase inhibitor, α_2-antichymotrypsin) it binds to proteolytic enzymes such as trypsin, chymotrypsin and elastase and inactivates them [47, 48]. In contrast to C-reactive protein, decreased levels of α_2-macroglobulin have been found in acute pancreatitis, and appear to be related to severity [49]. Decreased α_2-macroglobulin levels are related to clearance of the antiprotease-protease complex by cells of the reticuloendothelial system and other cell types [47, 48].

Radiological tests in the diagnosis of gallstone pancreatitis

Plain films of the abdomen are usually unhelpful in the diagnosis of acute pancreatitis. A 'sentinel loop' of small bowel in the vicinity of the pancreas or evidence of large bowel pseudo-obstruction with a cut-off at the distal transverse colon may rarely be seen. Their main value, however, may lie in outruling other causes of an acute abdomen, such as a perforated viscus or intestinal obstruction. Other radiological investigations may be useful in both confirming the diagnosis of pancreatitis and identifying gallstones and other biliary tract disorders as an aetiological factor.

Oral cholecystography is generally not helpful in acute pancreatitis as the gallbladder may fail to opacify in over 50% of patients [50]. Intravenous cholangiography is also unhelpful in the diagnosis of gallstones associated with acute pancreatitis [51]. These investigations fail because the contrast material is not absorbed orally, there is a decrease in circulating bile salts and the biliary tract may be obstructed due to stones. Because of difficulties in the above tests radionuclide scanning using ^{99m}Tc HIDA has been used to detect gallstones associated with acute pancreatitis [52]. Neoptolemos and colleagues, however, found that radionuclide biliary imaging was normal in up to 50% of patients with gallstone pancreatitis whereas ultrasonagraphy was accurate in up to 67% of patients with gallstones [53]. The use of real time ultrasonagraphy as in this study has been found to be more accurate than earlier studies using grey scale ultrasound [54]. Non-visualization of the gallbladder, however, remains a major problem with ultrasonography and cannot be taken as an indicator of gallbladder disease. If initially negative or if the gallbladder is not visualized with ultrasonography repeated testing is advisable as sensitivity and specificity increase with repeated examinations, identifying up to 80% of patients with gallstones [53, 55].

Although ultrasonography has gained an important role in the early diagnosis of pancreatitis because of its ability to detect gallstones and examine the common bile duct, its use in visualizing the pancreas however, is frequently limited because of associated ileus and bowel gas. For this reason computed tomography (CT) scanning is the radiological investigation of choice for examining the pancreas [56] (Table 15.3). CT scanning is, however, no more useful in detecting gallstones than ultrasonography [57]. In addition to pancreatic enlargement, CT scanning will demonstrate pancreatic necrosis and abscess and pseudocyst formation. Contrast-enhanced tomography gives the best resolution; the presence of pancreatic enhancement and preservation of peripancreatic tissue planes allows differentiation between mild and severe pancreatitis. [58]. This will be discussed in the section dealing with assessment of severity in acute pancreatitis.

Table 15.3 Radiological investigations in the diagnosis of gallstone pancreatitis

Plain abdominal film
Oral cholecystography
Intravenous cholangiography
Radionuclide scanning
Ultrasonography
Computed tomography (CT) scanning
Percutaneous transhepatic cholangiography (PTC)
Endoscopic retrograde cholangiopancreatography (ERCP)

In certain cases of pancreatitis where gallstone disease is suspected and cannot be identified by the tests described, more invasive radiological investigations may be required. Percutaneous transhepatic cholangiography (PTC) has been proposed as a safe and effective means of demonstrating stones in the biliary tree although it is not widely used in this regard [59]. Endoscopic retrograde cholangiopancreatography is more readily available and has the added attraction of allowing therapeutic options such as allowing sphincterotomy and common bile duct stone extraction. The role of ERCP in the management of gallstone pancreatitis will be discussed later in this chapter.

Assessment of severity of gallstone pancreatitis – multiple scoring systems

Because the spectrum of gallstone pancreatitis ranges from a mild self-limiting disease to multiple organ failure and death, efforts have been made to examine clinical, biochemical and radiological parameters in an attempt to predict severity of disease. This would allow closer monitoring and earlier intervention, possibly altering outcome.

Although the elevation in serum amylase remains the cornerstone in diagnosis, it is apparent that amylase levels do not correlate with severity of disease [60]. Likewise clinical examination at presentation may also be unreliable, unless the situation is extreme and the patient is shocked. As isolated laboratory values may also be imprecise, various scoring systems have been developed based on multiple laboratory criteria. Clinical experience indicates that these systems are useful in discriminating between mild and acute attacks of acute pancreatitis. One drawback remains, however, in that collections of the laboratory values may take up to 48 hours.

Ranson and coworkers developed the first prognostic scoring system which has become widely used [61]. The eleven signs indicative of a poor prognosis are listed in Table 15.4. If less than two of these signs were present the patient was unlikely to die, mortality was 15% if more than three signs were present, 40% with five or six signs and nearly 100% with over seven signs present.

A similar scoring system was developed by Imrie and colleagues in Glasgow. In this system, three of eight prognostic criteria present within 48 hours of admission indicated a severe acute pancreatitis [6]. Unlike the system devised by Ranson in the USA, this system was developed in an older population with a preponderance of gallstone-induced pancreatitis. The Glasgow system, however, was altered by dropping age and doubling the AST threshold to strengthen its prognostic value (Table 15.5) [62].

These systems pose problems in that time is required for collection of the data and hence may be of limited use in the early assessment of the patient. Furthermore, they provide a static 'once off' assessment which does not provide for sequential measurement. Since the introduction of the Ranson and Glasgow scoring systems in acute pancreatitis use of prognostic scoring systems have also been introduced for the management of the trauma patients. One of the most comprehensive trauma scoring systems is the acute physiology and chronic health evaluation (APACHE) illness grading system first introduced by Knaus and coworkers in 1981 [63]. The original system provided weightings for 34 potential physiological and laboratory measurements in addition to scoring the patients current health status. This original classification was considered too cumbersome for widespread or routine use. A simplified APACHE II scoring system was introduced in 1985 which utilizes 12 routinely available physiological and laboratory variables (Table 15.6) [64]. This system was also found to correlate with risk of hospital death.

Various workers have examined the usefulness of APACHE II scoring in acute pancreatitis. Larvin and McMahon compared APACHE II with other multiple scoring systems. APACHE II correctly predicted 63% of severe attacks [65]. After 48 hours, outcome was correctly predicted in 88% of cases, in comparison to 69% for Ranson scoring and 84% for Glasgow scoring. In another prospective study Wilson and

Table 15.4 Prognostic criteria in acute pancreatitis (Ranson) [9]

Criteria present on presentation	
1	Age >55 years
2	WCC >16 000/mm³
3	Blood glucose >10 mmol/L
4	Serum LDH >350 iu/L
5	Serum AST >250 iu/L
Criteria developing within the first 48 hours	
6	Haematocrit fall >10%
7	Blood urea (BUN) >8 mg/dL
8	Serum Ca^{++} <8 mg/dL
9	Arterial P_{O_2} <8 kPa
10	Base deficit >4 mmol/L
11	Fluid sequestration >6 L

Table 15.5 Prognostic criteria in acute pancreatitis (Glasgow)

1	WCC >15 000 mm³
2	Blood glucose >10 mmol/L
3	Blood urea >16 mmol/L (post-hydration)
4	LDH >600 iu/L
5	AST >200 iu/L
6	Plasma albumin <32 g/L
7	Uncorrected plasma Ca^{++} <2 mmol/L
8	Arterial P_{O_2} >8 kPa

Table 15.6 Prognostic criteria in acute pancreatitis (APACHE II)

1	Temperature (rectal)
2	Mean arterial pressure
3	Heart rate (ventricular response)
4	Respiratory rate (ventilated or non-ventilated)
5	Oxygenation (A_{aDO_2} or P_{aO_2})
6	Arterial pH
7	Serum sodium
8	Serum potassium
9	Serum creatinine (Double score for ARF)
10	Haematocrit
11	WCC
12	Glasgow Coma Scale

Scoring is based on a scale depending on the degree of abnormality of that parameter A_{aDO_2}, alveolar-arterial oxygen difference; P_{aO_2}; arterial partial pressure of oxygen; ARF, acute renal failure.

colleagues compared APACHE II to the Ranson and Glasgow scoring systems in 160 patients with acute pancreatitis [66]. APACHE II could discriminate between uncomplicated, complicated and fatal attacks of pancreatitis within a few hours of admission. Peak APACHE II scoring within the first 72 hours was more accurate than either of the other two systems for gallstone-associated pancreatitis. Ranson's criteria interestingly, however, performed better for alcohol-associated pancreatitis, which presumably reflects that fact that the Ranson system is based on a population with a predominance of alcohol-associated pancreatitis. Patients dying within that hospital admission demonstrated a rising score with the APACHE II system, whereas those with an uncomplicated course demonstrated falling scores. Because of the ability for repetitive scoring with the APACHE system, it allows monitoring of disease progression and response to treatment.

Assessment of severity of gallstone pancreatitis – single prognostic factors

Several single biochemical markers have been examined in an attempt to identify a simple early marker of outcome in acute pancreatitis. Arterial hypoxia on admission predicted 50% of severe attacks of acute pancreatitis in a study by Cooper and colleagues [67]. Single plasma biochemical parameters also examined include a_2-macroglobulin and C-reactive protein. C-reactive protein appears to be the most promising single factor so far examined. Wilson and colleagues compared C-reactive protein levels with other acute phase reactants and complement components, in addition the Ranson and Glasgow scoring systems in acute pancreatitis [46]. C-reactive protein showed the best discrimination between mild and severe acute pancreatitis. Complicated acute pancreatitis gave rise to more prolonged and greater elevations in C-reactive protein levels. Either peak or seventh day C-reactive protein levels were comparable in accuracy to either of the multiple scoring systems, particularly for gallstone-associated pancreatitis. Beger and colleagues have argued that persistent elevation of C-reactive protein or lactate dehydrogenase (LDH) both of which are simple and inexpensive tests allows discrimination between oedematous and necrotizing pancreatitis with a high degree of sensitivity and specificity [68].

Fluid taken from the peritoneum by peritoneal lavage on admission is also a useful indicator of severity in acute pancreatitis. The risk of inadvertent damage is small and is less than 1%. Meyer and colleagues carried out peritoneal lavage in patients with acute pancreatitis and using a colour chart for examination of the peritoneal fluid they identified 72% of severe cases and 90% of patients who died [69]. Since this does not allow serial examination and because of its invasive nature this procedure has never become widely performed.

Assessment of severity of gallstone pancreatitis – radiological assessment

CT scanning is the only radiological procedure which is useful in assessing the degree of severity of acute pancreatitis. Its accuracy in assessing the pancreas has been shown to be superior to that of ultrasonography [56]. This is in addition to the detection of complications such as abscess and pseudocyst formation allowing early surgical management.

Nordestgaard and colleagues prospectively evaluated CT in 51 patients with acute pancreatitis on a mean of 4 days post-admission. A good correlation was found between extent of pancreatitic inflammation, based on degree of pancreatitic enlargement and extension into surrounding tissues, with local complications and clinical course [70]. Balthazar and colleagues also compared CT scanning with multiple prognostic criteria prospectively in 83 patients with acute pancreatitis [71]. Acute pancreatitis was graded by CT into grades A to E depending on severity. Based on these grades five of the six deaths and 88.8% of all abscesses occurred within grades D and E whereas no abscesses occurred within grades A or B. All patients with a CT grade A had a mild clinical course. While the authors of this study conclude that early CT is a useful prognostic indicator of outcome many of these patients were preselected in that only 48% of patients had CT performed within 72 hours of admission; the sickest patients being scanned first.

Clavian and coworkers evaluated the prognostic value of CT in 176 patients with acute pancreatitis [72]. This study also demonstrated a high degree of CT diagnostic specificity (92%) and sensitivity (100%). The authors attribute their good results to early CT scanning, within 36 hours of admission for the majority of patients and the high proportion of severe pancreatitis (17.6% of patients developed pancreatic abscesses) in their study population. However, while CT gradation into severe pancreatitis (i.e., phlegmonous extrahepatic spread extending into three or more areas) was predictive of local complications, the addition of multiple clinical and prognostic criteria were required to predict the likelihood of death.

Prediction of severe pancreatitis and local complications have also been examined in a prospective study of 126 patients with acute pancreatitis by London and colleagues [58]. Pancreatitic size index (multiplication of the maximum anterioposterior measurement of the pancreatitic body and head) had a sensitivity of 73% in identifying patients who developed local complications. Specificity, however, was only 68% which casts doubt on the usefulness of CT in excluding patients with local problems. In this study contrast-enhanced abdominal CT scanning was also compared with multiple prognostic criteria in the prediction of acute pancreatitis [58]. Patients were scanned within 72 hours of admission and loss of pancreatitic enhancement and peripancreatic tissue planes were greater in patients with severe pancreatitis. Pancreatitic size index (maximum anteroposterior measurement of the head and body multiplied together), which was measured retrospectively, correlated best with degree of severity. Overall, however, CT scanning did not improve on a modified Glasgow criteria for the prediction of disease severity (Table 15.7).

Interpretation of CT scanning studies in acute pancreatitis is rendered difficult by aetiological differences in patient populations, pre-selection of ill patients for early scanning and lack of quantitative data for reporting and comparisions between series. While in some series CT scanning appears to be useful in identifying patients early who develop complications and allows sequential examination, little is gained over multiple prognostic criteria in the prediction of severity or death.

Table 15.7 CT findings in acute pancreatitis

Enlargement of gland
Ill-defined margins
Abnormal enhancement
Thickening of peripancreatic planes
Blurring of fat planes
Intra- and retroperitoneal fluid collections
Pleura effusions
Pancreatic gas indicative of necrosis/abscess formation
Pseudocyst formation

Management of patients with gallstone pancreatitis

The management of patients with gallstone pancreatitis rests on supportive treatment to maintain organ function during the period of pancreatic inflammation, surgical treatment of local complications of the disease and definitive management of the underlying gallstones. These supportive features have altered little in recent years and will not be discussed further. The discussion will now focus on the management of the precipitating biliary calculi where treatment changes have occurred with the availability of ERCP and laparoscopic surgery.

Surgical treatment of associated biliary calculi

Previously, definitive treatment for gallstones associated with acute pancreatitis was to allow the acute attack to settle, discharge the patient and at a later date perform an elective cholecystectomy and possible exploration of the common bile duct. This policy has altered for two main reasons. One, it is clear that a significant proportion of patients returned with a recurrent attack of acute pancreatitis prior to their elective readmission. Secondly, the advent of ERCP, with subsequent laparoscopic cholecystectomy has allowed a relatively non-invasive, albeit not without risk, approach to the retrieval of ductal calculi and sphincterotomy.

Osborne and colleagues examined rates of recurrent pancreatitis prior to elective readmission in patients discharged with acute gallstone pancreatitis [62]. Twenty of 78 patients had further attacks of acute pancreatitis during this interval. A more recent report from the same unit indicates that a small proportion of patients managed in this manner in fact suffer a fatal attack of pancreatitis during this period [73]. Other authors report recurrent attacks of acute pancreatitis in up to 50% of patients discharged prior to elective readmission [74, 75].

Since the realization that delayed elective surgery exposes patients to greater risks many centres now advocate biliary surgery for gallstone associated pancreatitis during the presenting hospital admission. This is safe once the clinical picture is stable and serum amylase and other biochemical indicators have returned to normal. The exact timing of this surgery, however, remains contentious. Acosta and colleagues were the first to propose that operative intervention should be carried out within 48 hours of admission [12]. In a group of 46 consecutive patients the mortality was 2%, this was in contrast to a group of historical controls in which the mortality was 16%. Acosta supported this policy on the basis that 75% of patients presenting for surgery early had stones impacted at the ampulla, this fell to 45% at 2–4 days and 25% after 4 days. He proposed that disimpaction allowed rapid decompression of the pancreatic duct and resolution of the inflamed pancreas.

Other authors have agreed with this policy. Mercer and colleagues operated on 34 patients for gallstone pancreatitis within 48 hours of admission, with no major morbidity or mortality [76]. However, only 12 patients in this series required common bile duct exploration, of which four had impacted ampullary stones, implying that the majority of patients within this group may have had a mild pancreatitis. Stone and colleagues also supported this policy with results of a randomized trial in which 36 patients were operated on within 72 hours of admission and 29 others operated on electively three months following acute presentation [15]. As mentioned previously a greater proportion of the group undergoing early surgery had ductal calculi. Outcome was similar in both groups with one death in the early group and two in the delayed group. The authors refer to the economic benefits of avoiding a second hospital admission with this policy. Apart from economic benefits advocates of this approach stress the importance of biliary decompression early to avoid conversion of an oedematous pancreatitis into haemorrhagic pancreatitis. Stone emphasises the importance of sphincterotomy and septotomy of the terminal 1 cm of pancreatic duct which results in a sudden 'gush' of pancreatic juice at sphincteroplasty during early surgery.

Because of difficulties in confirming the early diagnosis of gallstones associated with acute pancreatitis, identification of patients at risk of progression to haemorrhagic pancreatitis and doubt about the outcome of early surgical intervention, not all authors agree with the policy described above. Ranson reported on 74 patients who presented with gallstone pancreatitis [9]. Mortality amongst 22 patients who underwent early surgery was 23% whereas there were no deaths among 37 patients undergoing delayed operation during the same hospital admission, the other 21 patients were discharged without biliary surgery. Twenty-three patients within the study had severe pancreatitis, as defined by Ranson multiple criteria. Nine of this group underwent early surgery of which four died whereas none of 14 patients with severe pancreatitis treated conservatively in the first instance died. The fifth patient who died in this study was one of 13 patients operated on for mild pancreatitis. Ranson concluded that while early surgery for mild pancreatitis is safe, early surgery for severe pancreatitis is hazardous and should be deferred until the pancreatitis has subsided.

Other authors have also stressed the high mortality of early surgery. Tondelli and colleagues reported on a 31% mortality rate in patients undergoing early surgery for gallstone pancreatitis in comparison to a 2% mortality for delayed operation. Kelly and Wagner prospectively randomized 165 patients into early and delayed surgery [77, 78]. Of interest patients with mild pancreatitis had a low mortality when operated on early. Those with severe pancreatitis had a 48% mortality in comparison to a 12% for delayed surgery. However, in this study surgery involved supraduodenal common bile duct (CBD) exploration and T-tube drainage whereas the patients in the reports by Acosta [12] and Stone [15] underwent transduodenal sphincterotomy and release of impacted ampullary stones.

These latter studies indicate that early laparotomy following predicted severe gallstone pancreatitis may lead to a poor outcome. This problem, however, is difficult to resolve because of the small number of studies, few of which are prospective and randomized and because of lack of stratification of patients into mild and severe pancreatitis. This issue is of historical interest now as the availability of ERCP offers a safer approach to disimpaction of stones in the ampullary region during acute gallstone pancreatitis.

ERCP and endoscopic sphincterotomy (ES) in the treatment of associated biliary calculi

Since the late 1970s many small trials have demonstrated that urgent ERCP and ES is both feasible and safe in the management of patients with acute pancreatitis (Table 15.8). Initially all these trials were small and had inherent problems of patient selection, grading of severity of attack and timing of ERCP. To date, however, only two randomized trials comparing urgent ERCP and ES with conventional management have been reported [79, 80].

Neoptolemos and colleagues prospectively randomized 121 patients with acute gallstone pancreatitis into urgent ERCP ± ES within 72 hours of admission, or conservative treatment in which ERCP was offered 5 days following admission if still indicated [79]. Fifty-nine patients were randomized to the ERCP ± ES group and 62 patients into the conventional management arm. There were fewer complications in those treated

Table 15.8 Results of ERCP ± EP for CBD stones in patients with gallstone pancreatitis

Author	Patients (no.)	Complications	Mortality
Classen 1978 [81]	17	0	0
Safrany 1981 [82]	29	3	2
Schott 1982 [83]	32	2	0
Kautz 1982 [84]	21	1	1
Riemann 1984 [85]	15	0	0
Rosseland 1984 [86]	29	2	1
Neoptolemos 1986 [87]	10	0	0
Van der Spuy 1991 [93]	29	0	0
Randomized trials			
Neoptolemos *et al.* 1988 [79] (59 randomized to ERCP ± ES)	121	10	1
Fan *et al.* 1993 [80] (97 randomized to ERCP ± ES)	195	36	5

After Carr-Locke [88].

with early ERCP ± ES (18.6% complication rate and one death (1.7%)) in comparison to the conventionally treated group (43.6% complication rate and five deaths (8.1%)). These differences, however, were confined to those with predicted severe pancreatitis, as assessed using a modified Glasgow system. A criticism of this study is the small number of patients with CBD stones in the ERCP ± ES group requiring ES (12 in total) [89]. Despite this no major complications or mortality occurred in this group who conventionally would be expected to have a high incidence of major morbidity.

Fan and coworkers also undertook a randomized trial to examine whether earlier ERCP with or without sphincterotomy 24 hours following admission improved outlook in patients with gallstone pancreatitis [80]. In this study 127 patients ultimately proved to have biliary stones. Ninety-seven patients underwent ERCP ± EP and 98 were entered into the control arm. Mortality and major complications were unchanged with ERCP ± EP, however, the incidence of biliary sepsis was significantly reduced in the patients with severe pancreatitis undergoing early ERCP intervention (0 of 41 patients versus 8 of 40 patients). Of the 41 patients predicted to have severe pancreatitis in the ERCP ± EP group only 19 had ductal calculi. This is an important point to note when considering both of these randomized studies as a total of only 60 patients from both studies predicted to have severe pancreatitis were subsequently found to have ductal calculi at ERCP. Hence, the number of patients expected to have a poor outlook is small and, therefore, the results must be interpreted with this in mind.

What these trials do demonstrate clearly is that early ERCP ± ES appears to be safe in patients with gallstone pancreatitis and also may decrease complications and mortality. Further studies are needed, however to more accurately define the most appropriate timing for this procedure. It is also important to note that ERCP performed during acute pancreatitis itself carries a small morbidity and mortality, although with experience this should be small. This is demonstrated by a recent collective series of ERCPs preformed in a collective European series of gallstone pancreatitis which reported a 2% mortality and 6% morbidity related to the procedure [90]. It is essential, however, that a skilled ERCP endoscopist is available.

A further advantage of this approach is that following ERCP and sphincterotomy frail and elderly patients can be treated non-surgically leaving their gallbladder *in situ*. Reports indicate that only a small proportion of patients with symptomatic ductal calculi treated in this manner will encounter further problems and require elective cholecystectomy [91–93]. Ingoldby and colleagues have shown that less than 10% of poor risk patients with gallstones require cholecystectomy following ERCP and EP over a two to three year follow-up period [91]. However, only a minority of these patients have gallstone pancreatitis, hence it is unclear whether this approach is appropriate for all of this subgroup of patients.

For young fit patients elective cholecystectomy is recommended following acute gallstone pancreatitis as further problems may be expected because of their projected survival. For these patients the advent of laparoscopic cholecystectomy necessitates the importance of pre-operative imaging of the CBD. This is because peroperative cholangiography may be difficult or may not be routinely used at laparoscopic surgery and furthermore identification of unsuspected ductal calculi at laparoscopic cholecystectomy poses a dilemma regarding management. The ideal situation is for pre-operative imaging to be carried out with ERCP with the advantage of sphincterotomy and stone retrieval if necessary. The other imaging option is intravenous cholangiography (IVC). With modern contrast media IVC is a safe investigation and offers good quality images with the use of tomography [94].

Although routine peroperative cholangiography may not be necessary for patients undergoing laparoscopic cholecystectomy for uncomplicated gallstones [95]. Peroperative CBD imaging should be mandatory for those with a history of gallstone pancreatitis in whom preoperative duct imaging has not been performed. With experience the success rate of laparoscopic cholangiography is 80–90%. A percutaneous approach with a polyethylene sheath for the introduction of the cholangiocatheter as originally described by Petelin [96] or the use of a catheter introduced into the cystic duct via one of the trocars [97] both give satisfactory results.

Experience with laparoscopic CBD exploration may be difficult to accumulate because with appropriate pre-operative assessment the necessity for laparoscopic duct exploration should be rare. This is demonstrated by McMahon's group from Leeds who reported on 60 patients with CBD calculi [98]. Eighty five per cent of these patients were treated by ERCP and ES and laparoscopic cholecystectomy if symptoms related to the gallbladder. Only six patients underwent laparoscopic duct exploration of which one was converted to open exploration. Rhodes and colleagues reported on 16 consecutive patients with acute gallstone pancreatitis [99]. All of these patients were treated with ERCP and ES and staged laparoscopic cholecystectomy indicating the success of this strategy without the need to resort to common bile exploration by conventional or laparoscopic means.

The management of ductal calculi identified following peroperative cholangiography depends on technical expertise and equipment availability. Laparoscopic exploration of the CBD is in its infancy, no doubt however, the general expertise in this area will improve with wider availability of laparoscopically aided choledochoscopy with dormia and balloon extraction of stones. The use of a flexible choledochoscope inserted into a CBD enterotomy has been successfully reported by Stoker and colleagues in five patients; ductal calculi were extracted with the aid of a dormia basket, local irrigation and a balloon embolectomy catheter [100]. Petelin has amassed considerable experience with CBD exploration at laparoscopy via either the cystic duct or choledochotomy [96]. Using a combination of choledochoscopic dormia and Fogarty balloon extraction Petelin reported laparoscopic common bile duct exploration in 22 patients with convertion to open exploration in one patient, leaving residual stones in two patients. Another approach to CBD stone clearance is that reported by Cuschieri and Berci on the use of the ultrathin (2–3 mm) flexible choledocholscope inserted through the cystic duct in conjunction with laser lithotripsy [101]. The added expense and logistics of laser use in a congested theatre setting may, however, limit this technique.

If laparoscopic CBD stone extraction is not feasible another reasonable option is to leave the stones *in situ* and arrange staged ERCP and sphincterotomy. Finally, conversion to open cholecystectomy and CBD exploration should be seriously considered if ERCP or ES is deemed difficult because of anatomical considerations, such as previous upper gastrointestinal surgery or the size of the calculi preclude reasonable success at ERCP extraction. It must be re-emphasized that with adequate pre-operative imaging of the biliary tree and subsequent ES and stone extraction few patients should 'slip through the net' and require laparoscopic stone extraction.

Given the available data we would propose the following management plan for patients with acute gallstone pancreatitis (Fig. 15.1). Those patients with mild disease can be managed conservatively, with subsequent imaging of their biliary tree and semi-elective laparoscopic cholecystectomy within their hospital admission. Identified ductal calculi in this group should be managed with ERCP and ES prior to cholecystectomy. Those patients with severe disease should undergo urgent ERCP with ES if necessary. In the elderly or frail this may be adequate treatment, for those younger or patients with recurrent problems laparoscopic cholecystectomy should be undertaken either on that admission or as a staged procedure. The most appropriate timing for cholecystectomy in this group remains known.

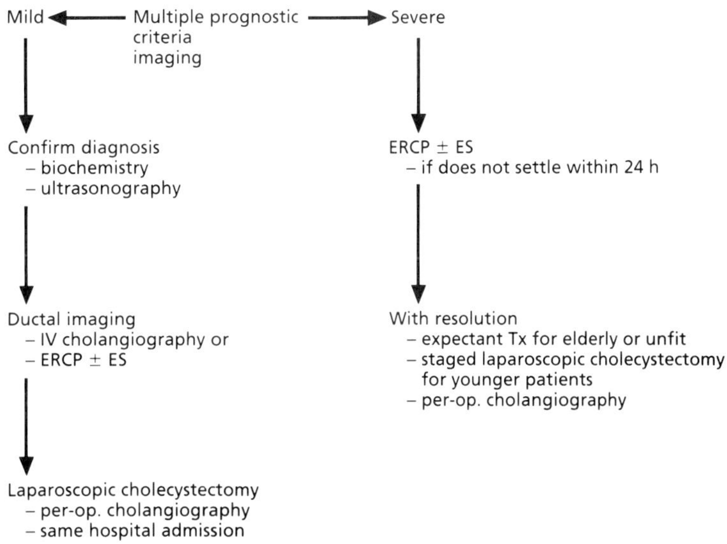

Fig. 15.1 Management plan for patients with acute gallstone pancreatitis.

References

1 Blamey S, Osborne D, Gilmore W, O'Neill J, Carter D, Imrie C. The early identification of patients with gallstone associated pancreatitis using clinical and biochemical factors only. *Ann Surg* 1983;**198**:574.
2 Ranson J. Acute pancreatitis, In: *Surgery of the Pancreas*. Philadelphia: Saunders, 1983:146–81.
3 Mero M. Changing aetiology of acute pancreatitis. *Ann de Chir et Gynaecol* 1982;**71**:126.
4 Svensson J, Norback B, Bokey E, Edlund Y. Changing patterns in aetiology of pancreatitis in an urban Swedish area. *Br J Surg* 1979;**66**:159.
5 Cornfield A, Cooper M, Williamson R. Acute pancreatitis: a lethal disease of increasing incidence. *Gut* 1985;**26**:724–9.
6 Imrie C, Benjamin I, Ferguson J *et al*. A single-centre double blind trial of Trasylol therapy in primary acute pancreatitis. *Br J Surg* 1978;**65**:337.
7 DeBolla A, Obeid M. Mortality in actue pancreatitis. *Ann Roy Coll Surg End* 1984;**66**:184.
8 Opie E. The aetiology of acute haemorrhagic pancreatitis. *Bull Johns Hopkins Hosp* 1901;**12**:182–8.
9 Ranson J. The timing of biliary surgery in acute pancreatitis. *Ann Surg* 1979;**189**:654–63.
10 Moreau J, AR Z, Melton L *et al*. Gallstone pancreatitis and the effect of cholecystectomy: a population based cohort study. *Mayo Clinic Proc* 1988:**63**:466.
11 Banks P. Acute pancreatitis. *Gastroenterology* 1971; **61**:382–97.
12 Acosta J, Rossi R, Galli O, Pellegrini C, Skinner D. Early surgery for acute gallstone pancreatitis: Evaluation of a systematic approach. *Surgery* 1978;**83**:367–70.
13 Acosta J, Ledesma C. Gallstone migration as a cause of acute pancreatitis. *N Engl J Med* 1974;**290**:484–7.
14 Kelly T. Gallstone pancreatitis: pathophysiology. *Surgery* 1976;**80**:488–92.
15 Stone H, Fabian T, Dunlop W. Gallstone pancreatitis: Biliary tract pathology in relation to time of operation. *Ann Surg* 1981;**194**:305–12.
16 Armstong C, Taylor T, Jeacock J, Lucas S. The biliary tract in patients with acute gallstone pancreatitis. *Br J Surg* 1985;**72**:551–6.
17 McMahon M, Shefta J. Physical characteristics of gallstones and the calibre of the cystic duct in patients with acute pancreatitis. *Br J Surg* 1980:**67**:6–9.
18 Taylor T, Rimmer S, Holt S, Jeacock J, Lucas S. Sex differences in gallstone pancreatitis. *Ann Surg* 1991;**214**:667–79.
19 Cuschieri A, Hughes J. Pancreatic reflux during operative choledochography. *Br J Surg* 1973;**60**:933.
20 Guelrud M, Mendoza S, Vicent S *et al*. Pressures in the sphincter of Oddi in patients with gallstones, common duct stones, and recurrent pancreatitis. *J Clin Gastroenterol* 1983;**5**:37.
21 Chiari H. Uber die Selbstverdauung des Menschlichen Pankreas. *Zeitschrift für Heilkunde* 1896;**17**:69.
22 Armstrong C, Taylor T. Pancreatic-duct reflux and acute gallstone pancreatitis. *Ann Surg* 1986;**204**:59–64.
23 Ofstad E. Formation and destruction of plasma kinins during acute pancreatitis in patients with migrating gallstones. *Scand J Gastroenterol* (Suppl.) 1970;**5**:1.
24 Harvey M, Wedgewood K, Austin J, Reber H. Pancreatic duct pressure, duct permeability and acute pancreatitis. *Br J Surg* 1989;**76**:859–62.
25 McCutcheon A. A fresh approach to the pathogenesis of pancreatitis. *Gut* 1968;**9**:296.
26 Armstrong C, Taylor T, Torrance H. Ionic flux and mucosal ultrastructure in the rat bile-pancreatic duct. *Dig Dis Sci* 1987;**32**:861.
27 Broe P, Cameron J. Experimental gallstone pancreatitis. Pathogenesis and response to different treatment modalities. *Ann Surg* 1982;**195**:566–73.
28 Sanfey H, Sarr M, Buckley G, Cameron J. Oxygen-derived free radicals and acute pancreatitis: a review. *Acta Physiol Scand* 1986;**548** (Suppl.):109–18.
29 MacGowan S, Bouchier-Hayes D, Broe P. Experimental pancreatitis: the effect of allopurinol. *Gut* 1987;**28**:A368.
30 Gough D, Boyle B, Joyce W *et al*. Free radical inhibition and serial chemiluminescence in evolving experimental pancreatitis. *Br J Surg* 1990;**77**:1256–9.
31 Wedgewood K, Farmer R, Reber H. A model of hemorrhagic pancreatitis in cats. Role of 16, 16-dimethyl Prostaglandin E2. *Gastroenterology* 1986; **90**:32–40.
32 Elman R, Arneson N, Graham E. Value of blood amylase estimation in the diagnosis of pancreatic disease: A clinical study. *Arch Surg* 1929;**19**:943–6.
33 Clavian P, Burgan S, Moossa A. Serum enzymes and other laboratory tests in acute pancreatitis. *Br J Surg* 1989;**76**:1234–43.
34 Lott J, Speicher C, Nemesansky E. Is serum amylase an absolute test in the diagnosis of acute pancreatitis. *Arch Pathol Lab Med* 1985;**109**:314–15.
35 Brooks F. Testing pancreatic function. *N Eng J Med* 1972;**286**:300–3.
36 Weaver D, Bouwmann D, Walt A, Clink D, Resto A, Stephany J. A correlation between clinical pancreatitis and isoenzyme patterns of amylase. *Surgery* 1982;**9**:576–80.
37 Moossa A. Diagnostic tests and procedures in acute pancreatitis. *N Eng J Med*. 1984;**311**:639–43.
38 Koehler D, Eckfeldt JH, Levitt M. Diagnostic value of routine isoamylase assay of hyperamylasemic serum. *Gastroenterology* 1982;**82**:887–90.
39 McMahon M, Pickford I. Biochemical prediction of gallstones early in an attack of acute pancreatitis. *Lancet* 1979;**ii**:541–3.
40 Ventrucci M, Pezilli R, Gullo L, Plate L, Sprovieri G, Barbara L. Role of serum pancreatic enzyme assays in diagnosis of pancreatic disease. *Dig Dis Sci* 1989;**34**:39–45.
41 Croton R, Warren R, Stott A, Roberts N. Ionized

calcium in acute pancreatitis and its relationship with total calcium and serum lipase. *Br J Surg* 1981;**68**: 241–4.

42 Satake K, Chung Y, Umeya K. Serum elastase-1 levels in pancreatic disease. *Am J Surg* 1982;**144**:239–42.

43 Bird N, Goodman A, Johnson A. Serum phospholipase A2 activity in acute pancreatitis: and early guide to severity. *Br J Surg* 1989;**76**:731–2.

44 Gronroos J, Hietaranta A, Nevalainen T. Renal tubular cell injury and serum phospholipase A2 activity in acute pancreatitis. *Br J Surg* 1992;**79**:800–1.

45 Kushner I. The phenomenon of the acute phase response. *Ann NY Acad Sci* 1989;**559**:39–46.

46 Wilson C, Heads A, Shenkin A, Imrie C. C-reactive protein, antiproteases and complement factors as objective markers of severity in acute pancreatitis. *Br J Surg* 1989;**76**:177–81.

47 Van Leuyen F, Cassiman J, Van den Bergue H. Demonstration of an alpha 2-macroglobulin receptor in human fibroblasts absent in tumor cell lines. *J Bio Chem* 1979;**254**:5155–60.

48 Barret A, Starkey P. The interaction of alpha 2-macroglobulin with proteinases. Characteristics and specificity of the reaction and a hypothesis concerning its molecular mechanism. *Biochem J* 1973;**133**:709–24.

49 Dubick M, Mar G, Mayer D, Majumder A McMahon, MJ, Geokas M. Digestive enzymes and protease inhibitors in plasma from patients with acute pancreatitis. *Pancreas* 1987;**2**:187–94.

50 Kaden V, Howard J, Doubleday L. Cholecystographic studies during and immediately following acute pancreatitis. *Surgery* 1955;**38**:1082.

51 Freund H, Pfefferman R, Durst A, Rabinovici N. Gallstone pancreatitis. *Arch Surg* 1976;**111**:1106.

52 Fonseca C, Greenberg D, Rosenthall L *et al.* ^{99m}Tc-IDA imaging in the differential diagnosis of acute cholecystitis and acute pancreatitis. *Radiology* 1979;**130**: 525–7.

53 Neoptolemos J, Hall A, Finlay D, Berry J, Carr-Locke D, Fossard D. The urgent diagnosis of gallstones in acute pancreatitis: a prospective study of three methods. *Br J Surg* 1984;**71**:230–3.

54 McKay A, Imrie C, O'Neill J, Ducan J. Is an ultrasound scan of value in acute pancreatitis? *Br J Surg* 1982;**69**:369–72.

55 Goodman A, Neoptolemos J, Carr-Locke D, Finlay D, Fossard D. Detection of gallstones after acute pancreatitis. *Gut* 1985;**26**:125.

56 Silverstein W, Isikoff M, Hill M, Barkin J. Diagnostic imaging of acute pancreatitis: a prospective study using CT and sonography. *Am J Roentgenol* 1981; **137**:497–502.

57 Wang S, Lin X, Tsai Y *et al.* Clinical significance of ultrasonography, computed tomography, and biochemical tests in the rapid diagnosis of gallstone-related pancreatitis: a prospective study. *Pancreas* 1988;**3**:153–8.

58 London N, Neoptolomos J, Lavelle J, Bailey I, James D. Contrast-enhanced abdominal computed tomography scanning and prediction of severity of acute pancreatitis: a prospective study. *Br J Surg* 1989;**76**: 268–72.

59 Coppa G, LeFleur R, Ranson J. The role of Chiba-needle cholangiography in the diagnosis of possible acute pancreatitis and cholelithiasis. *Ann Surg* 1981; **193**:393.

60 Williamson R. Early assessment of severity in acute pancreatitis. *Gut* 1984;**25**:1331–9.

61 Ranson J, Rifkind K, Rosen D *et al.* Prognostic signs and the role of operative management in acute pancreatitis. *Surg Gynecol Obstet* 1974;**139**:69–81.

62 Osborne D, Imrie C, Carter D. Biliary surgery in the same admission for gallstone-associated acute pancreatitis. *Br J Surg* 1981;**68**:758–61.

63 Knaus W, Zimmerman J, Wagner D, Draper E, Lawrence D. APACHE–acute physiology and chronic health evaluation: a physiologically based classification system. *Crit Care Med* 1981;**9**:591–7.

64 Knaus W, Draper E, Wagner D, Zimmerman J. APACHE II: a severity of disease classification system. *Crit Care Med* 1985;**13**:818–29.

65 Larvin M, McMahon M. APACHE II score for assessment and monitoring of acute pancreatitis. *Lancet* 1989;**ii**:201–4.

66 Wilson C, Heath D, Imrie C. Prediction of outcome in acute pancreatitis: a comparative study of APACHE II, clinical assessement and multiple factor scoring systems. *Br J Surg* 1990;**77**:1260–4.

67 Cooper M, Williamson R, Pollock A. The role of peritoneal lavage in the prediction and treatment of severe acute pancreatitis. *Ann Roy Coll Surg Eng* 1982;**64**:422–5.

68 Beger H. Management of pancreatic necrosis and pancreatic abscess. In: *Pancreatitis*. Edinburgh: Churchill Livingstone, 1989.

69 Mayer D, McMahon M. The diagnostic and prognostic value of peritoneal lavage in patients with acute pancreatitis. *Surg Gynecol Obstet* 1985;**160**:507–12.

70 Nordestgaard A, Wilson S, Williams R. Early computerized tomography as a predictor of outcome in acute pancreatitis. *Am J Surg* 1986;**152**:127–32.

71 Balthazar E, Ranson J, Naidich D, Megibow A, Caccavale R, Cooper M. Acute pancreatitis: prognostic value of CT. *Radiology* 1985;**156**:767–72.

72 Clavian P, Hauser H, Meyer P, Rohner A. Value of contrast-enhanced computerized tomography in the early diagnosis and prognosis of acute pancreatitis. *Am J Surg* 1988;**155**:457–66.

73 Wilson C, Imrie C, Carter D. Fatal acute pancreatitis. *Gut* 1988;**29**:782.

74 Kelly T. Gallstone pancreatitis: the timing of surgery. *Surgery* 1980;**88**:345.

75 Paloyan D, Simonowitz D, Skinner D. The timing of biliary tract operations in patients with pancreatitis

associated with gallstones. *Surg Gynaec Obstet* 1975; 141:737.
76 Mercer L, Saltzstein E, Peacock J *et al.* Early surgery for biliary pancreatitis. *Am J Surg* 1984;**148**:749.
77 Tondelli P, Stutz K, Harder F, Schuppisser J, Allgower M. Acute gallstone pancreatitis: best timing for surgery. *Br J Surg* 1982;**69**:709–10.
78 Kelly T, Wagner D. Gallstone pancreatitis: a prospective randomized trial of the timing of surgery. *Surgery* 1988;**104**:600.
79 Neoptolemos J, Carr-Locke D, London N, Bailey I, James D, Fossard D. Controlled trial of urgent endoscopic retrograde cholangiopancreatography and endoscopic sphincterotomy versus conservative treatment for acute pancreatitis due to gallstones. *Lancet* 1988;**ii**:979–83.
80 Fan S, Lai E, Mok F, Lo C, Zheng S, Wong J. Early treatment of acute biliary pancreatitis by endoscopic papillotomy. *N Engl J Med* 1993;**328**:228–32.
81 Classen M, Ossenberg W, Wurbs D, Dammerman R, Hagen-muller F. Pancreatitis: An indication for endoscopic papillotomy? (Abstract) *Endoscopy* 1978; **10**:223.
82 Safrany L. Controversies in acute pancreatitis. In: Hollender LF. ed. *Controversies in Acute Pancreatitis* New York: Springer-Verlag 1982:214.
83 Schott B, Neuhaus B, Portacarrero G, Krause S, Safrany L. Endoskopische Papillotomie bei akuter billärer Pankreatitis. *Klinikarzt* 1982;**II**:52.
84 Kautz G, Kohaus H, Keferstein R, Bunte H. Zur Pathogenese und Endoskopischen Therapie der akuten biliären Pankreatitis. *Klinikarzt* 1982;**II**:1202.
85 Riemann JF, Lux G. Therapeutische Stratagie bei der akuten Pankreatitis. *Fortschr Med* 1984;**102**:179.
86 Rosseland AR, Solhaug JH. Early or delayed endoscopic papillotomy (EPT) in gallstone pancreatitis. *Ann Surg* 1984;**199**:165.
87 Neoptolemos JP, London N, Slater D *et al.* A prospective study of ERCP and endoscopic sphincterotomy in the diagnosis and treatment of gallstone actue pancreatitis. *Arch Surg* 1986;**121**:697.
88 Carr-Locke D. Acute gallstone pancreatitis and endoscopic therapy. *Endoscopy* 1990;**22**:180–3.
89 Anonymous. Obstruction or reflux in gallstone-associated pancreatitis. *Lancet* 1988;**i**:915–17.
90 Winslet M, Imray C, Neoptolemos J. Biliary acute pancreatitis. *Hepatogastroenterology* 1991;**38**:120–3.
91 Ingoldby C, el Saadi J, Hall R, Denyer M. Late results of endoscopic sphincterotomy for bile duct stones in elderly patients with gall bladders in situ. *Gut* 1989;**30**:1129–31.
92 Cotton P. Two to nine year follow up after sphincterotomy for stones in patients with gallbladder *in situ*. *Gastrointest Endosc* 1986;**32**:157.
93 Van der Spuy S. Endoscopic retrograde cholangiopancreatography and endoscopic sphincterotomy in the management of suspected gallstone pancreatitis. *S Afr Med J* 1991;**79**:16–18.
94 Joyce W, Keane R, Burke G, Daly M, Drumm J, Egan T, Delaney P. Identification of bile duct stones in patients undergoing laparoscopic cholecystectomy. *Br J Surg* 1991;**78**:1174–6.
95 Grace P, Qureshi A, Burke P *et al.* Selective cholangiography in laparoscopic cholecystectomy. *Br J Surg* 1993;**80**:244–6.
96 Petelin J. Laparoscopic approach to common duct pathology. *Surg Lap aroscop Endosc* 1991;**1**:33–41.
97 Hunter J. Laparoscopic transcystic common bile duct exploration. *Am J Surg* 1992;**163**:53–8.
98 Martin I, Curley P, McMahon M. Minimally invasive treatment for common bile duct stones. *Br J Surg* 1993;**80**:103–6.
99 Rhodes M, Armstrong C, Longstaff A, Cawthorn S. Laparoscopic cholecystectomy with endoscopic retrograde cholangiopancreatography for acute gallstone pancreatitis. *Br J Surg* 1993;**80**(247).
100 Stoker M, Leveillee R, McCann J, Maini B. Laparoscopic common bile duct exploration. *J Laparoendosc Surg* 1991;**1**:287–93.
101 Cuschieri A, Berci G. *Laparoscopic Biliary Surgery.* Oxford: Blackwell Scientific Publications, 1990:94pp.

Chapter 16
Operative management of common bile duct stones

P.M. Murchan, J. Stewart & T.G. Brennan

Choledocholithiasis is responsible for much of the serious morbidity and mortality of gallstone disease. Stone-induced jaundice, cholangitis, pancreatitis and biliary stricture may ensue, if appropriate and expeditious action is not taken following the discovery of ductal calculi. Over the past 2 decades, few areas of surgical gastroenterology have seen such change as the management of common bile duct stones. Once the domain of the general surgeon, the management of choledocholithiasis has to some extent been claimed by medical endoscopists and interventional radiologists. Moreover, from the vast literature reporting excellent results from such specialties, it might appear that the future of ductal stone treatment may move even further from the surgical arena. However, such claims are poorly substantiated in as much as surgery still offers the only definitive and probably the most durable option in the management of ductal stones. The abdominal surgeon must, therefore, be able to diagnose and deal with duct calculi both at the time of gallbladder surgery and subsequent to a previously performed cholecystectomy. This chapter outlines the surgical techniques employed to treat choledocholithiasis and gives an account of some of the current controversies associated with the management of common bile duct stones.

Surgical anatomy of the common bile duct

Before embarking on exploration of the common bile duct (CBD), it is mandatory to be fully aware of the exact anatomy and possible structural variants of the duct system likely to be encountered during surgery. While the complete network of intrahepatic duct architecture is beyond the scope of this chapter, the extrahepatic ducts are described below. The common hepatic duct is formed by the union of the left and right hepatic ducts. This junction usually occurs in the *porta hepatis* but can rarely occur lower down within the free edge of the lesser omentum. Beyond the confluence of the cystic and common hepatic duct, the duct name changes to the CBD. The cystic duct junction is at an angle to the common bile duct in the vast majority of cases but can run parallel and even spiral around it, in a significant minority of patients (Fig. 16.1).

The CBD then passes in the free edge of the lesser omentum parallel to the gastro-hepatic artery and in front of the portal vein. Its blood supply has special importance to the surgeon and should be remembered. A network of small vessels which encapsulate the duct, arise from the nearby vessels; above from the right and left hepatic arteries, below from branches of the gastro-duodenal and retro-duodenal arteries. These vessels usually lie along the lateral border of the duct and an injudicious siting of a choledochotomy or use of diathermy may seriously impair the blood supply resulting in an ischaemic stricture. The venous drainage from the CBD is via an epicholedochal venous plexus which drains to the portal vein. The lymphatic drainage is to the coeliac plexus.

The CBD passes obliquely behind the first part of the duodenum, approaching the second part while lying on the posterior surface of the pancreas. The duct now lies within the bile duct-pancreatic groove and is usually separated from the duodenum by a thin layer of connective tissue only. If the duct is covered by a tongue of pan-

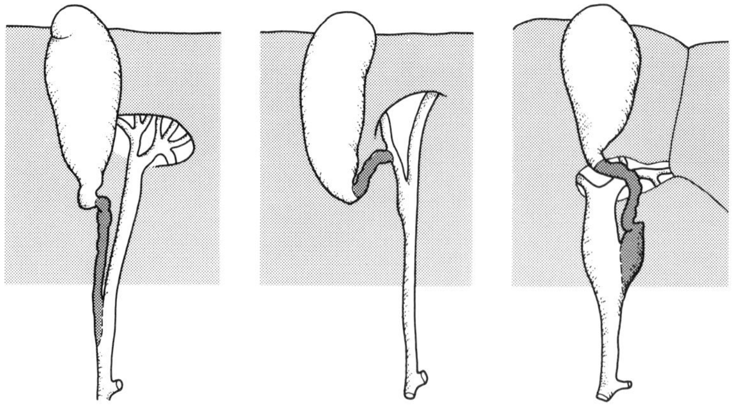

Fig. 16.1 Variations in the length and course of cystic duct.

creatic tissue arising from the left side of the groove, a plane of cleavage is always present and facilitates duct palpation from the right side. As it runs adjacent to the wall of the second part of the duodenum, the lumen of the duct begins to narrow and is associated with a corresponding thickening of its wall, the sphincter of Oddi. This narrow segment is of variable length ranging from 8–25 mm and gives the distal duct a characteristic radiological appearance, not to be confused with a biliary stricture. In some instances, an eccentric position of the distal duct in relation to its proximal segment gives rise to difficulties during blind instrumentation at exploration and can result in a false passage. Occasionally, localized areas of dilatation of the common duct immediately proximal to the narrow segment occur and stones may lodge within these pseudo-diverticulae. Not surprisingly, calculi can, therefore, be missed on blind exploration as instruments merely slide past. Post-exploration cholangiography or choledochoscopy, however, minimizes this risk.

A precise understanding of the sphincter mechanism and its relationship to the pancreatic duct opening is necessary to avert disaster during transduodenal biliary duct exploration. The main pancreatic duct (of Wirsung) runs transversely through the pancreas and turns sharply down to approach the distal as it lies in the CBD-pancreatic groove. The two ducts run adjacently for 1–2 cm. In approximately 75% of patients the pancreatic and the bile ducts unite and form a common channel, ranging in length from 5–20 mm. When this common channel is present, the pancreatic duct joins the distal CBD postero-medially and is usually observed in the 5 o'clock position at transduodenal exploration. However, other configurations can occur and should be noted (Fig. 16.2).

Detection of stones in the CBD

Common bile duct calculi present three diagnostic dilemmas: detection before or at the time of cholecystectomy; failure to identify stones during exploration of the CBD; and identification of residual common duct stones left behind after a previous exploration. The search for improved methods of stone detection has resulted in the introduction of a variety of pre-operative and intra-operative diagnostic techniques [1].

Pre-operative assessment

In patients with gallbladder stones awaiting cholecystectomy, the search for calculi in the CBD begins pre-operatively. From patient interview, it is important to establish a history of jaundice or any of its associated features such as dark coloured urine or pale stool. Similarly, a previous history of pancreatitis in a patient with established gallstones but no other apparent cause for pancreatic inflammation suggests a some-time diag-

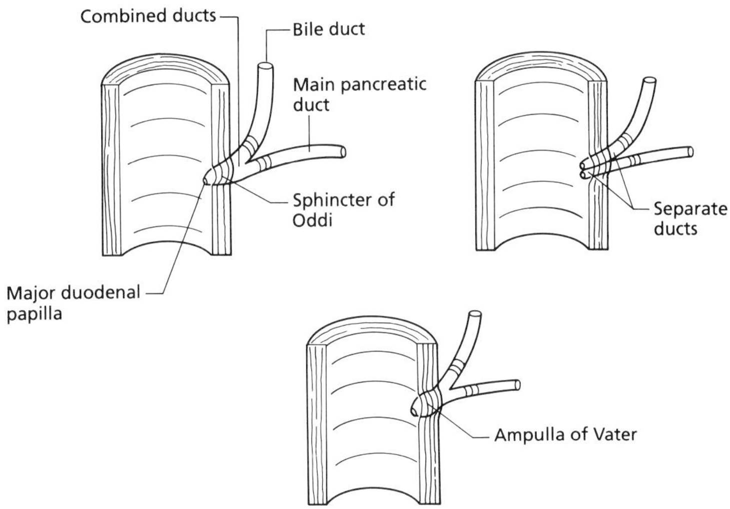

Fig. 16.2 Three common variations of terminations of bile and pancreatic ducts.

nosis of choledocholithiasis. The clinical symptoms of jaundice, rigors and right-upper quadrant abdominal pain known as Charcot's triad often denotes the presence of ductal stones, however, the vast majority of patients with common duct stones do not present with classical symptoms [2]. Careful physical examination may sometimes reveal stigmata of unresolved jaundice. Clinical assessment of the patient however is not sufficiently accurate to assess the extrahepatic biliary tree. In a series of 500 consecutive cystic duct cholangiograms performed to assess common duct pathology, Farha and Pearson found that relying on clinical criteria alone led to a negative duct exploration rate of 50% [3]. Clearly, investigations other than clinical assessment are necessary to assess the biliary tract. Urinalysis, which can be performed easily in the outpatient clinic or on the ward, can be useful in detecting an obstructive jaundice. Hepatic and pancreatic enzyme assays are always a necessary investigation, as an elevated alkaline phosphatase or bilirubin level often alerts the surgeon to an otherwise occult stone in the biliary ducts. However, unobstructing stones in the duct may well result in normal biochemistry.

Clinical assessment is augmented by some useful radiological procedures to aid in the diagnosis of ductal stones. Ultrasound remains the investigation of choice in gallbladder disease, detecting gallstones and gallbladder wall inflammation with ease [4]. It is both specific, sensitive, and reproducible. Ultrasound is also accurate in measuring CBD diameter but unfortunately its role in detecting common duct stones is less defined. The usual ultrasonic shadow cast by gallstones lying in the gallbladder is often absent with CBD calculi and the gas in the duodenum and adjacent intestinal loops may mask the typical acoustic profile of stones in the duct. Some studies record a sensitivity of only 15% [4]. Although such high false-negative rates fall greatly in patients with jaundice [5], it is an insufficiently powerful tool to predict stones within the duct. Bismuth and his co-workers studied common duct diameter in conjunction with clinical symptoms and biochemistry and formulated a prediction value for each parameter [6]. He reported that a duct diameter greater than 12 mm, plus either a raised alkaline phosphatase, past history of jaundice or a marginally elevated bilirubin gave a 90–100% positive predictive value for ductal stones in patients not obviously jaundiced. Dilated common ducts are not infrequently displayed on pre-operative ultrasound scans but do not always result from duct calculi. In addition to stone disease, Lygdikas found that dilatation of the CBD was related to patient age, presence or absence of previous biliary surgery, biliary infection and duration of history [7]. In this study, while common duct stones were found in 93% of patients with a CBD diameter greater than 15 mm, 6% of patients with stones had a duct of normal calibre. Undoubtedly, delay between radiological examination and operation is an important factor, the bile duct having the ability to alter diameter over a short time span [8]. It is likely that this phenomenon results from stone passage into the bowel before the patient gets to surgery, but may also be a feature of biliary dyskinesia. At any rate, CBD dilatation is not always due to stone blockage and conversely duct stones frequently occur without any increase in duct diameter. Cameron has reported a series of patients with ductal stones in whom there was no pre- or peri-operative evidence of duct dilatation [9].

Endoscopic retrograde cholangiography remains the most accurate pre-operative method to assess the CBD. It also allows the therapeutic option of sphincterotomy with stone extraction when indicated and permits concomitant pancreatic assessment in patients in whom the exact pathology is unclear [10]. Some patients harbour other common duct pathology which can mimic stones and in this respect endoscopic cholangiography is superior to all other tests in delineating biliary obstruction. However, even in expert hands there is a small but serious morbidity and recorded mortality with this invasive procedure [11]. Therefore, it probably has no role in routine screening of the bile ducts for stone disease in non-jaundiced patients with gallstone disease. Its principle use is in jaundiced patients to establish the level and cause of obstruction.

Iodine-based dye contrast studies of the biliary tract still have a place in the investigation of suspected duct stones and good quality intravenous cholangiography can often delineate duct blockage. Pre-operative intravenous cholangiography is favoured by many French surgeons with good results [12]. Percutaneous transhepatic cholangiography is an excellent imaging technique of the biliary tree. However, it is an invasive procedure with a morbidity of 5% or more and like retrograde cholangiography has no place in routine assessment [13]. In jaundiced patients with dilated ducts and in whom endoscopic evaluation of the duct is not possible, the percutaneous route may be preferred. Other modalities of pre-operative assessment of the extrahepatic biliary anatomy include liver excretion scintigraphic scanning, computed tomography (CT) and trans-nasal biliary manometery, none of which are commonly employed.

Peri-operative assessment

Despite the many advances in radiological technology, pre-operative suspicion of ductal stones is quite often only confirmed at operation. An obvious dilated duct frequently results in a palpable stone within its lumen. If calculi are suspected, then a formal mobilization of the second part of the duodenum and thorough palpation of the intra-enteric, as well as supraduodenal segments, of the duct is necessary if distal stones are not to be missed. The practice of operative cholangiography was until recently time-honoured and performed either routinely or for strict criteria by most surgeons, not only to delineate the presence of ductal stones, but also to identify the biliary anatomy and thereby effect safe surgery. The technique was first described by Mirrizzi in 1932 [14] and was modified subsequently by several others. Since then, many papers have emphasized the importance of cholangiography in detecting common duct stones that would have otherwise been overlooked. In brief, the examination is carried out by inserting a soft catheter into the cystic duct via a small ductotomy and passing it into the CBD. Care is taken to ensure that no air enters the duct, so the catheter is flushed with sterile saline prior to insertion. Occasionally, the spiral valve in the cystic duct renders insertion difficult and gentle dilatation of the duct is required. A distal ligature on the cystic duct secures the catheter *in situ*. Flow is tested by gently flushing some saline into the bile duct. Before taking the films, all instruments are removed from the operation field as are any swabs containing radio-opaque markers. The operating table is tilted 15° to the right to minimize the image superimposition over the vertebral column. A sterile towel is placed over the abdomen and the centre of the exposure is marked by a drop of saline. The X-ray machine or image intensifier, if available, is placed in position, preferably from the patient's left side. A 20 mL syringe containing 25% sodium diatrizoate replaces that containing saline. Again it is important to ensure that no air bubbles get into the lumen at this stage. Mechanical ventilation is momentarily interrupted while the films are exposed after slow injection of 3–5 mL and subsequently a second injection of 10–12 mL of dye. If the common duct is greatly dilated then it may be necessary to increase the volume accordingly. However, it is critical that only a small volume is injected initially, as the image of the lower part of the duct may be obscured by contrast and as a result, small filling defects can be missed. Figure 16.3 illustrates an operative cholangiogram with an obstructed common bile duct. Advances to the technique of cholangiography include the use of small dental films placed behind the second part of the duodenum to detect distal calculi. Although the technique has certain theoretical advantages over conventional cholangiography, it too has failed to eliminate the problem of retained stones.

The advent of laparoscopic cholecystectomy has effected a change in the practice of operative cholangiography [97, 98, 103]. Most laparoscopic biliary surgeons do not now perform routine cholangiography. Cuschieri reported on the European experience with the technique and found surgeons were using routine cholangiography in only 25% of cases [12]. A more selective policy of duct imaging has been adapted by the majority of surgeons and in the absence of certain predictive factors most surgeons forego the procedure. As in open cholecystectomy, endoscopic retrograde cholangiography in patients awaiting laparoscopic surgery is indicated in selected patients but has no role in the routine evaluation of the duct system [99–101] despite the therapeutic advantage of sphincterotomy to treat any calculi encountered.

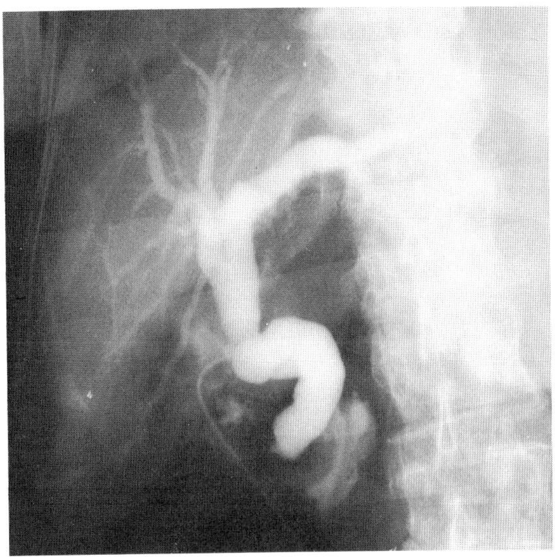

Fig. 16.3 Operative cholangiogram showing obstructed lower common bile duct due to impacted stone.

Intra-operative ultrasonic imaging to assess the status of the bile duct has also been evaluated in open cholecystectomy and the early results of the method are so far encouraging [15, 16]. The technique has further evolved and recently, it has been employed to assess the integrity of the bile duct during laparoscopic procedures [17, 18]. Both intra-luminal and transmural approaches have been described, but as yet there is insufficient data to comment properly on either system.

Surgical techniques

Laparoscopic surgery for gallbladder stone disease has almost relegated open cholecystectomy to the preceding era. The same cannot be said, however, for the problem of choledocholithiasis. Limited access to the lower segment of the duct, inability to feel stones within the duct, and the availability of relatively crude instrumentation for intra-duct visualization and stone extraction via the laparoscope has to date secured a role for open exploration of the bile duct. Undoubtedly, the rapid developments currently taking place in laparoscopic and endoscopic instrument technology will bring about a reversal of this situation, with open duct exploration ultimately reserved for the more complex problems and 'redo' procedures. In this section we describe the two techniques commonly employed to explore the bile duct at laparotomy. The supraduodenal route is favoured by most surgeons, though the transduodenal route has many advocates. As both techniques include the use of choledochoscopy, a technique which we believe is essential for proper duct exploration, an account of this procedure is also included.

Supraduodenal exploration

The patient is placed on an operating table which allows for on-table radiology. Sterile drapes are sutured to the skin rather than clipped, as this avoids any interference on the subsequent operative cholangiogram. The abdomen is opened through a midline, right paramedian or subcostal incision, depending on individual preference, and a full laparotomy is performed to exclude any other pathology. The gallbladder and the CBD are then palpated, particular attention being paid to the width, texture, thickness of the duct and whether any stones are present. The lower portion of the duct, the periampullary region, the duodenal papilla and the head of the pancreas can only be adequately assessed by fully mobilizing the second part of the duodenum as originally described by Kocher [102]. Having incised the peritoneum on the lateral border of the duodenum, the retro-duodenal plane is established using a dissecting scissors and the surgeon's hand is employed to extend this avascular plane to the left border of the aorta. When complete, the surgeon's hand can be introduced through the retro-duodenal space in front of the vena cava and aorta. The importance of this manœuvre is only fully appreciated when a choledochoscope is passed down the lower end of the duct to view the ampullary region. If cholangiography has not already been performed prior to cholecystectomy then it is obtained at this stage. Patients coming to surgery for retained stones following previous cholecystectomy often require a direct puncture of the bile duct as the cystic duct remnant can be difficult to find or utilize. If a recent endoscopic retrograde or percutaneous transhepatic cholangiogram is available and stones are adequately demonstrated, then some surgeons would forego operative cholangiography. The CBD is then explored. Two fine catgut sutures (4/0) are placed 5 mm apart into the anterior surface of the CBD and a 1 cm vertical choledochotomy is made between them using a no. 11 scalpel blade. Due care is taken to avoid the laterally placed vessels, which if damaged, may result in stricture formation at a later date. In order to facilitate subsequent introduction of a choledochoscope, the choledochotomy should be placed as near to the superior border of the duodenum as is safely possible. This is an important point because if the opening is more proximally placed, both the liver and the costal margin may make it difficult to introduce the choledochoscope into the distal duct, particularly if a rigid scope is used. A bile sample should be sent for microbiological culture at this stage. Routine exploration of the biliary tree is then carried out.

A variety of instruments are available for the removal of any stones including Desjardins forceps, Moynihan's malleable scoop, biliary balloon catheter, and 'Dormia'-type stone baskets. Individual preference will dictate which instruments are used, but as with all blind instrumentation, great care must be exercised to avoid damage to the ducts. This particularly applies to the lower end and the periampullary regions, where injudicious use of instruments such as Bake's dilators may result in the creation of a false passage or damage to the ampulla with subsequent stenosis. Routine exploration is completed by saline lavage of the biliary tree following which choledochoscopy is carried out. This is the sequence employed by most surgeons, although pre-exploratory endoscopy of the biliary tree has been reported. We advocate the use of the flexible choledochoscope as it allows greater manœuvrability within the duct system [67]. It is necessary to firstly establish a satisfactory irrigation system with the choledochoscope and we routinely use normal saline in 1 L bags, pre-warmed to slightly above body temperature and connected to the endoscope. It is important that the surgeon can control the flow of irrigation fluid by either an inbuilt tap on the instrument or ensuring the gate tap of the giving set remains sterile and is in his operation field. Some authors stress the importance of a constant pressure to maintain flow and recommend the use of a pressure infusor. We have found, however, that adequate flow and visualization are achieved by elevating the container of saline to a height of 80 cm above the patient. The total volume of saline needed varies, but the average is between 1–1.5 L. Before commencing choledochoscopy, it is necessary to take steps to retrieve the irrigating fluid. Failure to do so can lead to dissemination of potentially contaminated bile through the peritoneal cavity and unwelcome saturation of the surgical gowns and drapes. A Poole's type suction should be employed and large sterile gauze packs are suitably placed to isolate the duct from the peritoneal cavity.

To facilitate introduction of the end of the instrument into the CBD, the assistant places gentle traction on the stay sutures thus opening the choledochotomy. The main operating light is now switched off and the light source of the choledochoscope is switched on, as is the irrigation. Sometimes the choledochotomy is too large, resulting in excessive irrigation flow. This can be reduced by crossing over the stay sutures. Irrespective of choledochoscope type used, the surgeon holds the instrument in his right hand and the left hand is used to guide it inside the ducts. With the flexible instrument, the thumb of the right hand manipulates the directional control.

The initial view obtained is often red and hazy, but as the irrigation continues, bile, blood, fibrin and 'mud' are washed away and a clear view is obtained. The operator quickly learns to compensate for the distortion caused by magnification by altering the lens in relation to the site under observation. The greatest distortion occurs when the tip of the instrument is closest to the observed area, and the normal size relationship exists when the distance between the lens and the object under view is 1–2 cm. It is important that the complete lumen of the duct is constantly seen. With the flexible instrument this is achieved by combination of the directional control together with the rotation of the instrument about its long axis. The rigid choledochoscope can also be rotated about its long axis, but in addition it can be tilted in any direction.

The proximal ducts are explored first. The choledochoscope is slowly passed up the common hepatic duct. This usually has the appearance of an oval tube, with a pale yellow mucous membrane, through which a sparse submucosal vascular network can be seen. (Plate 16.1, opposite page 182.) The glandulae mucosae appear as minute pits in the mucous membrane 1–2 mm in size. As the instrument is advanced the bifurcation into the right and left hepatic ducts is observed and is easily identified by a vertical septum 0.5–1.2 cm in length, the carina. The right duct is explored first. It is usually 1–2 cm in length and has a characteristic reddish-yellow mucous membrane. It bifurcates into ventro-cranial, passing to the right and the dorso-caudal branches which further branches into two subdivisions. This carina can usually be seen. This is the usual configuration but other variants are known. An attempt is then made to advance the choledochoscope into the tertiary ducts, often difficult and at times impossible. Success requires manipulation of the instrument and where the flexible choledochoscope is used, this entails rotating it about its long axis in combination with judicious control of the directional control. Manipulation of the rigid instrument by its very nature is more limited and we have regularly been able to advance the flexible choledochoscope more proximally than the rigid one, where both have been used in the same patient. We have also found that the more experienced the operator, the more proximal can the instrument be advanced, so that not infrequently, the tertiary ducts are reached, particularly if they are dilated. The instrument is now removed and as with most forms of endoscopy, the best views are obtained on withdrawal and therefore requires careful and slow extraction.

The left hepatic duct is now examined and as it enters the common hepatic duct anteriorly it may be missed unless looked for. It is wider than the right and has prominent glandulae mucosae. It is well recognized that the left duct is often the place where stones are displaced during blind instrumentation and it is all the more important therefore that it is examined thoroughly. (Plate 16.2, opposite page 182.) Having done so, examination of the proximal biliary tree is complete and the instrument is withdrawn to the choledochotomy, great care being taken to keep the lumen in view at all times.

The choledochoscope is next inserted into the distal CBD. In the case of the rigid instrument, the liver and costal margin tend to hinder its proper insertion and manœuvrability and again we stress the importance of as distally placed choledochotomy as safety allows. Examination of the lower duct and periampullary region is facilitated if the surgeon stands on the patient's left side. Holding the instrument in his right hand, he controls the duodenum and the head of the pancreas with his left in the retro-duodenal space, thus straightening out the bile duct (Fig. 16.4). The choledochoscope is again slowly advanced towards the ampullary region with similar manœuvres to the proximal examination. The appearances of the distal duct are like those seen proximally with a yellowish-red mucosa and a sparse submucosal vascular network. The lumen gradually narrows and there is a transformation to the typical pattern of the ampullary mucosa. The sphincteric portion has a stellate appearance which can assume a variety of shapes depending on the peristaltic activity. Some workers inject methylene blue as a bolus through

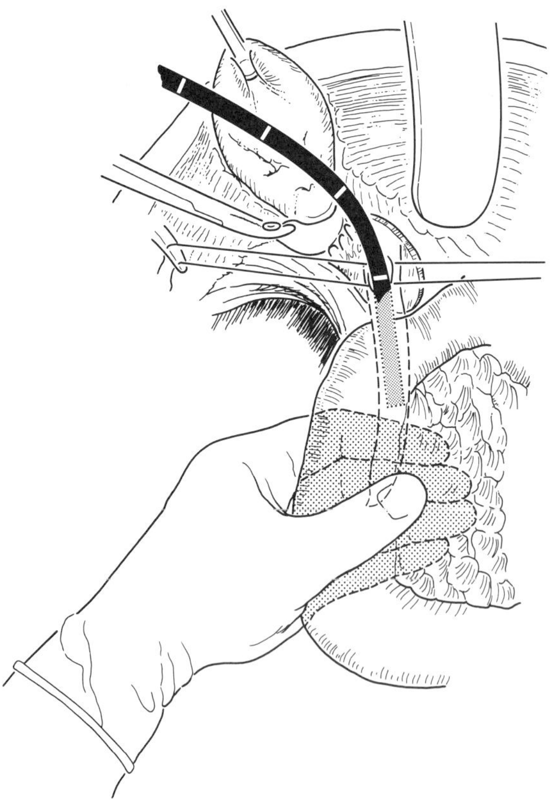

Fig. 16.4 Control of choledochoscope by left hand in retro-duodenal space.

the irrigation port of the instrument to stain the sphincteric mucosa, in order to get better views of the sphincteric region. It is claimed that the stained mucosa makes it easier to identify the contraction of the sphincter and to determine whether sphincteroplasty is necessary. Having examined the ampullary region, an attempt is made to pass the choledochoscope through the sphincter and into the duodenum. This is often facilitated by the use of the left hand in the retro-duodenal space to direct the instrument to the right and anteriorly. Again great care and gentleness must be exercised, otherwise severe damage or a false passage may result. Failure to visualize the ampullary region or the passage of the instrument through the duodenum means that this part of the examination is incomplete. Most authors agree that it is the ampullary region where stones are most frequently missed following supra-duodenal bile duct exploration and choledochoscopy.

Where stones are found under direct vision, a variety of techniques may be used to extract them. (Plate 16.3, opposite page 182.) The choledochoscope can be removed and as in the initial pre-endoscopy exploration, further blind instrumentation employed. Most surgeons, however, prefer to remove them under direct vision. To this end, all modern choledochoscopes have a channel down which a variety of instruments may be passed. These include balloon catheters, 'Dormia'-type stone baskets, stone grasping forceps and stone crushing forceps. We have found the balloon catheter both easy to use and effective and have successfully employed the no. 3 and no. 4 Fogarty biliary catheters. The choice of catheter is governed by the size of the stone and its position in the biliary tree. The catheter is passed slowly down the instrument port and is advanced until the tip and balloon segment have passed beyond the stone. The balloon is inflated with the required volume of saline, following which the instrument and catheter are slowly withdrawn from the biliary tree as a unit. Care should be taken that it is the surgeon who controls the balloon pressure and the withdrawal process himself. Failure to do so can result in the balloon being inflated to a diameter greater than that of the bile duct, which may result in damage to the wall. Conversely, if the diameter of the balloon is too small from insufficient pressure, then the stone will slide past and remain in the duct.

The 'Dormia'-type stone basket is also very effective particularly for the slightly larger stone. It is passed down the instrument port in similar manner to the balloon catheter and is advanced until the basket segment lies beyond the stone. The basket is opened and under direct vision the stone is engaged. The basket is closed and removed together with the choledochoscope. From time to time, stones become impacted either high up in the biliary tree, or low down at the ampulla in such a way that they are impossible to remove using either of the two described techniques. In this situation the crushing or grasping forceps are of particular value in fragmenting the stone. The residual stone debris can then be flushed out following removal of the choledochoscope. Reintroduction of the instrument identifies any remaining stone debris which can be further dealt with by any of the methods described. In the past few years contact shock wave lithotripsy has also been evaluated and used regularly in cases of impacted stones. The probe is passed down the bile duct and approximated to the stone and the resulting mechanical shock waves generated result in complete or partial fragmentation of stone [112].

During the course of the exploration a variety of other abnormalities may be encountered. On rare occasions, a stricture or duct neoplasm may be seen and these can be biopsied under direct vision. More commonly, cholangitis is present and the appearance of this can vary depending on the severity of the inflammation.

When the exploration is completed, the choledochotomy is closed with interrupted 2/0 catgut sutures around a latex rubber T-tube. The size of this tube is determined by the size of the bile duct but also on the relative success of the procedure. If the exploration is incomplete or the surgeon is unable to extract an impacted stone the largest T-tube possible should be placed. The minimal size of T-tube employed should not be less than a 14 F and more preferably a 16 F. When the T-tube track matures, subsequent access to the biliary tree is possible so that postoperative choledochoscopy or fluoroscopic-guided instrumentation can be performed. The abdomen is then closed with or without drainage of the sub-hepatic space and the T-tube is brought through the abdominal wall laterally and away from the main wound and in as direct route as is possible.

Transduodenal exploration of the CBD: sphincterotomy and sphincteroplasty

The position of the patient on the operating table, the incision and the assessment of the biliary tree is identical to the supra-duodenal operation. Having decided to proceed with the transduodenal technique, the first step is to identify the duodenal papilla, which can usually be palpated as a small nipple on the medial wall of the second part of the duodenum. This can often be quite difficult and requires a degree of experience. Once again we stress the importance of full mobilization of the second part of the duodenum and the head of the pancreas. A more simple and reliable method is to advance the cannula used for the operative cholangiogram down the duct and into the duodenum. We recommend a soft 6 F gauge Portex cannula which has been introduced via the cystic duct or if the patient has had a cholecystectomy previously, via the cystic duct remnant. With the soft cannula easily palpable within the duodenal lumen, the surgeon can now select the appropriate site for duodenotomy. This is achieved via a 1 cm vertical incision made between two catgut stay sutures on the anterior wall of the second part of the duodenum. Incisions on the lateral surface of the duodenum result in a higher incidence of duodenal leak and fistulae.

The cannula is delivered through the duodenotomy and with appropriate retraction, the duodenal papilla is easily identified. Stay sutures are next placed through the anterior wall of the papilla at 9 o'clock and 1 o'clock positions. For these we use 2/0 chromic catgut. A grooved probe is then inserted into the CBD to facilitate the sphincterotomy and we recommend that the cholangiogram catheter may be used to guide its insertion. The probe is introduced into the lumen of the Portex cannula, both of which are then withdrawn back into the lower duct. Attempts to insert the cannula blindly and without guidance from above should be avoided as it can result in formation of a false passage and not infrequently, pancreatic duct cannulation and possible damage. With the grooved probe safely in the intra-duodenal segment of the duct and using it as a guide, a 1.5 cm sphincterotomy is made in the 11 o'clock position between the stay sutures. The sphincterotomy is started with a fine pointed no. 11 blade and completed with a Pott's angled scissors. The incision is made at 11 o'clock in order to avoid damage to the pancreatic duct, which is usually at the 5 o'clock position. The opening of the pancreatic duct can be seen to secrete clear juice and its position can be confirmed by inserting a fine metal probe. If difficulty is encountered with its identification, some authors recommend intravenous injection of secretin to stimulate flow of pancreatic juice. When the pancreatic duct has been accurately localized, a safe sphincteroplasty can then be performed. This is done by suturing the duct mucosa to the duodenal wall with interrupted 4/0 ethibond sutures. Particular care is required at the apex of the sphincterotomy where the walls of the bile duct and duodenum diverge. Failure to accurately approximate them might result in this area being disrupted at subsequent instrumentation. It is for this reason that we recommend the sphincteroplasty be complete before exploration and choledochoscopy are carried out. The instruments used to explore the CBD by the transduodenal route are the same as those used in the supra-duodenal exploration and once again stones are removed using Moynihan's malleable scoop, Desjardin's forceps and various biliary balloon catheters. Routine exploration is completed by irrigating the biliary tree with normal saline via a Jaques catheter.

As in the supra-duodenal approach, choledochoscopy usually follows routine exploration. However, in the transduodenal approach to the bile ducts, reversing this sequence confers some theoretical advantages, in that blind instrumentation might result in stones easily accessible in the common bile and common hepatic ducts being pushed higher into the liver and therefore rendered relatively inaccessible from the duodenum. Should choledochoscopy be performed initially, these stones could be seen lower down and easily removed under direct vision. The set up of the choledochoscope and its accessories is identical to that described earlier. The surgeon stands on the patient's right side and with the assistant gently retracting stay sutures of the sphincteroplasty, the choledochoscope is easily introduced into the CBD. The main operating light is switched off and the instrument light source connected and irrigation commenced. As before, care is taken to collect all the irrigation fluid and in order to minimize the volume used the surgeon should ensure that the cystic duct has been ligated. As the instrument is being advanced excellent views of the lower end of the bile duct are obtained. The first anatomical landmark to be seen is the junction of the cystic duct and the common hepatic duct. The distance travelled to this junction is variable depending on the level at which the cystic duct joins the hepatic duct. The cystic duct opening is carefully inspected and if dilated, the scope should be carefully advanced up its lumen as high as possible. Stones can sometimes lodge at this point and may subsequently enter the main duct to produce symptoms. Difficulty can sometimes be encountered in advancing the instrument beyond this junction, and particularly if the cystic duct is dilated, the scope tends to selectively enter the lumen of the duct. This can be overcome by manipulating the choledochoscope with the left hand placed behind the duodenum and the CBD. Once past the cystic duct, the appearances of the biliary tree and the techniques employed to negotiate the intrahepatic branches are as described under supra-duodenal exploration. Again, care is taken to ensure that the lumen is kept constantly in view, both as the instrument is being introduced and as it is being withdrawn. The appearances of both normal and abnormal duct findings are as described and stones seen can be removed under direct vision by instruments passed down the choledochoscope.

One aspect of technique which we have found particularly helpful with transduodenal exploration and choledochoscopy relates to the size of balloon and basket which can be accommodated by the instrument channel on the choledochoscope. The largest Fogarty catheters (or equivalent sized stone basket) which will pass down the instrument port is no. 4. Frequently, where the bile duct is dilated the inflated balloon on this size of catheter does not fill the diameter and allows the stone to slip between the wall and the balloon. This problem is overcome by using much bigger catheters (no. 5 and no. 6) and passing them along the side of the choledochoscope, a manœuvre which still allows instrumentation under direct vision.

When choledochoscopy is completed the duodenotomy is closed in two layers of continuous catgut and interrupted linen. A drain of the surgeon's choice is placed into the sub-hepatic space and the abdomen is closed in the routine manner. A latex T-tube is not usually employed in this technique. On rare occasions a stone may be seen impacted high up in the liver but all attempts at its removal fail. A 14 F–16 F gauge T-tube should then be inserted into the supra-duodenal duct to provide a mature T-tube track through which postoperative instrumentation can later take place.

Natural history of common bile duct stones

Surgical doctrine has traditionally highlighted the adverse natural history of a non-operative policy to stones in the CBD. Surgical and more recently, endoscopic stone extraction have been recommended to obviate the complications of choledocholithiasis. Evidence has come to light of a sub-population of asymptomatic patients harbouring common duct stones for years. As long ago as 1941, Millbourn reported 38 patients with CBD stones who were either unfit for or declined surgery [19]. He found that in a 6-month to 13-year follow-up, 45% of these patients had no further symptoms attributable to their calculi. Since then it has become accepted that ductal stones are not always malevolent. Autopsy studies of patients dying from causes other than biliary tract diseases have shown that up to 25% of patients noted to have incidental gallstones also had asymptomatic ductal stones at the time of death [20, 21]. In one autopsy series, 23% of patients older than 60 years had cholelithiasis of whom more than 50% had asymptomatic common duct stones [113]. Moreover, it would appear that gallstones can not only lie dormant in the duct system for years but they can also pass from the bile duct into the duodenum without incident. In two separate studies, Acosta and Kelly both demonstrated that a significant number of patients with gallstone pancreatitis have gallstones in their faeces. Of more interest, however, is the observation that gallstones are also present in the faeces of 12% of control patients without pancreatitis, confirming their benign natural history in some patients [22, 23]. Evidence that stones can pass without incident from the duct into the gut is also seen in patients known to have retained stones following surgery of the bile duct and confirmed by post-exploration T-tube cholangiography. By the time of the interval T-tube cholangiogram, usually 7–10 days following surgery, approximately 20% of retained stones will have passed into the duodenum without deleterious effect [24]. In general, it should be remembered that most stones that pass spontaneously are small and tend not to obstruct the duct.

The majority of patients with ductal stones do not have an uneventful outcome, however, with approximately 75% of patients with choledocholithiasis ultimately developing symptoms [25]. As with gallbladder stones, the incidence of ductal stones increases with age and duration of gallstone disease, suggesting that the migration of stones into the duct is also time-dependent [26]. Because life expectancy has increased over the past few decades, elderly patients with cardiorespiratory problems frequently present with gallstone disease. With the increased morbidity encountered in this subset of patients, surgeons are not infrequently reluctant to perform cholecystectomy on them [27]. The consequences of this are that patients are even older by the time complications of choledocholithiasis occur. Over 40 000 cholecystectomies are performed for calculous disease each year in the UK [28] and it is estimated that between 500 000 and 700 000 patients undergo removal of the gallbladder in the USA annually [29]. The incidence of cholecystectomy in Scandinavia is probably higher than in this country, with 5 000 per million population requiring gallbladder surgery for stones [114]. One in every nine patients will require attention for concomitant common duct stones and of these, one-third are older than 65 years. In patients older than 80 years with gallstones, there is an even greater incidence of ductal stones with as many as 33% requiring ductal surgery — this in an age group where between 25–48% will develop serious complications [30]. In the UK, approximately 4 000 bile duct explorations are performed annually, but again this is not an accurate reflection of the incidence of choledocholithiasis, as many patients will be treated by endoscopic surgery or alternative modalities [65]. Nonetheless, it is widely accepted that the presence of a stone within the duct is generally an indication for its removal, only the method and timing of extraction remain controversial.

Supra-duodenal or transduodenal exploration: for and against

Surgery of the common duct has been practised for 100 years. Supra-duodenal exploration was described in 1884 [31] and apart from the developments in cholangiography and choledochoscopy, the procedure has changed little since then. It is the technique most favoured by biliary surgeons worldwide in operative management of ductal stones. Transduodenal removal of an impacted stone in the ampulla of Vater was first reported by McBurney in 1891 [32], who 7 years later described six further cases in which formal sphincterotomy was performed [33].

The principal criteria which govern the relative success of any operation include the degree of morbidity associated with it and the durability of the procedure in preventing disease recurrence. Failure to attain one or both of these mitigates strongly against the technique. Of the two surgical methods of CBD exploration, it should be noted that neither operation is easy to perform and both can give rise to serious complications, even in experienced hands. Technically, the transduodenal approach is more difficult and as already described, requires certain precise attention to detail, particularly in correct identification and protection of the pancreatic duct orifice. The procedure has its firm proponents however and it is apparent that exploration across the ampulla of Vater has much to recommend it. In supra-duodenal exploration, a complication encountered with a worrying degree of frequency is damage that can result from blind instrumentation of the intraduodenal segment of the duct. This can result in a false passage or distal duct perforation, the consequences of which may be disastrous. Furthermore, in the supra-duodenal approach to the CBD, the axis of catheter or instrument insertion is at a right angles to both the choledochotomy and course of the bile duct. Attempts to negotiate this angle may predispose to longitudinal tears along the choledochotomy or even perforation of the wall. Such injuries have been again cited as a potential cause of late bile duct stricture in patients, particularly with non-dilated ducts requiring exploration [9]. Also it is well recognized that the most common site for retained stones is at the periampullary end of the duct, as seen when completion cholangiography or choledochoscopy are employed [9]. This is the least accessible region from a supra-duodenal approach whereas transduodenal exposure allows both direct access to this site and also avoids blind instrumentation of the intraduodenal segment of the duct. Concomitant sphincteroplasty, an integral part of the transduodenal procedure, also permits this narrowest part of the duct to be dilated and facilitates delayed passage of the rare missed or non-recoverable stones into the duodenum. This appears to be confirmed in at least one large follow-up series in which the incidence of symptomatic retained stones following transduodenal exploration was only 1% [34]. The corresponding figure seen with supra-duodenal exploration is between 4 and 22% [35–38]. An almost constant feature of supra-duodenal exploration is that the duct is closed over a T-tube which unless the duct is particularly dilated can further compromise the internal diameter of the duct. Not only may the patient be then predisposed to short-term obstructive complications or in some instances the development of late strictures, but also where a small tube is used in a non-dilated duct, difficulty in postoperative mechanical retrieval of retained stones through a narrow tube tract may be experienced. Another infrequent but not rare complication of supraduodenal exploration and not seen with transduodenal surgery is devascularization injury to the duct. As described in the anatomy section of this chapter, the blood supply to the middle-third of the common duct is scant and injudicious use of diathermy or of stripping clean the duct can lead to the development of late ischaemic strictures.

Evolution of bile duct surgery

There have been several significant landmarks in the perfection of open common duct exploration as practised today. An excellent and detailed account of the history of the procedures has been written by Longmire [39]. Although the surgical procedures have changed little, the intra-operative techniques to assess the extent of stone disease and minimize the incidence of retained calculi have flourished. Intra-operative post-exploratory cholangiography has been shown to reduce significantly the incidence of retained stones [40]. With choledochoscopy, this incidence has fallen even further [41]. One series in which both modalities of assessment were used prospectively in patients having either supra- or transduodenal exploration found no retained stones as determined by subsequent T-tube cholangiography [42].

The remarkable evolution of endoscopic biliary surgery and stone extraction techniques over the past 15 years, however, has transformed the management of biliary duct calculi. Once the mainstay of treatment, surgery is now often reserved for complicated cases and failed endoscopic procedures. In the early days of endoscopic surgery, the technique was confined only to those patients who had undergone previous removal of the gallbladder or already had a duct exploration and were subsequently noted to have recurrent stones. Additionally, the procedure was deemed quite suitable for patients considered to be medically unfit for major surgery [43–49]. Since then, applications of the procedure have broadened widely and today, young patients awaiting laparoscopic or open cholecystectomy with stones suspected or confirmed within the duct are readily submitted to endoscopic evaluation and subsequent sphincterotomy with stone extraction where necessary. Several European and North American centres have virtually abandoned surgical exploration of the duct and now routinely use the endoscopic route as the treatment of choice in the management of ductal stones [50–53].

The indications for cholecystectomy after successful endoscopic extraction of stones when life expectancy is short need to be closely reexamined. In a recently published series, 191 elderly and infirm patients were treated endoscopically for ductal stones, the gallbladder being left *in situ* [54]. Subsequently, only 5% of these patients underwent cholecystectomy for further acute symptoms. Although 25% of the group died within 3 years, none of the deaths were attributable to biliary complications. It was concluded that this group of patients did not need further gallbladder surgery. A similar Swedish study found that over a median observation period of 42 months, only 11% of 148 mainly elderly patients treated by sphincterotomy alone developed gallbladder symptoms, necessitating cholecystectomy. The life-table probability of remaining free from cholecystectomy-requiring symptoms or biliary-related complication was 0.87 in this three- and a half-year period [55]. In another study from Sweden, Rosseland followed 75 patients for up to 8 years and found only 12 eventually required cholecystectomy [51]. Worthley and Toouli, in Australia, also observed 20 debilitated and elderly patients who had sphincterotomy without subsequent cholecystectomy [56]. Interestingly, they found that of eight patients shown to have an obstructed cystic duct, six developed acute cholecystitis and three of these patients died. They concluded that the presence of cystic duct occlusion at initial endoscopic cholangiography, as reflected by non-filling of the gallbladder with contrast medium, is an indication for removal of the viscus. Their findings are supported by results in a similar Japanese study [57]. The consensus is that the less invasive procedure of endoscopic sphincterotomy may be prudent in selected elderly patients. However, it must be acknowledged that if such a policy is to be applied to all patients presenting with choledocholithiasis, up to 50% of younger patients treated by sphincterotomy and stone extraction without subsequent cholecystectomy may ultimately develop biliary-induced pancreatitis [58].

In the past 2 decades, other non-operative approaches to the management of CBD stones such as direct contact and extra-corporeal shock wave lithotripsy, dissolution therapy and percutaneous transhepatic stone removal have broadened the alternatives to both conventional and endoscopic surgery. Most recently, significant advances have been made in the field of laparoscopic surgery, with procedures on the bile duct to extract stones now commonplace in some centres. Petelin [59], Carroll *et al.* [60], Zucker [61] and others [104, 105], have all independently reported success with laparoscopic extraction of common duct stones. The procedure does not yet enjoy popular use but as technological and surgical skills in laparoscopic surgery develop, it is likely that this technique will become widely accepted.

Outcome of biliary tract surgery for stones

The increased mortality observed with addition of either supra- or transduodenal exploration to cholecystectomy is seen in all patient groups but particularly so in the older subgroup. Patients having emergency operations or surgery in the presence of acute cholecystitis are also at considerably higher risk of developing complications. The true mortality in patients over 60 years, who are complicated by jaundice, cholangitis, stricture, undergoing re-operation or other serious illnesses probably lies between 5% and 28% [62]. McSherry and Glenn have reported a mortality rate of 8% in unfit patients [63]. Houghton *et al.* have also reported a worrying 20% death-rate in elderly patients and recommended that the procedure only be performed by experienced surgeons and in low-risk patients [64]. Despite these discouraging figures, large series of patients with low or no mortality have been reported for both supra- and transduodenal procedures and are to be commended. Menzies and Motson reported no operation-related deaths in a series of 108 patients having supra-duodenal duct exploration [65]. Kramling recently reported an admirable death-rate of only 1% in 420 patients undergoing supra-duodenal duct exploration [10]. McEntee *et al.* have published work recording one death in 56 patients with transduodenal exploration; with no mortality in a further 81 consecutive supra-duodenal explorations, and advocated a return to the latter technique [66].

In a previous paper from this department (at the St James University Hospital, Leeds), we have reported an operation-related mortality of 2% in 100 consecutive transduodenal explorations of the common duct, with no mortality recorded in patients under 60 years [67]. In the largest review of transduodenal sphincteroplasties reported to date, Stefanini *et al.* recorded an impressive 1.1% mortality in 712 consecutive procedures, with only one death resulting from pancreatitis [68]. Similarly, in the USA, Cameron reported no deaths in patients having transduodenal exploration with ductal stones but non-dilated ducts, and recommended the procedure for this subgroup [69] In their paper on bile duct surgery for stone disease, Hardy and Davenport reported a 1.7% mortality rate in 101 patients undergoing transduodenal exploration of the duct [69]. Disappointingly however, the same authors recorded an 11% mortality rate in a further 208 patients as part of a subsequent report [70]. The reasons for this were not clear, but it was believed that the second series included a greater proportion of elderly and infirm patients. In general, the relative risk of mortality in supra-duodenal duct surgery is approximately 2%, a rate slightly lower than usually seen with transduodenal exploration.

A vogue for using a combined technique has been advocated in some situations, particularly where distal impaction of a calculus occurs in patients having had an unsuccessful supra-duodenal procedure. Aubrey and Edwards reported no deaths in a series of 42 consecutive cases with only one case of postoperative pancreatitis [71]. Vellacott and Powell, however, have had a different experience using combined procedures, with one-third of all patients not surviving [72]. Only 12 patients of a series of 122 having duct surgery for stones had both transduodenal and supra-duodenal exploration, of whom four died. In all, nine patients died, with the combined procedures accounting for almost one-half of all deaths but only 10% of all operations.

A number of authors have found that a negative exploration of the duct did not increase the overall mortality or significant morbidity from the procedure. McSherry has shown that negative exploration is not harmful in younger, relatively fit patients, with one death out of 221 negative explorations [63]. At the time of the study, this was the same mortality for elective cholecystectomy alone in the author's own institution. However, in a more recent review of 42 474 open cholecystectomies performed in the USA, the overall mortality rate recorded was less than 0.03% for patients younger than 65 years and it is against such current yardsticks that mortality figures for laparoscopic cholecystectomy must be measured [28].

Non-fatal morbidity is not an infrequent consequence of duct exploration and has influenced the acceptance of these surgical procedures over the past few decades. The specific complications of most concern are pancreatitis, intra-abdominal sepsis, and haemorrhage. Cardio-respiratory compromise can also arise in certain older patients requiring prolonged anaesthesia for difficult biliary surgery. A complication unique to the transduodenal approach is lateral duodenal fistulae which alone carries a mortality as high as 5%. As with many intra-abdominal operations, complications are encountered with a greater frequency in the emergency setting, including acute cholecystitis. Postoperative pancreatitis may complicate any operation on the biliary tract, particularly if it is protracted but usually follows surgery on the sphincter [73–76]. In 214 transduodenal explorations performed over an 8-year period, Cave-Bigley reported an 18% incidence of pancreatitis [70]. Unfortunately, there is a problem in accurately assessing the incidence of pancreatitis in the postoperative patient. Serum amylase alone may be a misleading investigation and a diagnosis should not be made on the basis of the biochemical findings alone. Keighley and Graham showed an elevation of the serum amylase level in over 30% of patients undergoing exploration of the CBD, most of whom had no symptoms to support a pancreatitis attack [77]. In the Leeds series, we found that 50% of patients had hyperamylasaemia within the first 5 days post-surgery, yet only 6% of the group were considered to have pancreatitis [67]. Previous episodes of pancreatitis also greatly increase the risk of further post-exploratory inflammation and as a result Peel *et al.* have recommended that a prior attack of pancreatitis should be considered an absolute contraindication to transduodenal exploration [78]. For the same reasons, Imrie *et al.* have concluded that supra-duodenal duct exploration is always preferable to the transduodenal approach in patients presenting initially with pancreatitis [79]. Sheridan *et al.* [80] have reported an alarming overall morbidity of 46% in a series of patients undergoing supra-duodenal duct exploration, with a similar experience documented at Johns Hopkins, where a 28% non-fatal morbidity was recorded for patients having transduodenal exploration of the common bile duct [9]. Despite these figures, overall morbidity for duct exploration is between 10–20%.

Surgery or sphincterotomy?

Unfortunately, an almost constant feature in many of the studies cited is that almost all are retrospective reviews, making meaningful interpretation of their data difficult. They are further flawed in that mortality and morbidity rates recorded are more often related to the debilitated condition of patients with jaundice, sepsis and cardiorespiratory disease who require ductal surgery, rather than the influence of the additional procedure. It is important, therefore, to analyse critically each study presenting results on exploration of the CBD, as several important differences in patient populations frequently exist. Patients having duct exploration for stones found incidentally during cholecystectomy cannot be compared with patients having biliary decompression for cholangitis and sepsis who also undergo concomitant cholecystectomy, although the operative procedures are essentially identical. Argument against open surgery in favour of endoscopic sphincterotomy and stone extraction has been supported by a stated lower mortality and incidence of non-fatal complications in the latter technique. In a worthwhile review of the literature on the complications associated with endoscopic biliary surgery, Thornton and Axon have questioned whether the procedure is actually safer than surgery [11]. With a procedure-related mortality of less than 1% and a morbidity of around 7% [82, 83], therapeutic endoscopy certainly compares favourably with the mortality and morbidity of open surgery for common duct stones [84]. Nonetheless, significant haemorrhage [83], acute pancreatitis [82, 85], and endoscope introduced or induced infection have been frequently recorded [86–90]. In the Middlesex Hospital series of 1 000 endoscopic sphincterotomies performed, the incidence of haemorrhage was 3.6%, with transfusion required in 0.6% [83].

As the complication rate is less than that experienced with open exploration, it would seem logical that in patients with known ductal stones, open cholecystectomy following a pre-operative endoscopic sphincterotomy and stone extraction should present an attractive alternative to open surgical duct exploration. Indeed, the results of several retrospective studies have indicated that such a staged treatment policy of CBD stones may be better than open surgical duct exploration alone [47, 50, 91, 92]. Furthermore, with the recent graduation to laparoscopic surgery several authors have already discovered pre-operative endoscopic sphincterotomy to be an excellent technique in dealing with suspected or confirmed ductal stones [10, 61]. Surprisingly, there have been only a few properly constructed trials comparing directly the efficacy of a precholecystectomy endoscopic sphincterotomy versus surgical exploration of the duct plus concomitant cholecystectomy. Neoptolemos, having randomized patients to such a study, found no benefit in having precholecystectomy-endoscopic procedures and in fact noted a less favourable outcome and greater morbidity in those having this additional procedure [93]. In a similarly constructed and more recent study from Los Angeles, Stain has confirmed the findings of the Leicester group. In other words, surgery alone was more efficacious in clearing the bile duct than pre-operative endoscopic clearance followed by surgery [94]. Other prospective but non-randomized studies also support a non-endoscopic approach to the management of ductal stones. Toouli has directly compared endoscopic with open procedures prospectively and while his findings favour an endoscopic approach in the elderly, he has concluded that an operative policy was more suitable for the young patient [95]. The Austrian experience of Schwab *et al.*, comparing patients having endoscopic sphincterotomy or open surgery was similar [27]. There was no difference in the mortality rate between groups and the incidence of retained stones was significantly lower in the group that underwent surgical treatment. The resultant failure of attempted endoscopic clearance of the common duct to confer benefit to patients undergoing cholecystectomy in randomized and controlled settings is disappointing, as the technique has many potential benefits for the patient. Successful removal of the ductal stones makes the subsequent operation safer and simpler by avoiding surgery on the duct. Secondly, in jaundiced patients or in the presence of cholangitis successful endoscopic sphincterotomy permits deferral of cholecystectomy until the condition of the patient can be optimized. Furthermore, pre-operative endoscopic retrograde cholangiography also allows the surgeon to see the number and position of the stones within the duct and take notice of any biliary anomalies if present. Finally, in selected elderly patients, surgery may be postponed indefinitely with minimal risk of subsequent life-threatening complications from the *in situ* gallbladder.

Problem of retained and recurrent ductal stones

It is important to note the various terminologies used for stones found in the bile ducts following duct exploration. Retained stones are those detected in the duct usually by T-tube cholangiogram, in the immediate postoperative period and are likely to have been overlooked at the original operation. By convention surgeons have referred to these stones as residual stones. Rarely, stones can form primarily within the bile ducts following removal of the gallbladder and where these occur they are termed recurrent ductal stones [96]. If stones are detected within the bile duct within a 2-year period following exploration then it is accepted that calculi are residual rather than recurrent. Beyond this time, it is assumed that stones have formed *de novo* and are considered to be primary common duct stones. It is important to distinguish between the two conditions as continuous primary stone formation within the duct may require a permanent drainage procedure whereas residual stones can be adequately treated by extraction techniques alone.

Although most initial operations for calculous disease of the CBD are curative, concern has been expressed at the high incidence of retained stones. Factors bearing on the incidence of retained stones include the inexperience of the surgeon and failure to use choledochoscopy or perform completion cholangiography. Supraduodenal exploration is associated with a retained stone rate between 4–30% [97], a lower incidence approaching 2% noted in patients undergoing transduodenal surgery [34, 67]. The incidence of retained stones seems to be related to the number of stones found in the duct at the original operation. In negative explorations of the duct the retained stone rate is only 1–4% but this figure rises to 30% if up to four stones were extracted initially [98].

Surgery for recurrent or residual stones is technically difficult and is best avoided. Biliary re-operation is associated with a further recurrence rate as high as 10% with an even higher recurrence rate for subsequent explorations [99]. The hazards of re-exploration is reflected in the number of papers supporting non-operative retrieval of retained calculi. It is not possible to describe in detail here the many alternatives to operative surgery for retained stones, which are dealt with in Chapters 17–20. Of these, endoscopic sphincterotomy has evolved as an excellent alternative to re-exploration. In skilled hands sphinc-terotomy can be performed in about 95% of cases and 90% of these will have a successful extraction of stones from the duct, giving an overall stone clearance figure of 85%. The incidence of failed clearance of the common duct for retained stones following endoscopic sphincterotomy is between 4–10% [106, 107]. Not surprisingly, the com-plication rate in patients having endoscopic extraction of retained stones is also higher when compared with patients undergoing a primary procedure. Retroperitoneal perforation, pancreatitis and haemorrhage are seen more frequently in procedures for retained stones and 1% of patients require an emergency laparotomy [62]. The mortality rate is 1.4% which is twice the normal for primary endoscopic sphincterotomy [62]. Comparative results following surgical re-exploration of the bile duct are available and vary between an 18–83% incidence of further stone retention, depending on the number of previous choledochotomies [108–110]. These figures are improved if an internal drainage procedure is performed. The mortality rate for 'redo' procedures may be as high as 5% which is two to three times greater than recorded for endoscopic sphincterotomy. Although endoscopic clearance may be preferable, it is sometimes not possible particularly where a stricture occurs below a retained stone or in the presence of a tortuous bile duct. Residual or recurrent large stones, greater than 20 mm in diameter, is also a frequent indi-cation for an operation approach. Today, surgery is often reserved for these selected groups of patients with retained stones who have failed endoscopic or an alternative method of stone removal.

If an operative policy is deemed appropriate then patients should undergo re-exploration 6–8 weeks after the primary procedure. Earlier than this makes the operation technically more difficult and the mortality rate is significantly higher if the second operation takes place within 3 weeks of initial surgery. The most straightforward approach is a supra-duodenal re-exploration with insertion of a T-tube to permit drainage of the duct. The disadvantage of this technique is the high recurrence rate of stones and particularly if the duct is still dilated. Way and his group recorded only a 60% success rate if the duct was greater than 20 mm in diameter, but were successful in non-dilated ducts [110]. Some surgeons leave the T-tube *in situ* for a 6–8-week period to allow a mature tract to form. Should the duct then be shown to contain further calculi, radiologically assisted extractions can then be performed [115].

Transduodenal sphincteroplasty is indicated in those patients with multiple small stones and a normal diameter duct. The procedure is exactly as described earlier in the chapter and again we stress the importance of careful choledochoscopy. Not infrequently, a residual stone will be impacted in the ampullary region, making the sphincterotomy part of the procedure easier to perform. Biliary-enteric anastomosis, either as choledochoduodenostomy or Roux-en-Y choledochojejunostomy is indicated in patients with very large multiple stones and a dilated duct. These procedures must also be considered for a second 'redo' procedure irrespective of the findings. Both procedures are difficult to perform in patients with a normal diameter duct. Choledochoduodenostomy can be constructed in either side-to-side or end-to-side fashion and although the latter technique theoretically minimizes the risk of a Distal Duct Sump Syndrome, this has yet to be confirmed. Some authors prefer to use a Roux-en-Y choledochojejunostomy with the bile duct anastomosed into a defunctioned segment of bowel. The operation itself is somewhat more extensive than a choledochoduodenostomy, requiring a second anastomosis, but it does confer the additional advantage of preventing enteric reflux into duct and perhaps minimizing biliary infection. It is also used following failure of choledochoduodenostomy, usually due to anastomotic stenosis.

References

1 Rubin JR, Beal JM. Diagnosis of choledocholithiasis. *Surg Gynecol Obstet* 1983;**156**:16 20.

2 Berk JE. Choledocholithiasis. *Am J Surg* 1941;55:96–104.

3 Farha GJ, Pearson RN. Transcystic duct operative cholangiography: Personal experience with 500 consecutive cases. *Am J Surg* 1976;131:228–31.

4 Cooperberg PL. High resolution real time ultrasound in the evaluation of the normal and obstructed biliary tract. *Clin Radiol* 1978;**129**:477–80.

5 Vallon AG, Lees WR, Cotton PB. Greyscale ultrasonography in cholestatic jaundice. *Gut* 1979;**20**:51–4.

6 Lacaine F, Corlette MB, Bismuth H. Preoperative evaluation of the risk of common bile duct stones. *Arch Surg* 1980;**115**:1114–16.

7 Lygdakis NJ. The incidence and significance of common bile duct dilatation in biliary calculous disease. *World J Surgery* 1984;**8**:327–34.

8 Mueller PR, Ferucci JT, Simeone JF, van Sonnenberg E, Hall DA, Wittenberg J. Observations on the distensibility of the common bile duct. *Radiology* 1982;**142**:467–72.

9 Ratych RE, Sitzmann JV, Lillemore KD, Yeo CJ, Cameron JL. Transduodenal exploration of the common bile duct in patients with nondilated ducts. *Surg Gynecol Obstet* 1991;**173**:49–53.

10 Kramling HJ, Lange V, Schildberg FW, Heberer G. Surgical intervention for bile duct stones. *Ballière's Clin Gastroenterol* 1992;**6**(4):819–31.

11 Thornton J, Axon A. Towards safer endoscopic retrograde cholangiopancreatography. *Gut* 1993;**34**(6):721–4.

12 Cuschieri A, Dubois F, Mouiel JM. The European experience of laparoscopic cholecystectomy. *Am J Surg* 1991;**161**:385–7.

13 Mueller PR, van Sonnenberg E, Simeone JF. Fine needle transhepatic cholangiography. Indications and usefulness. *Ann Int Med* 1982;**97**:567–72.

14 Mirrizzi PL. Operative cholangiography. *Surg Gynecol Obstet* 1937;**65**:702–10.

15 Siegel B, Coehlo JCU, Machi J *et al.* The application of real-time ultrasound imaging during surgical procedures. *Surg Gynecol Obstet* 1983;**157**:33–7.

16 Jakimowicz JJ, Rutten H, Jurgens PJ. Comparison of operative ultrasonography and radiography in screening of the common bile duct for calculi. *World J Surg* 1987;**11**:628–9.

17 Thompson H, Kisslo K, Farouk M, Chung K, Saperstein LA, Meyers WC. Technique of intraluminal biliary ultrasonography during laparoscopic surgery. *Am J Surg* 1993;**165**:265–9.

18 Ascher SM, Evans SR, Goldberg JA *et al.* Intraoperative bile duct sonography during laparoscopic cholecystectomy: Experience with a 12.5 MHz catheter-based probe. *Radiology* 1992;**185**:493–6.

19 Millbourn E. Klinische Studien über die Choledocholithiasis. *Acta Chir Scand* (Suppl. 65) 1941:86.

20 Crump C. The incidence of gallstones and gallbladder disease. *Surg Gynecol Obstet* 1931;**53**:623–30.

21 Lieber MM. Incidence of gallstones and their correlation with other diseases. *Ann Surg* 1952;**135**:394–405.

22 Acosta JM, Ledesma CL. Gallstone migration as a cause of acute pancreatitis. *New Eng J Med* 1974;**290**:484–7.

23 Kelly TR. Gallstone pancreatitis: Pathophysiology. *Surgery* 1976;80:488–92.

24 Bergdahl L, Holmund D. Retained bile duct stones. *Acta Chir Scand* 1976;**142**:145–49.

25 Sherman S, Hawes RH, Lehman GA. Management of bile duct stones. *Semin Liver Dis* 1990;**10**(3):205–21.

26 Marks JW. Natural history, clinical manifestations and diagnosis of cholelithiasis. In: Gitnick G, ed. *Principles*

and Practice of Gastroenterology and Hepatology. New York: Elsevier, 1988:912–36.

27 Schwab G, Pointner R, Wetscher G, Glaser K, Foltin E, Bodner E. Treatment of calculi of the common bile duct. *Surg Gynecol Obstet* 1992;**175**:115–20.

28 Britton BJ. The management of stones in the common bile duct. In: Taylor I, ed. *Progress in Surgery.* Vol 2. Edinburgh: Churchill Livingstone, 1987:86–98.

29 Roslyn JJ, Binns G, Hughes EFX, Saunders-Kirkwood K, Zinner MJ, Cates JA. Open cholecystectomy: A contemporary analysis of 42 474 patients. *Ann Surg* 1993;**218**:129–37.

30 Peel ALG. The challenge of the bile duct in 1990. *Ann Roy Coll Surg* 1990;**72**:165–7.

31 Langenbuch C. Einiges über Operationen am Gallensystem. 1884;**21**:809.

32 McBurney CL. Section of the intestine for removal of a gallstone. *New York State J Med* 1891;**53**:520.

33 McBurney CL. Removal of biliary calculi from the common duct by the duodenal route. *Ann Surg* 1898;**24**:481.

34 Carter AE. The transduodenal per-ampullary approach to the common bile duct. *Ann Roy Coll Surg* 1983;**54**:183–4.

35 Cranley B, Logan H. Exploration of the common bile duct–The relevance of the clinical picture and the importance of peroperative cholangiography. *Br J Surg* 1980;**67**:869–72.

36 Way LW, Aimirand WH, Dunphy JE. Management of choledocholithiasis. *Ann Surg* 1972;**176**:347–57.

37 Glenn F. Retained calculi within the biliary ductal system. *Ann Surg* 1974;**17**:528–39.

38 Corlette MB, Schatzki S, Ackroyd F. Operative cholangiography and overlooked stones. *Arch Surg* 1978;**113**:729–34.

39 Longmire WP. Historic landmarks in biliary surgery. *South Med J* 1982;**75**:1548–50.

40 Feeley TM, Peel ALG. A critical assessment of fluoroscopy in per-operative cholangiography–the use of modern radiologic techniques during surgery. *Ann Roy Coll Surg Eng* 1982;**64**:180–1.

41 Ashby BS, Motson RW. Biliary Endoscopy. In: Motson RW, ed. *Retained Common Duct Stones.* London: Grune & Stratton, 1985:37–58.

42 Leahy AL, Peel ALG. Choledochoscopy? Post-exploratory fluorocholangiography? Or both? *Ann Roy Coll Surg Eng* 1985;**67**:99–100.

43 Classen M, Safrany L. Endoscopic papillotomy and removal of gallstones. *Br Med J* 1975;**4**:371–4.

44 Koch H. Endoscopic papillotomy. *Endoscopy* 1975;**7**: 89–95.

45 Safrany L. Duodenoscopic sphincterotomy and gallstone removal. *Gastroenterology* 1977;**72**:338–43.

46 Cotton P, Vallon M. Duodenoscopic sphincterotomy for removal of bile duct stones in patients with gallbladders. *Surgery* 1982;**6**:628–30.

47 Reiter J, Bayer H, Mennicken C, Manegold B. A collective experience from endoscopic centres in West Germany. *World J Surg* 1978;**2**:505–11.

48 Hansell DT, Millar MA, Murray WR. Endoscopic sphincterotomy for bile duct stones in patients with intact gallbladders. *Br J Surg* 1989;**76**:856–8.

49 Ingoldby CJH, El-Saadi J, Hall RI, Denyer ME. Late results of endoscopic sphincterotomy for bile duct stones in elderly patients with gall bladders *in situ. Gut* 1989;**30**:1129–31.

50 Heinerman M, Boeckel O, Pimpl W. Selective ERCP and preoperative stone removal in bile duct surgery. *Ann Surg* 1989;**3**:267–72.

51 Rosseland R, Solhaug H. Primary EPT in patients with stones in the common bile duct and the gallbladder *in situ*: A 5–8 year follow up study. *World J Surg* 1988;**12**:111–16.

52 Summerfield JA. Biliary obstruction is best managed by endoscopists. *Gut* 1988;**29**:741–5.

53 Sahel I. Komplikationen nach endoskopischer Papillotomie Ergebnisse einer internationalen Umfrage. *Leber Magen Darm* 1987;**6**:364–70.

54 Hill J, Martin DF, Tweedle DEF. Risks of leaving the gallbladder *in situ* after endoscopic sphincterotomy for bile duct stones. *Br J Surg* 1991;**78**:554–7.

55 Kullman E, Borch K, Dahlin LG, Liedberg G. Long-term follow up of patients with gallbladder *in situ* after endoscopic sphincterotomy for choledocholithiasis. *Euro J Surg* 1991;**157**:131–5.

56 Worthley CS, Toouli J. Gallbladder non-filling: An indication for cholecystectomy after endoscopic sphincterotomy. *Br J Surg* 1988;**75**:796–8.

57 Tanaka M, Ikeda S, Yoshimoto H, Matsukoto S. The long term fate of the gallbladder after endoscopic sphincterotomy. *Am J Surg* 1987;**154**:505–9.

58 Windsor JA. Gallstone pancreatitis: a proposed management strategy. *Aust NZ J Surg* 1990;**60**:589–94.

59 Petelin JB. Laparoscopic approach to common duct pathology. *Surg Laparosc Endosc* 1991;**1**:33–41.

60 Carroll BJ, Phillips EH, Daykhovsky L *et al. J Laparoendosc Surg* 1992;**2**:15–21.

61 Zucker KA. Laparoscopic cholecystectomy and the patient with suspected or unsuspected choledocholithiasis. In: *Diseases of the Liver, Biliary tract and Pancreas.* Chicago: American College of Surgeons, Postgraduate Course, 1991:103–5.

62 Johnson AG, Hosking SW. Appraisal of the management of bile duct stones. *Br J Surg* 1987;**74**:555–60.

63 McSherry CK, Glenn F. The incidence and causes of death following surgery for non malignant biliary tract disease. *Ann Surg* 1980;**191**:271–5.

64 Houghton PWJ, Jenkinson LR, Donaldson LA. Cholecystectomy in the elderly: A prospective study. *Br J Surg* 1985;**72**:220–2.

65 Menzies D, Motson RW. Operative common bile duct imaging by operative cholangiography and flexible choledochoscopy. *Br J Surg* 1992;**79**:815–17.

66 McEntee GP, Mulvin DM, Peel ALG. A surgical audit of patients undergoing common bile duct exploration for stone. *Br J Surg* 1989;**76**:1136–8.

67 Finan PJ, Hegarty JH, Donaldson DR, Stewart J, Brennan TG. Transduodenal exploration of the common bile duct–A reappraisal. *J Roy Coll Surg Edin* 1985;30:34–8.

68 Stefanini P, Carboni M, Patrassi N, De Bernardinis G, Negro P, Lorgia P. Transduodenal sphincteroplasty–its use in the treatment of lithiasis and benign obstruction of the common duct. *Am J Surg* 1974;**128**:672–7.

69 Hardy EG, Davenport TJ. The transduodenal approach to the common bile duct. *Br J Surg* 1969; **56**:667–71.

70 Cave-Bigley DJ, Aukland P, Kane JF, Hardy EG. Transduodenal exploration of the common bile duct in a district general hospital. *Ann Roy Coll Surg Eng* 1984;**66**:187–9.

71 Aubrey DA, Edwards JL. The selective use of combined supraduodenal and transduodenal exploration of the common bile duct. *Br J Surg* 1978;**65**:246–51.

72 Vellacott KD, Powell PH. Exploration of the common bile duct: a comparative study. *Br J Surg* 1979;**66**: 389–91.

73 Schieber W. Duodenotomy with common duct exploration. *Arch Surg* 1962;**85**:944–7.

74 Cattell RB, Braasch JW. An evaluation of the long T-tube. *Ann Surg* 1961;**154**:252–4.

75 Warren KW. Surgery of pancreatic diseases. In: *Modern Trends in Gastroenterology*, 3rd edn. London: Butterworths, 264.

76 White TT, Morgan A, Hopton D. Postoperative pancreatitis. A study of 70 cases. *Am J Surg* 1970; **120**:132–7.

77 Keighley MRB, Graham NG. The aetiology and prevention of pancreatitis following biliary tract operations. *Br J Surg* 1973;**60**:149–52.

78 Peel ALG, Hermon-Taylor J, Ritchie HD. Technique of transduodenal exploration of the common bile duct. *Ann Roy Coll Surg Eng* 1974;**55**:236–44.

79 Imrie CW, McKay AJ, Benjamin IS, Blumgart LH. Secondary acute pancreatitis: aetiology, prevention, diagnosis and management. *Br J Surg* 1978;**65**:399–402.

80 Sheridan WG, Williams HOL, Lewis MH. Morbidity and mortality of common bile duct exploration. *Br J Surg* 1987;**74**:1095–9.

81 Jacobs JK, Cebul RD, Adamson TE. Acute cholecystitis. Evaluation of factors influencing common duct exploration. *Am Surg* 1986;**52**:177–82.

82 Ostroff JW, Shapiro HA. Complications of endoscopic sphincterotomy. In: Jacobsen I, ed. *ERCP: Diagnostic and Therapeutic Applications*. New York: Elsevier, 1989:61–73.

83 Vaira D, D'Anna L, Ainley C, Dowsett J, Williams S, Baillie J. Endoscopic sphincterotomy 1 000 consecutive patients. *Lancet* 1989;ii:431–4.

84 Winslet MC, Neoptolemos JP. The place of endoscopy in the management of gallstones. *Baillière's Clin Gastroenterol* 1991;**5**:99–129.

85 Hamilton I, Lintott DJ, Rothwell J, Axon ATR. Acute pancreatitis following endoscopic retrograde cholangiopancreatography. *Clin Radiol* 1983;**34**:543–6.

86 Motte S, Deviere J, Dumonceau J-M, Serruys E, Thys J-P, Cremer M. Risk factors for septicaemia following biliary stenting. *Gastroenterology* 1991;**101**:1374–81.

87 Cryan EM, Falkiner FR, Mulvihill TE, Keane CT, Keeling PWN. *Pseudomonas aeruginosa* infection following endoscopic retrograde cholangiography. *J Hosp Infect* 1985;**5**:371–6.

88 Classen DC, Jacobsen IA, Burke JP, Jacobsen JT, Evans RS. Serious pseudomonas infections associated with retrograde cholangiography. *Am J Med* 1988;**84**: 590–6.

89 Earnshaw JJ, Clark AW, Thon BT. Outbreak of *Pseudomonas aeruginosa* following endoscopic retrograde cholangiopancreatography. *J Hosp Infect* 1985;**6**:95–7.

90 Hatfield ARW. Palliation of malignant obstructed jaundice–surgery or stent? *Gut* 1990;**31**:1339–40.

91 Cotton P, Vallon M. Duodenoscopic sphincterotomy for removal of bile duct stones in patients with gallbladders. *Surgery* 1982;**6**:628–30.

92 Steigmann GV, Pearlmann NW, Goff JS, Sun JH, Norton LW. Endoscopic cholangiography and stone removal prior to cholecystectomy. *Arch Surg* 1989; **124**:787–90.

93 Neoptolemos JP, Carr-Locke DL, Fossard DP. Prospective randomized study of preoperative endoscopic sphincterotomy versus surgery alone for common bile duct stones. *Br Med J* 1987;**294**:470–4.

94 Stain SC, Cone H, Tsuishoysha M, Donovan AJ. Choledocholithiasis. Endoscopic sphincterotomy or common bile duct exploration. *Ann Surg* 1991;**213**: 627–34.

95 Worthily CS, Watts JMcK, Toouli J. Common duct exploration or endoscopic sphincterotomy for choledocholithiasis? *Aust NZ J Surg* 1989;**59**:209–15.

96 Clair DG, Carr-Locke DL, Becker JM, Brooks DC. Routine cholangiography is not warranted during laparoscopic cholecystectomy. *Arch Surg* 1993;**128**: 551–5.

97 Cooperberg PL, Burhenne HJ. Real-time ultrasonography. Diagnostic technique of choice in calculous gallbladder disease. *New Eng J Med* 1980;**302**: 1277–9.

98 Barkun JS, Fried GM, Barkun AN *et al.* Cholecystectomy without operative cholangiography. Implication for common bile duct injury and retained common bile duct stones. *Ann Surg* 1993;**218**: 371–9.

99 Franceschi D, Brandt C, Margolin D *et al.* The management of common bile duct stones in patients undergoing laparoscopic cholecystectomy. *Am Surg* 1993;**59**:525–32.

100 O'Rourke NA, Askew AR, Cowen AE, Roberts R, Fielding GA. The role of ERCP and endoscopic sphincterotomy in the area of laparoscopic chole-

cystectomy. *Aust NZ J Surg* 1993;**63**:3–7.
101 Cotton PB. Endoscopic retrograde cholangiopancreatography and laparoscopic cholecystectomy. *Am J Surg* 1993;**165**:474–8.
102 Kocher T. Ein Fall von Choledochoduodenostomia Interna wegen Gallensteines. *Korrespondenz-Blatt fur Auerzle* 1895;**7**:193.
103 Graham SM, Flowers JL, Scott TR *et al.* Laparoscopic cholecystectomy and common bile duct stones. The utility of planned perioperative endoscopic retrograde chol-angiography and sphincterotomy: Experience with 63 patients. *Ann Surg* 1993;**218**:61–7.
104 Jacobs M, Verdeja J-C, Goldstein HS. Laparoscopic choledocholithotomy. *J Laparoendosc Surg* 1991;**1**: 79–82.
105 Bailey RW, Zucker KA. Laparoscopic cholangiography and management of choledocholithiasis. In: Zucker KA, ed. *Surgical Laparoscopy*. St Louis: Quality Medical Publishing, 1991;201–25.
106 Rosch W, Rieman JF, Lux G, Linder HG. Long term follow-up after endoscopic sphincterotomy. *Endoscopy* 1981;**13**:152–3.
107 Excourrou G, Gordova JA, Lazorthes F, Frexinos J, Ribet A. Early and late complications after endoscopic sphincterotomy for biliary lithiasis, with and without the gallbladder *in situ*. *Gut* 1984;**25**:598–602.
108 Cotton PB, Vallon AG. Duodenoscopic sphincterotomy for removal of common bile duct stones in patients with gallbladders *in situ*. *Surgery* 1982;**91**: 628–30.
109 Sahiara PC, Zuidema GD, Cameron JL. Primary common duct stones. *Ann Surg* 1977;**185**:598–602.
110 Allen B, Shapiro H, Way LW. Management of recurrent and residual common duct stones. *Am J Surg* 1981;**142**:41–6.
111 Gadacz TR. Reoperation versus alternatives in retained biliary calculi. *Surg Clin N Am* 1991;**71**:93–108.
112 Callans LS, Gadacz TR. Fragmentation of human gallstones using ultrasound and electrohydraulic lithotripsy: Experimental and clinical experience. *Surgery* 1990;**107**:121–27.
113 Johnson G, Sprinkle. Autopsy incidence of cholelithiasis in a general hospital. *N Carol Med J* 1962;**23**:107–8.
114 Reitsma BJ. Common duct stones. A reappraisal of etiology and surgical management with special emphasis on operative biliary endoscopy. PhD thesis: Ricksuniversiteit Limburg te Maastricht, 1981.
115 Burhenne HJ. Nonoperative instrument extraction of retained bile duct stones. *World J Surg* 1978;**2**:439–45.

Chapter 17
Endoscopic approaches to common bile duct stones

S.C. Sydney Chung

Removal of common duct stones through an endoscopically created sphincterotomy has been one of the most significant advances in therapeutic endoscopy. Since endoscopic sphincterotomy was first described in the early 1970s by Japanese and German endoscopists, the technique has steadily gained acceptance as an alternative to open common duct exploration. In the beginning the technique was advocated for patients with retained ductal stones after surgery and for old and frail patients who were unfit for surgery. As the safety and longer term results of endoscopic sphincterotomy became established the indications for endoscopic stone removal have widened. With the recent advent of laparoscopic cholecystectomy the demand for endoscopic clearance of ductal stones has further increased.

Endoscopic extraction of stones from the bile ducts generally includes the following basic steps:
1 cannulation of the common bile duct and obtaining a retrograde endoscopic cholangiogram (ERC);
2 dividing the sphincter of Oddi using diathermy current through a sphincterotome;
3 delivery of the stones from the duct into the duodenum with or without prior fragmentation.

The technique of endoscopic retrograde cholangiopancreatography (ERCP), sphincterotomy and stone extraction is demanding and requires a long period of training and practice under supervision before acceptable success rates can be achieved. A trained biliary endoscopist also requires a certain case-load to maintain his expertise. In experienced hands sphincterotomy can be performed successfully in 90–95% of patients, and the duct cleared of stones in over 80% [1, 2]. The main complications of the procedure are pancreatitis, haemorrhage and perforation. These occur in approximately 10% of cases. Less than 20% of these complications require an operation to remedy the situation and the overall mortality is around 1.5% [3].

Techniques [4–6]

Because of the risk of inducing bacteremia during instrumentation within the bile duct, therapeutic ERCP should be covered with prophylactic antibiotics. A single intravenous dose of a second or third generation cephalosporin, given just prior to the procedure, should suffice in the absence of pre-existing cholangitis. Continuation of antibiotic treatment after the procedure is not necessary if the obstructing stone is removed and drainage of the biliary tree is adequate.

Cannulation

ERCP is usually performed with intravenous sedation. Most endoscopists use a combination of an opiate (such as pethidine or fantanyl) and a benzodiazepine (diazepam or mediazolam). Drugs such as Buscopan or glucagon are also necessary to eliminate duodenal peristalsis to make cannulation easier. A side-viewing duodenoscope is used. The patient is placed on the X-ray table in the left semi-prone position with the left arm behind the back. The passage of the endoscope through the pharynx is blind; with slight upward angulation an adequate view of the oesophagus is possible. The stomach can be examined completely if care is taken. Passage of the scope through the pylorus may be facilitated if the patient is temporarily returned to the left-lateral position. The pylorus is first brought into view by down angulation of the tip of the endoscope. To pass the pylorus, return the tip of the scope to neutral. This will result in the pylorus just disappearing from the field of vision, the so-called 'setting sun sign'. Gentle pushing at this stage should advance the scope into the first part of the duodenum.

The patient should now be returned to the prone position. The endoscope is further advanced, allowing a loop to form along the greater curvature of the stomach. The left/right control should now be turned fully to the right and the lock applied. The up/down control is turned fully to the up-position and the endoscope withdrawn slowly while rotating the shaft of the instrument to the right. A combination of these movements will advance the endoscope down the duodenum. This results from the paradoxical movement of the tip of the endoscope as the angulation of the bending section anchors it in the junction of the bend between the first and second part of the duodenum. With 60–65 cm of endoscope inside the patient, relaxation of the angulation controls should normally bring the papilla into view.

The landmark for identification of the papilla is a vertical mucosal fold in the second part of the duodenum. The papilla lies at the apex of the vertical fold, where the vertical fold meets a horizontal mucosal fold. Sometimes, the papillary opening is covered by the horizontal fold, which has to be pushed away with the cannula before cannulation. Juxta-papillary diverticula are not uncommon in elderly patients and in patients with ductal stones. Sometimes the papilla may be situated inside such a diverticulum, making cannulation much more difficult. Once cannulated, however, it is usually possible to lift it out of the diverticulum with the cannula or the papillotome. The risk of sphincterotomy is not increased by the presence of such diverticula.

With the endoscope in the straight position the angulation controls of the tip are more sensitive. Torque on the shaft is also much more easily transmitted to the tip. The patient is more comfortable and less likely to retch as there is no loop stretching the greater curvature of the stomach. The short-scope position is, therefore, the ideal position to start cannulation. Occasionally, because of distorted anatomy the papilla cannot be brought into a satisfactory position for cannulation in the short-scope position. It is then necessary to attempt cannulation in the semi-long or the long-scope position by advancing the scope further.

Careful positioning of the scope tip in relation to the papilla is the key to successful cannulation. The papilla should be placed en-face in the centre of the endoscopic view. This is achieved by fine adjustments of the up/down and left/right angulations, rotation of the endoscope shaft, advancement and withdrawal of the insertion tube and insufflation and suctioning of air in the duodenum. It is necessary to keep the angulation locks on during these adjustments. To start poking at the papilla before a good position is achieved is counter-productive. Bruising and oedema will only make the subsequent procedure more difficult.

A plain film should be taken prior to the injection of any contrast material to look for the calcification or presence of air in the biliary tree. Cannulae with rounded metal tips that can be seen easily on fluoroscopy should be used (Fig. 17.1). The cannula should be filled completely with contrast, lest air bubbles may be confused with stones on the cholangiogram. Cannulae that allow guidewires to pass through should be used, so that instruments such as wire-guided papillotomes, balloon catheters or naso-biliary drains can be exchanged over the wire if necessary.

In humans the bile duct and pancreatic duct share the same papillary opening. The pancreatic duct travels perpendicularly from the papilla and is more easily cannulated. The bile duct travels cephalad from the roof of the papilla in the 11 o'clock direction. To enter the bile duct it is necessary to approach the papilla from below (with the tip of the scope deeper into the duodenum) and to use the elevator to lift the cannula into the roof of the papilla.

Reliable selective cannulation of the common bile duct is the most important prerequisite of sphincterotomy and stone extraction. If cannulation with the metal tipped cannula is unsuccessful a papillotome may be used. By applying

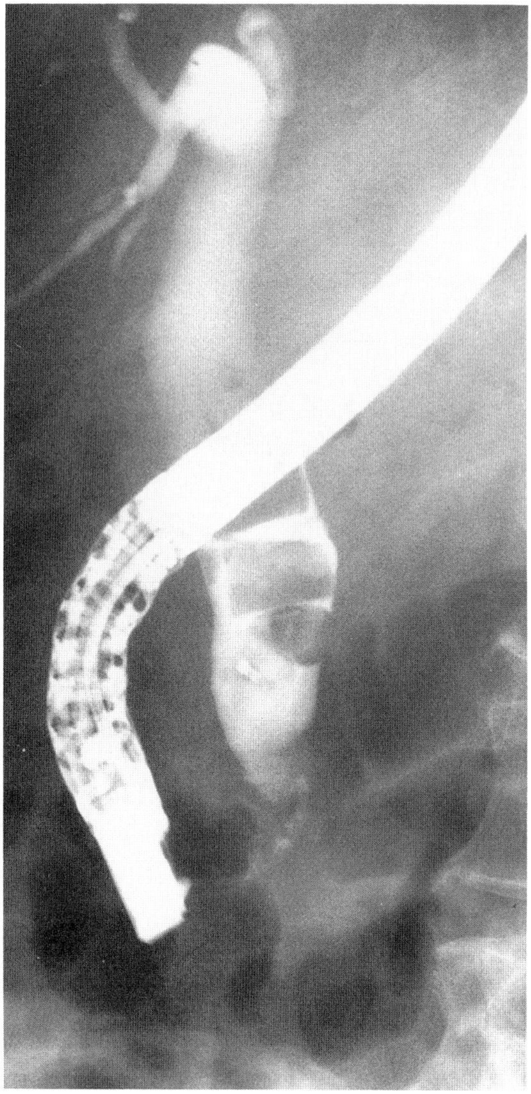

Fig. 17.1 ERCP showing multiple common duct stones. The metal tip of the cannula can be seen in the bile duct.

tension on the wire the papillotome can be bowed to achieve the cephalad angle needed for bile duct cannulation. If the presence of stones is strongly suspected one may commence cannulation with a papillotome instead of a cannula. Alternatively, a guidewire/papillotome combination, using a papillotome that can take a guidewire, may be useful in achieving bile duct cannulation.

Full strength contrast (Conray 280 or 60% Urograffin) should be used for the initial cannulation. Injection of contrast should always be under fluoroscopic control. Over filling of the pancreatic duct is likely to result in pancreatitis. Dense contrast may obscure stones in the bile duct; half strength contrast (diluted 50/50 with saline) should be used when filling a dilated bile duct or if small stones are suspected.

Endoscopic sphincterotomy

Endoscopic sphincterotomy (EST) refers to the division of the muscles of the biliary sphincter using diathermy current through a sphincterotome inserted through the channel of a duodenoscope. Although the terms endoscopic sphincterotomy and endoscopic papillotomy (EPT) are often used interchangeably, sphincterotomy is the more appropriate term as the sphincter muscles of the distal common duct beyond the papilla are also divided.

The sphincterotome consists of a Teflon catheter containing a wire. A segment of the wire near the distal end of the catheter is exposed to act as the cutting edge. Many designs are available, varying in the length of catheter beyond the exposed wire (the nose) and the length of the exposed wire (Fig. 17.2). Wire-guided sphincterotomes have a separate lumen for passage of a guidewire. These are a significant advance since they can be railroaded over a previously inserted wire without losing bile duct cannulation.

It is essential to achieve deep cannulation of the bile duct before sphincterotomy. The position of the sphincterotome in the bile duct should be checked fluoroscopically before commencing the cut. The exposed wire is brought into contact with the roof of the papilla by a combination of tension on the wire and upward lifting of the elevator. Keeping about 0.5 cm of wire in the papilla, blended current is applied with the wire in the 11 o'clock direction. Short bursts of current is used to achieve a graded, controlled cut. Most endoscopists prefer to use blended current for sphincterotomy.

Judging how far to cut requires experience. In

general, if one cuts along the direction of between 11 and 12 o'clock and does not extend the cut beyond the horizontal fold perforations do not occur. (Plate 17.1, opposite page 183.) If one strays from this direction perforations are likely. When the sphincter muscles are divided a gush of bile may appear. The size of the sphincterotomy may also be judged by passing a bowed sphincterotome in and out of the sphincterotomy. When a bowed sphincterotome can pass freely the sphincterotomy is adequate. The maximum limit of a safe sphincterotomy depends on the anatomy of the distal common duct and varies from case to case.

Stone retrieval

With an adequate sphincterotomy most stones under 1 cm will pass spontaneously. Most endoscopists however favour an active policy of stone extraction to avoid stone impaction, biliary obstruction and cholangitis.

Common duct stones of under 1.5 cm in size can be removed using standard accessories such as Dormia baskets and balloon catheters (Fig. 17.3). Larger stones need to be fragmented before they can be extracted. Mechanical lithotripsy is the preferred method of breaking up stones before removal.

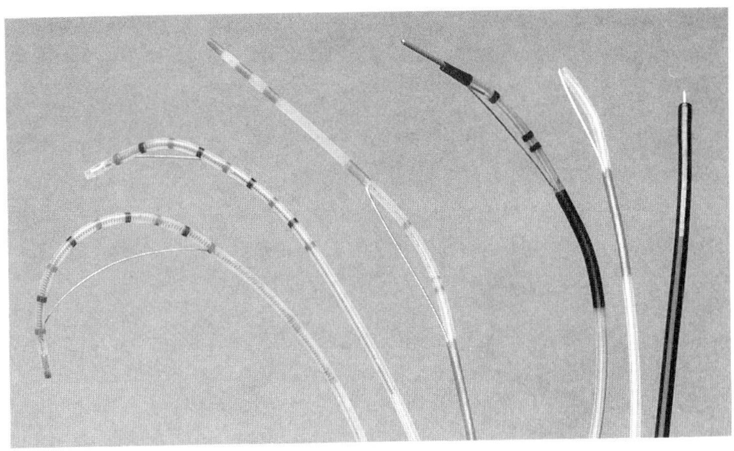

Fig. 17.2 Various types of sphincterotomes. From left: long wire, short wire, long nose, wire-guided, pre-cut and needle type.

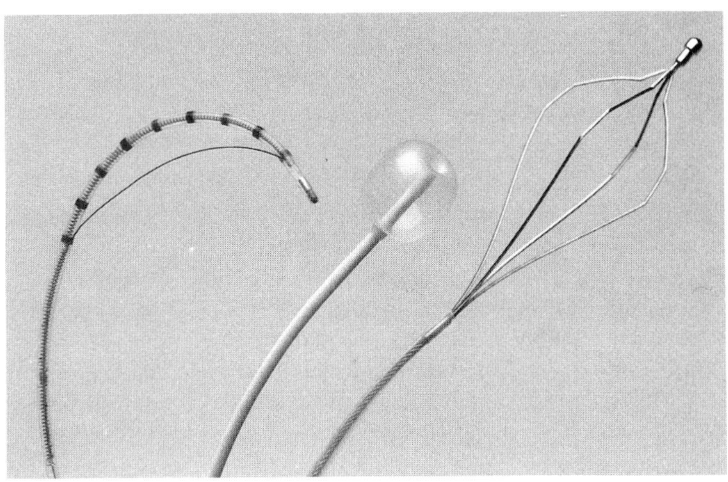

Fig. 17.3 Accessories for endoscopic sphincterotomy and stone removal: sphincterotome, balloon catheter and Dormia basket.

The use of balloon catheters for stone retrieval does not carry the risk of basket impaction. Pulling hard on a stone, however, is likely to cause the balloon to burst. If more than one stone is present the lowest one should be removed first. The balloon catheter is inserted and the balloon inflated above the lowest stone. The stone is then pulled out from the duct by traction on the basket. Balloon catheters are also useful for advancing stones from the intrahepatic ducts into the common duct; if the balloon is inflated in the common duct and then withdrawn slowly, the partial vacuum created will often suck the stone into the common duct.

Most endoscopists prefer Dormia baskets to balloon catheters as it is easier to entrap the stone in the basket and more force can be applied to pull the stone out. After insertion into the duct the basket should be opened a little and contrast injected to visualize the stones. Care should be taken not to push the stones up into the intrahepatic ducts. This may make subsequent entrapment very difficult. The closed basket is then advanced past the stone and opened. The stone is engaged by withdrawing the basket and shaking it. It is not necessary to close the basket onto the stone. Removal of the stone from the duct is effected by pulling the catheter tight until the tip of the endoscope lies against the papilla. The tip of the endoscope is then angled down and the scope rotated to the right at the same time. A combination of these movements pulls the stone out through the ampulla in the direction of the bile duct. The stone may then be dropped in the duodenum and the procedure repeated for other stones in the duct.

At the completion of the procedure a cholangiogram is performed to confirm that all the stones have been removed. After sphincterotomy contrast may not be retained in the duct. It is necessary to use a balloon catheter to occlude the lower end of the duct to achieve adequate filling. Sometimes it is impossible to be sure that the duct is clear after a prolonged procedure because a lot of air has entered the duct. It may then be prudent to insert a nasobiliary drain and perform a nasobiliary cholangiogram to confirm duct clearance at a subsequent date.

Special problems

Cholangitis

Cholangitis results when bacterial infection occurs in an obstructed biliary tree. When there is biliary pathology the bile rapidly becomes colonized by enteric organisms. The mere presence of bacteria in the biliary tree is insufficient to produce symptoms. Even with more than 10^5 organisms per mL in the bile, patients remain asymptomatic unless there is obstruction. Clinical cholangitis occurs only when bacteria and endotoxin reflux into the blood stream consequent upon a rise in the intraductal pressure. There are direct communications between terminal bile duct cannaliculi and liver sinusoids. When biliary pressure rises above 25 cm of water, reflux of bile into the blood occurs.

Classically cholangitis presents with epigastric or right upper quadrant pain, spiking fever and jaundice (i.e., Charcot's triad). Other clinical features include chills and rigors, tea coloured urine, epigastric tenderness and a palpable liver. In severe cases septic shock may occur suddenly. Confusion and hypotension in addition to Charcot's triad constitutes Reynolds' pentad. This occurs in patients with complete obstruction of the common bile duct and has been described as 'acute obstructive cholangitis'. Without urgent intervention to decompress the biliary system the outcome is fatal [7].

Patients without complete obstruction may respond to conservative measures, which should include nothing by mouth, intravenous fluids and broad spectrum antibiotics. In view of the possible development of renal shutdown, aminoglycosides should be avoided if possible. A second or third generation cephalosporin is the antibiotic of choice.

For patients who do not show rapid clinical response and for those who develop signs of septic shock urgent decompression of the biliary tree is mandatory. This may be achieved by open surgery and T-tube insertion, percutaneous transhepatic biliary drainage (PTBD) or by the retrograde endoscopic route. PTBD carries a risk of bile leakage and bleeding related to the liver puncture.

Surgery in these acutely ill patients carries a mortality of up to 40%. If endoscopic expertise is available, the treatment of choice is endoscopic drainage.

Endoscopic decompression of the biliary tree may be achieved by endoscopic sphincterotomy and stone removal, nasobiliary drainage or insertion of an indwelling stent. For relatively stable patients sphincterotomy and stone extraction solves the problem at one session and is the procedure of choice. Stenting may be used as a semi-long term option for unfit patients with a large stone.

Nasobiliary drains can be inserted without a papillotomy. (Plate 17.2, opposite page 183.) It is particularly useful for acutely ill patients in whom the coagulation indices are deranged and prolonged instrumentation is to be avoided. In these patients it is important not raise the intra-ductal pressure and worsen the septicaemia by injecting too much contrast. A minimal amount of contrast is used to outline the duct. After deep cannulation of the duct a guidewire is passed through the cannula. The cannula is then removed, leaving the guidewire in place. The nasobiliary drain can then be threaded through the channel of the endoscope over the guidewire. It is advanced until its tip is hooked into one of the intrahepatic ducts. The endoscope is then removed, with the endoscopist threading the drain into the patient while the nurse-assistant eases the scope out of the patient's mouth. The position of the drain is monitored by fluoroscopy. The procedure requires close co-operation between the endoscopist and the assistant. Bile is then aspirated from the drain to decompress the biliary tree. The procedure is then completed by bringing the drain out through the nose. This is achieved by passing a catheter through the nose, retrieving the other end through the mouth and then railroading the nasobiliary drain through the catheter. Care should be taken to avoid kinking the catheter in the pharynx and to check the position of the nasobiliary drain by fluoroscopy at the end of the procedure.

In patients with acute cholangitis, the material aspirated is often frank pus with little or no bile pigment. The bile drained from the nasobiliary tube only regains its normal green colour as the patient recovers and the secretory function of the liver recovers. (Plate 17.3, opposite page 183.) The effect of biliary decompression is often very dramatic; the pain disappears as soon as the biliary tree is decompressed and the fever subsides rapidly. Once the sepsis is controlled another ERCP can be performed for sphincterotomy and stone extraction.

The place of ERCP in acute cholangitis is now firmly established. In a series of 105 patients with severe cholangitis from Hong Kong, endoscopic drainage was successfully instituted in 102. Eight per cent of patients had sphincterotomy and stone extraction, 27% had nasobiliary drain alone and 66% had both sphincterotomy and nasobiliary drainage. Sepsis was rapidly controlled in those successfully drained. The overall mortality was 4.8%, which is much lower than the surgical mortality for similar patients [8]. In another study from Hong Kong endoscopic drainage was compared with surgical treatment in a randomized trial. Major complications occurred in 34% of patients in the endoscopy group and 66% in the surgery group. Statistically significant reduction in mortality was also demonstrated in the endoscopy group; 10% of patients in the endoscopy group and 32% in the surgery group succumbed [9].

Pancreatitis

In the past endoscopists were loath to perform ERCP during the acute phase of pancreatitis for fear of exacerbating the pancreatic inflammation. Recent evidence indicates that this fear is unfounded and ERCP during acute pancreatitis is safe, provided over injection of the pancreatic ductal system is avoided.

Endoscopic sphincterotomy and stone extraction has been compared with conventional treatment in patients with acute gallstone pancreatitis. Common duct stones were found in ERCP in 63% of those with severe attacks but only 26% of those with mild attacks. Complications of pancreatitis were significantly less frequent in the group who had early ERCP, the benefit was more marked in those with severe pancreatitis. This study demonstrated that ERCP could be safely undertaken in acute pancreatitis and that there was significant benefit in removing the stone early, especially in those with severe attacks [10].

Our present policy is to perform ERCP on an emergency basis for patients who have severe biliary pancreatitis (3 or more positive Ranson's criteria). We aim for selective biliary cannulation only and do not make an attempt at obtaining a pancreatogram. The plan is to perform sphincterotomy and remove the offending stone if one is found. Patients with mild attacks are scheduled for ERCP on the next list. After endoscopic clearance of the duct (or demonstration of a clear CBD) laparoscopic cholecystectomy is performed on the next day.

Whether cholecystectomy can be avoided in patients presenting with biliary pancreatitis if endoscopic sphincterotomy is performed is an interesting question [11]. After endoscopic sphincterotomy should further stones migrate from the gallbladder into the common duct, passage through the papilla should be uneventful. A case could be made for elective endoscopic sphincterotomy to prevent recurrent pancreatitis in high-risk patients with gallbladder stones, regardless of whether ductal stones are present at the time of ERCP. This approach seems logical, but documentary evidence in support of its efficacy is scant.

Large stones

The technical difficulty of endoscopic stone extraction increases with the size of the stone. Because of the risks of perforation and bleeding there is a limit to the size of the sphincterotomy that can be made. Stones less than 1.5 cm can usually be extracted using standard techniques. Larger stones require fragmentation before removal [12].

Fortunately very large common duct stones are usually of the brown pigment variety which are easily fragmented. In some cases it is possible to 'slice through' such stones by closing the Dormia basket forcibly around it [13]. (Plate 17.4, opposite page 183.) In other cases, this approach will result in the stone getting stuck in the basket. The Soehendra lithotripter is very useful in this situation (Figs 17.4 and 17.5). When stone impaction occurs the handle of the basket is cut off. The endoscope and the outer Teflon outer sheath of the basket is then removed. The metal sheath of the lithotripter is threaded onto the wires of the basket and the wires tightened onto the sheath using the handle. The stone, trapped in the basket is drawn tight onto the metal sheath and broken. The Soehendra lithotripter is indispensable for endoscopists who deal with stone disease. It is no

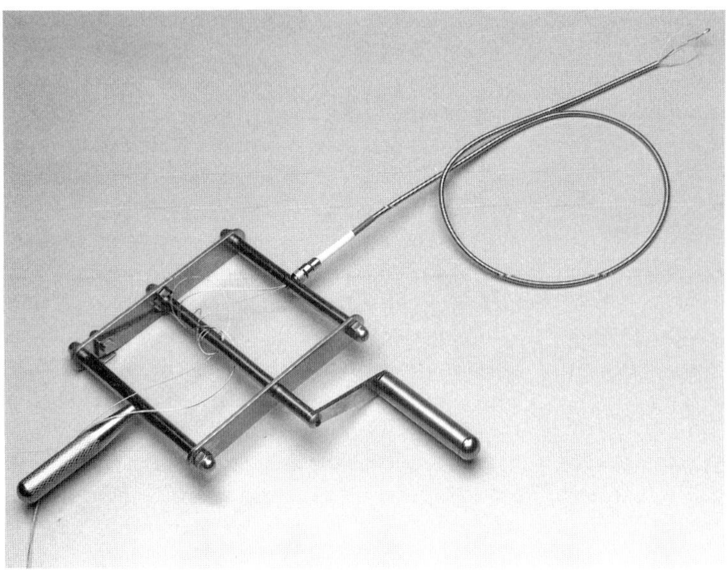

Fig. 17.4 The Soehendra lithotripter: retrieves a trapped basket but the basket has to be sacrificed.

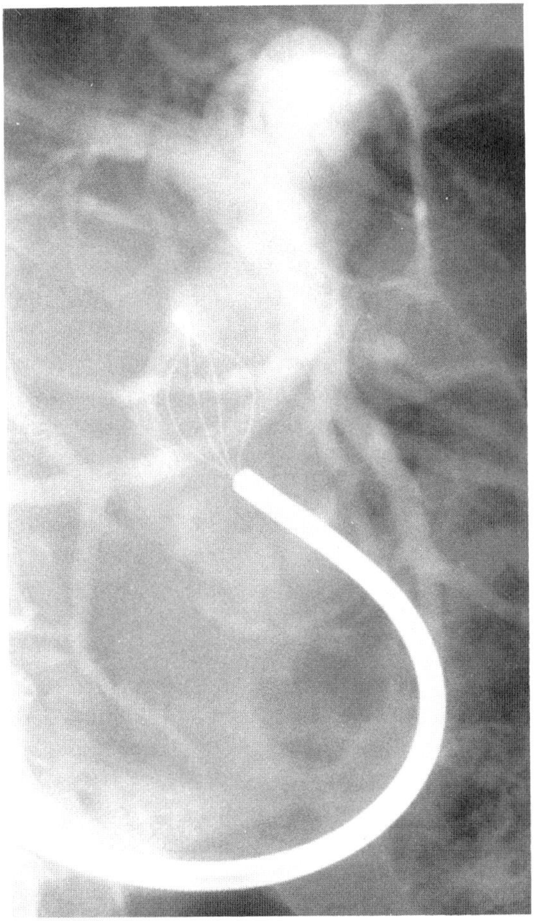

Fig. 17.5 The metal sheath of the Soehendra lithotripter railroaded onto the impacted stone before the handle is tightened.

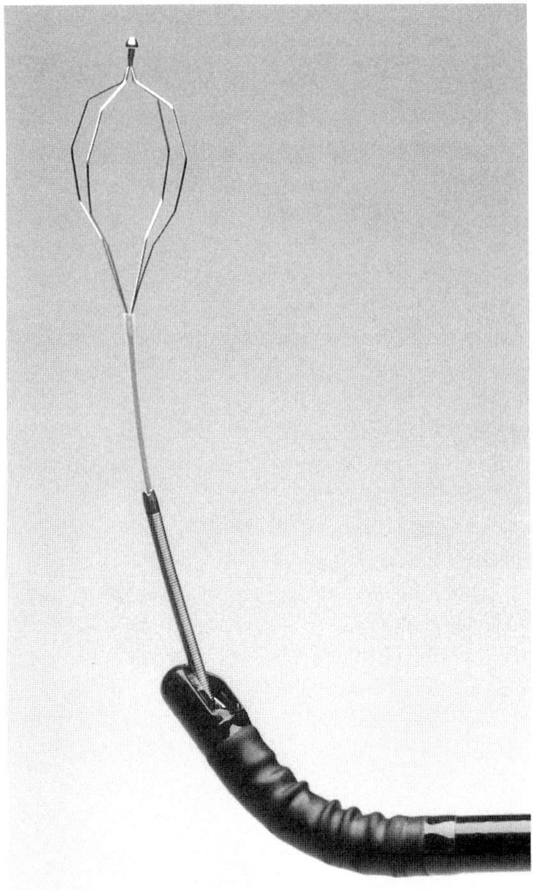

Fig. 17.6 Mechanical lithotripter that can pass through the channel of the endoscope.

longer necessary to operate on patients with trapped baskets if such a device is available. The disadvantage is that the Dormia basket is destroyed. The procedure can become very expensive if several stones need to be broken up using this method.

Mechanical lithotripters that can pass through the instrument channel of the endoscope have made breaking up large common duct stones much easier. The device consists of a strong 4-wire basket within a Teflon sheath, a flexible metal sheath and a handle (Fig. 17.6). An endoscopic sphincterotomy, performed previously or at the same session, is necessary before the lithotriptor basket can be inserted into the bile duct. The basket, within the Teflon sheath, is inserted above the stone. The basket is then opened and the stone engaged in the basket by a combination of withdrawal and gentle shaking. Once the stone is firmly engaged the metal sheath is advanced onto the basket to crush the stone (Fig. 17.7). In our experience mechanical lithotripsy using such basket lithotripters can deal with 80% of stones too large to be removed by standard means [14].

For mechanical lithotripsy to succeed the stone must first be trapped in the basket. In patients with very large stones there may be no room to open the basket in a duct filled with stones. Such

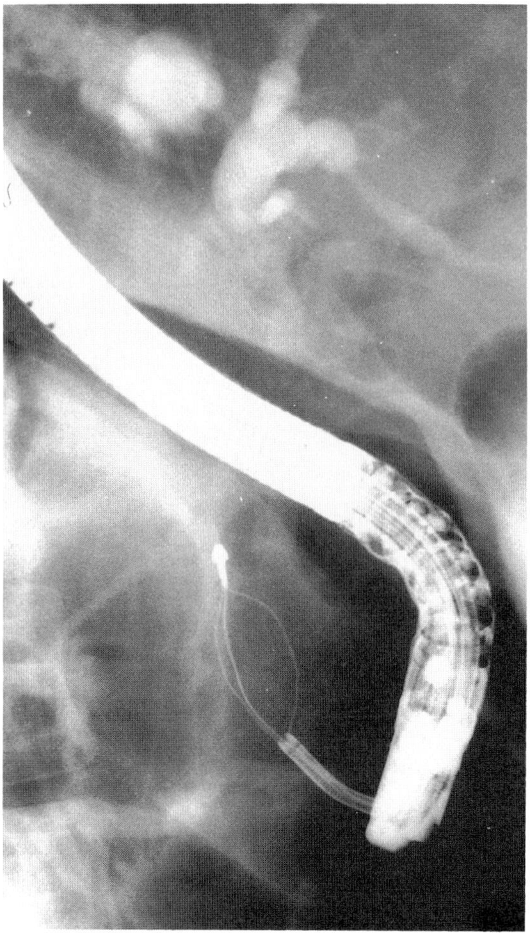

Fig. 17.7 Mechanical lithotripsy: the metal sheath is tightened onto the stone trapped in the basket.

stones may be broken up with extra-corporeal shock-wave lithotripsy, using contrast introduced through a nasobiliary catheter to target the stones.

Alternatively, electrohydraulic lithotripsy can be used to break up the stone. Electrohydraulic lithotripsy utilizes the principle of high pressure shock waves generated by a high voltage discharge. If the probe is fired directly at the bile duct wall, duct damage and even perforation can result. It is, therefore, necessary to visualize the tip of the probe during lithotripsy. The 'mother' endoscope is an extra large duodenoscope. It has an instrument channel which admits a 'baby' endoscope which has a working channel. Insertion of the baby endoscope requires a sphincterotomy, which is best performed a few days before. A nasobiliary catheter is also necessary for irrigation to clear away debris generated during lithotripsy [15] (Fig. 17.8).

For patients in whom stone fragmentation is not successful and for acutely ill or frail patients who tolerate prolonged manipulation poorly an indwelling stent is a very good option [16]. The stent will keep the stone from impacting, preventing cholangitis (Fig. 17.9). The stent may be used as a long-term measure; stent clogging will occur but does not result in obstruction as the function of the stent is to stop the stone from impaction. Alternatively, the patient may be brought back for another attempt at stone removal when he has regained his strength. Often the stone will be smaller and more easily engaged in the lithotripsy basket. Why this is so is not certain. Possible mechanisms include physical rubbing of the stent on the stone and altered bile composition after sphincterotomy and stent insertion.

Unsuccessful cannulation

Even in expert hands bile duct cannulation may prove impossible in around 5% of patients. If there are strong reasons to avoid surgery these patients may be managed by a combined percu-taneous/endoscopic approach or by pre-cut sphincterotomy.

In the combined method [17] (the so called 'rendezvous method') a percutaneous transhepatic puncture is made and a guidewire inserted through the percutaneous catheter, the guidewire is manipulated past the stone and through the sphincter of Oddi into the duodenum. The endoscope is then passed into the duodenum. The guidewire is retrieved through the instrument channel of the endoscope. A wire guided sphincterotome is then railroaded over the guidewire into the bile duct. Endoscopic sphincterotomy can then be carried out in the normal manner.

Precut sphincterotomy refers to sphincterotomy without selective bile duct cannulation. This may be performed by using a precut sphincterome

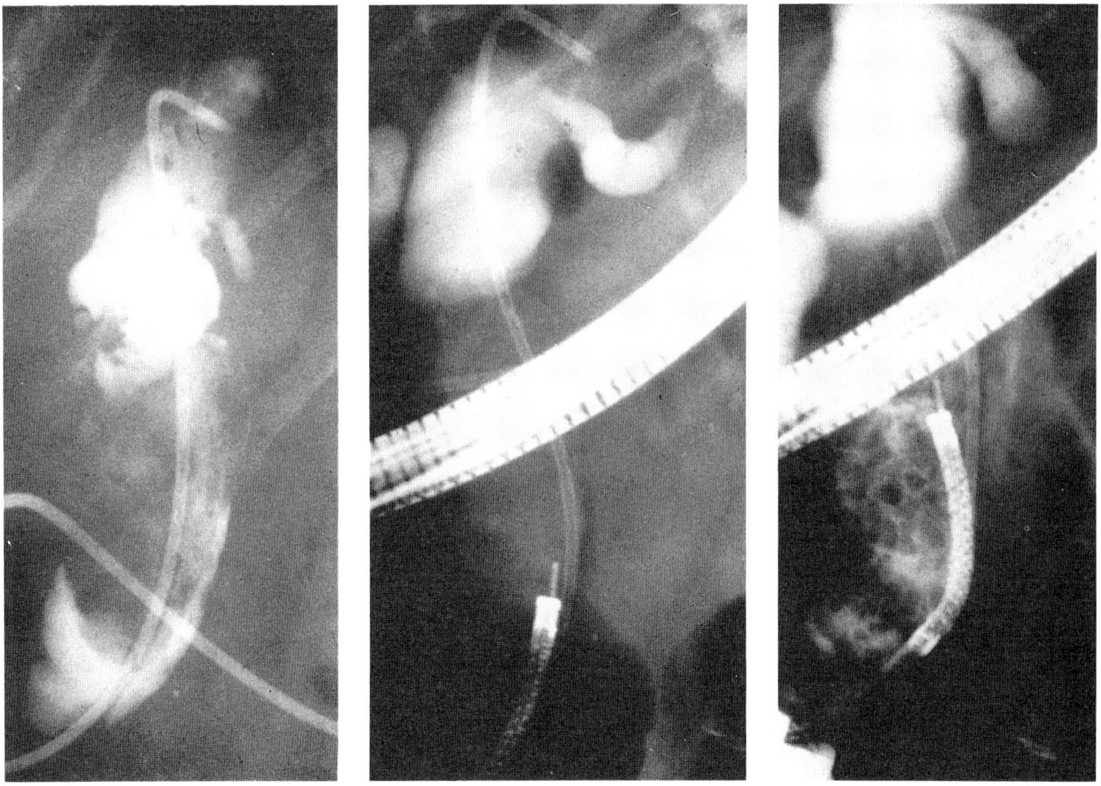

(a) (b) (c)

Fig. 17.8 Electrohydraulic lithotripsy with the mother and baby scope. (a) Nasobiliary cholangiogram showing a large stone; (b) lithotripsy in progress; and (c) partially fragmented stone.

which has no 'nose' or a 'needle knife' (see Fig. 17.2). The intramural part of the sphincter is divided free-hand until the bile duct is entered. Pre-cut sphincterotomy is a relatively uncontrolled procedure; its success depends on the endoscopists having a mental image of the direction of the bile duct.

Precut sphincterotomy carries higher complication rates than sphincterotomy using standard techniques. It should only be used by experts and only for patients in whom there is a strong indication for a therapeutic procedure [18]. One such situation is a patient with an impacted stone at the lower end of the common bile duct causing the ampulla to bulge into the lumen of the duodenum. In this situation it is safe to cut down onto the stone with a needle knife papillotome [19]. Completion of the papillotomy is easy using standard techniques once the stone is extruded.

Intrahepatic stones

Intrahepatic stones, especially those behind strictures, represent a challenge to the endoscopist. It is possible to dilate the strictures with balloon catheters and then extract the stones (Fig. 17.10). These procedures are technically demanding, principally because of the difficulties in directing accessories into the desired liver segment [20]. An alternative approach is to perform a transhepatic puncture, allow the tract to mature and then to remove the stones through the tract—with or without prior fragmentation [21]. In patients where the stones are confined to the left lobe and the affected lobe is already atrophic, the best

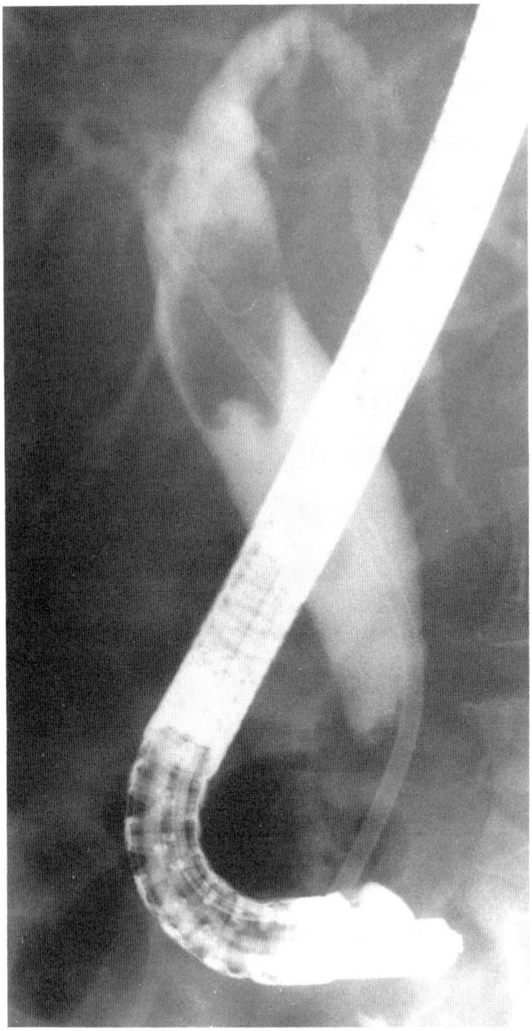

Fig. 17.9 Indwelling stents are good temporizing methods for unfit patients with difficult stones.

long-term results are obtained by surgical resection of the affected lobe.

Gallbladder stones

It is possible to negotiate a catheter via the endoscopic retrograde route through the cystic duct into the gallbladder. Cholesterol stones in the gallbladder can then be dissolved using methyl tert-butyl ether. Transcystic duct drain can also be inserted endoscopically for patients with acute cholecystitis [22]. These techniques have been eclipsed by the rapid development of laparoscopic cholecystectomy.

Complications [3]

Complications of endoscopic sphincterotomy include bleeding, perforation, pancreatitis and sepsis. These complications occur in about 10% of patients after sphincterotomy. Less than 20% of these complications require surgery and the overall mortality is about 1.5%.

Bleeding occurs in 2.5–5% of patients and has a mortality of about 0.3%. Bleeding is more likely when the sphincterotomy is performed for a papillary tumour and papillary stenosis. The risk is also higher for patients with portal hypertension and when a sphincterotomy is extended. Significant, even life threatening, bleeding may present several days after sphincterotomy.

Retroperitoneal perforation occurs in about 1% of patients and is more likely when the cut strays from the recommended direction. The diagnosis is made at the time of sphincterotomy if air or contrast is seen outside the confines of the bile duct and duodenum. If the diagnosis is made early most patients can be managed conservatively with nothing by mouth, antibiotics, nasogastric suction and nasobiliary drainage.

Post-ERCP pancreatitis is more likely if there has been repeated injection of contrast into the pancreatic duct, especially if the pancreatic duct is filled under pressure and 'acinarization' (filling of the pancreatic parenchyma) results. This complication is more likely in patients who undergo ERCP for dysfunction of the sphincter of Oddi.

Cholangitis after ERCP usually occurs in patients with an obstructed biliary system which is inadequately drained at the end of the procedure. Bacteria are introduced into the obstructed system and sepsis may flare up several days after the procedure. Post-ERCP sepsis may be minimized by meticulous disinfection of the endoscope and accessories, avoiding injection of contrast under pressure, and providing adequate drainage by nasobiliary drain or stents if the obstruction cannot be removed.

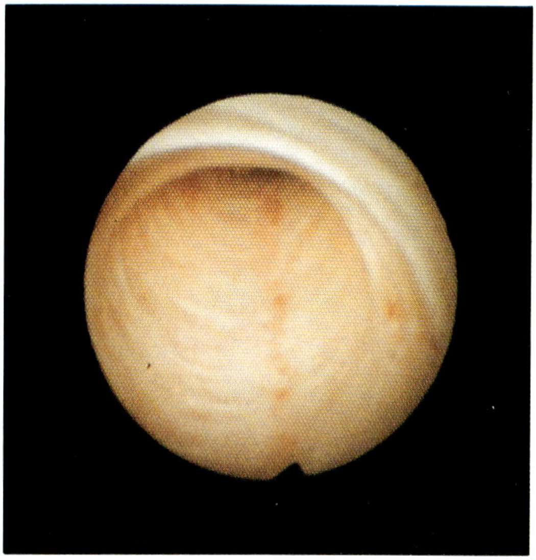

Plate 16.1

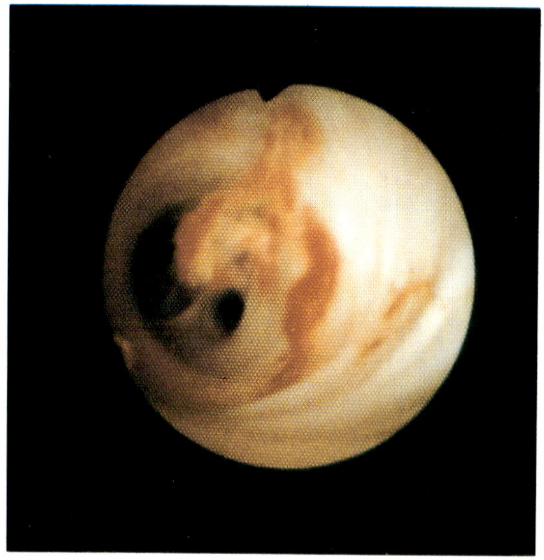

Plate 16.2

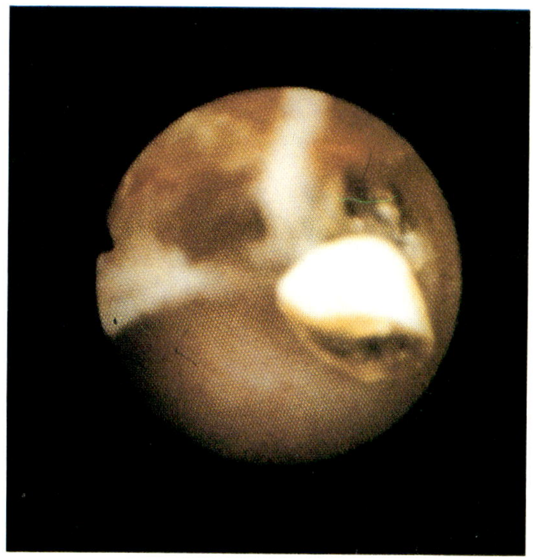

Plate 16.3

Plate 16.1 Proximal common bile duct as viewed through flexible choledochoscope.

Plate 16.2 Left hepatic duct with displaced stone fragments.

Plate 16.3 Distal common bile duct with stone.

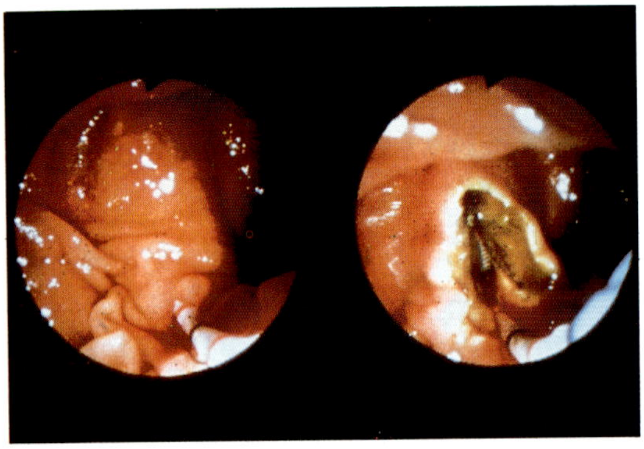

Plate 17.1 Endoscopic sphincterotomy: the cut may be extended safely to the horizontal fold.

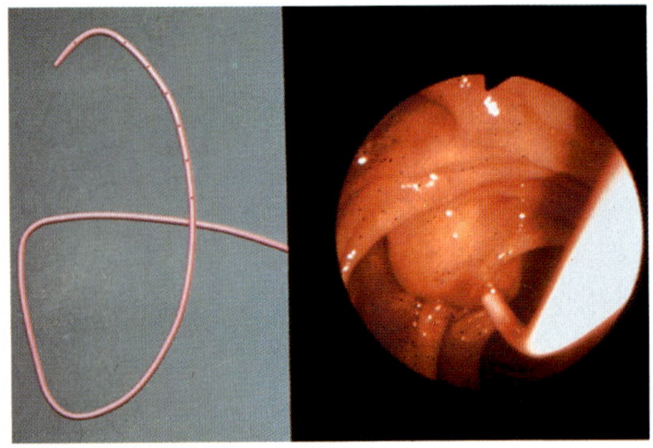

Plate 17.2 A nasobiliary drain can be inserted without a sphincterotomy.

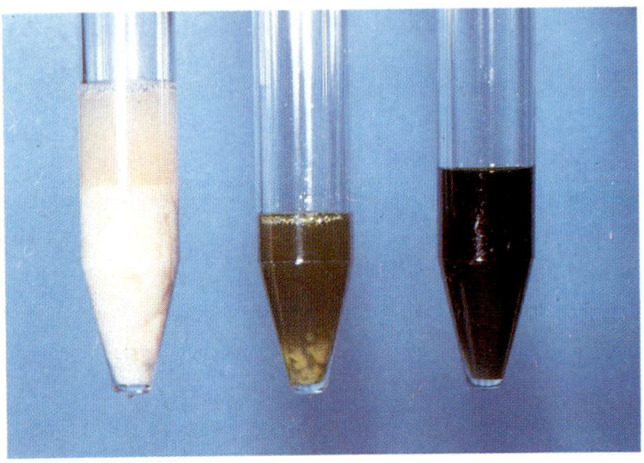

Plate 17.3 Bile obtained from a nasobiliary drain in a patient with acute cholangitis at the time of ERCP, 12 and 24 hours later.

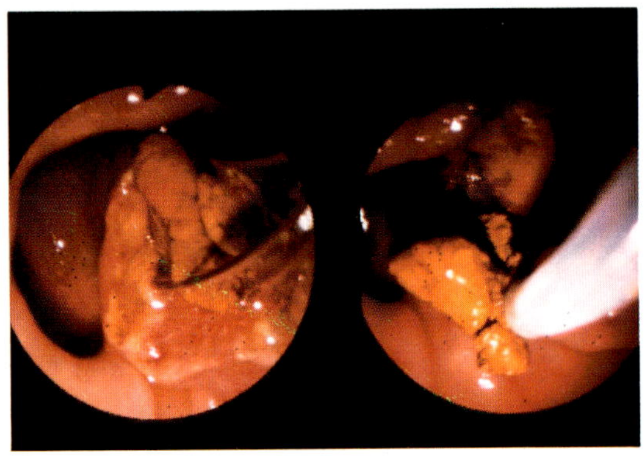

Plate 17.4 Soft pigment stones may be sliced through by closing Dormia baskets through them.

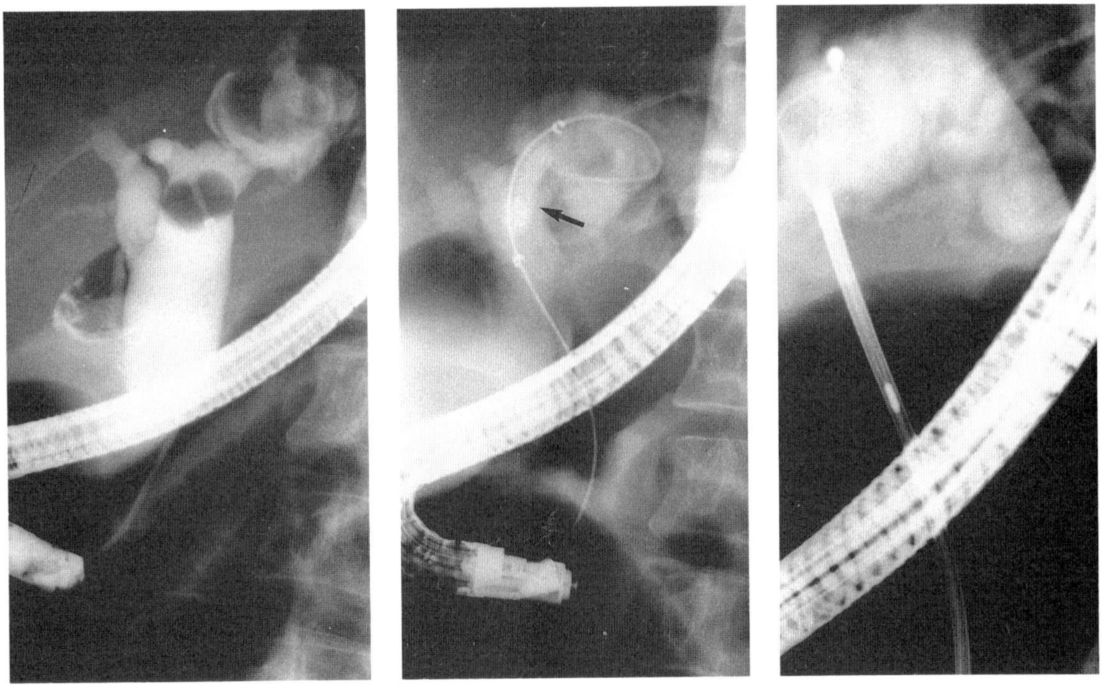

Fig. 17.10 Intrahepatic stones. Left: occlusion cholangiogram showing left intrahepatic duct stones behind a stricture. Centre: balloon dilatation of the stricture (arrow shows the balloon filled with contrast). Right: mechanical lithrotripsy prior to extraction.

In the era of laparoscopic cholecystectomy

The advent of laparoscopic cholecystectomy has revolutionized the management of gallstone disease. Within a short period of time laparoscopic cholecystectomy has replaced open surgery as the treatment of choice for patients with gallbladder stones. Because of this new technique the approach to patients with concomitant gallstones and common duct stones is also undergoing radical changes.

When laparoscopic cholecystectomy was not available, patients with concomitant gallbladder stones and common duct stones had a laparotomy, cholecystectomy and an operative cholangiogram. If common duct stones are confirmed on the operative cholangiogram the common duct is explored and the stone removed. Most surgeons would insert a T-tube after such a procedure. It is possible to remove the common duct stone through an endoscopic sphincterotomy before the operation. A randomized controlled trial comparing these approaches, however, showed that apart from a shortened hospital stay removing the stone pre-operatively did not confer any benefit [23]. The equation is changed with the arrival of laparoscopic cholecystectomy.

If common duct stones are found during laparoscopic cholecystectomy, the surgeon may:

1 abandon laparoscopic cholecystectomy and convert to open duct exploration;
2 explore the common duct laparoscopically;
3 proceed with laparoscopic cholecystectomy and perform postoperative ERCP and sphincterotomy.

Alternatively, ERCP can be performed pre-operatively in at risk patients and the common duct stones removed before laparoscopic cholecystectomy.

The common bile duct may be explored laparoscopically [24, 25]. This may be performed either through the cystic duct or through an incision in the common bile duct itself. Both techniques have certain limitations.

Transcystic exploration

Transcystic duct common duct exploration may be performed under fluoroscopic or endoscopic control. After dissection of Calot's triangle an operative cholangiogram is performed. If ductal stones are detected the cystic duct is cannulated with a catheter containing a wire basket and the common duct trawled for stones under fluoroscopic guidance. The cystic duct may have to be dilated with a balloon catheter over a guide wire beforehand. Pulling larger stones via this route runs a risk of avulsing the cystic duct. Alternatively, a •fine choledochoscope may be inserted through one of the ports into the cystic duct and thence into the common bile duct. The choledochoscope is attached to a video camera. Either two camera systems, or a picture-in-picture monitor, is used so that both the intra-abdominal and the intraductal view can be obtained at the same time. The stones may be trapped with baskets inserted through the choledochoscope and removed through the cystic duct, or they may be broken up using electro-hydraulic or pulsed-dye laser lithotripsy. At the moment transcystic exploration is only suitable for stones below the cystic duct junction as instruments (and scopes) cannot be manipulated upstream. The other drawbacks are the expense of the additional equipment, the prolonged operation time and that the expertise for laparoscopic duct exploration is not presently widely available.

Laparoscopic choledochotomy

Laparoscopic choledochotomy is suitable for patients with dilated common ducts containing large stones. After the placement of a stay suture on the common bile duct the duct is incised and the stone removed. A choledochoscope can be inserted to aid stone removal and to confirm clearance of the biliary tree. A T-tube is then inserted and the choledochotomy closed using intracorporeal suturing and knotting techniques. A drain is inserted into the subhepatic space at the end of the procedure. Stones above or below the cystic duct junction can be dealt with in this manner. The main drawbacks are that laparoscopic suturing is technically demanding and using a T-tube (and drain) prolongs the hospital course, defeating the purpose of laparoscopic cholecystectomy.

ERCP

The role of ERCP and endoscopic stone removal in patients undergoing laparoscopic cholecystectomy has been the subject of heated debate [26].

Intra-operative ERCP during laparoscopic cholecystectomy has been reported. Laparoscopic cholecystectomy is performed with the patient supine while ERCP is best performed with the patient prone. Inflating air into the gut during ERCP is likely to distend the bowel and make subsequent laparoscopy impossible. Because of these technical difficulties, and the logistic difficulties of bringing the laparoscopic team and the endoscopic team (and their equipment) into the same oper-ating room at the same time, intra-operative ERCP is unlikely to become popular.

Pre-operative ERCP and removing common duct stones endoscopically prior to laparoscopic cholecystectomy is an attractive option. The demand for pre-operative ERCP has increased since the introduction of laparoscopic cholecystectomy. Potential disadvantages of this approach are that:
1 some patients may have to undergo an unnecessary ERCP and may suffer complications, principally pancreatitis;
2 endoscopic sphincterotomy is not without complications;
3 stones may migrate into the duct from the gallbladder in the interval between ERCP and laparoscopic cholecystectomy.

Postoperative ERCP. Another approach is to perform ERCP in the immediate postoperative period if stones are detected on the operative cholangiogram. This avoids unnecessary ERCP for patients without stones. However, if endoscopic stone extraction is unsuccessful the patient requires another operation under general anaesthesia.

How patients with gallbladder stones and possible common duct stones should be managed is an unresolved question. Future research will be focussed on formulating criteria for pre-operative ERCP, developing and disseminating the skills of laparoscopic duct exploration and exploring methods of removing ductal stones without sphincterotomy. In the mean time the best clinical results in each individual hospital will be obtained by utilizing the available expertise, be it endoscopic sphincterotomy, laparoscopic duct exploration or open cholecystectomy and common duct exploration.

References

1 Vaira D, D'anna L, Ainley C *et al.* Endoscopic sphincterotomy in 1000 consecutive patients. *Lancet* 1989;ii:431–3.
2 Lambert ME, Betts CD, Hill JD, Faragher EB, Martin DF, Tweedle DEF. Endoscopic sphincterotomy, the whole truth. *Br J Surg* 1991;78:473–6.
3 Cotton PB, Lehman G, Vennes J *et al.* Endoscopic sphincterotomy complications and their management: an attempt at consensus. *Gastrointest Endosc* 1991;37:383–93.
4 Cotton PB, Williams CB. *Practical Gastrointestinal Endoscopy*, 3rd edn. Oxford: Blackwell Scientific Publications, 1990:85–156.
5 Waye J, Geenen JE, Fleischer D, Venu RP. *Techniques in Therapeutic Endoscopy*, 2nd edn. Philadelphia: Saunders, 1992.
6 Baillie J. *Gastrointestinal Endoscopy*. Oxford: Butterworth-Heinemann, 1992.
7 Reynolds BM, Dargan EI. Acute obstructive cholangitis—a distinct clinical syndrome. *Ann Surg* 1958; 150:299–303.
8 Leung JWC, Chung SCS, Sung JY, Banez VP, Li AKC. Urgent endoscopic drainage for acute suppurative cholangitis. *Lancet* 1989;1:1307–9.
9 Lai ECS, Mok FPT, Tan ESY *et al.* Endoscopy biliary drainage for severe acute cholangitis. *N Engl J Med* 1992;**326**:1582–6.
10 Neoptolemos JP, Carr-Locke DL, London NJ *et al.* Controlled trial of urgent endoscopic retrograde cholangio-pancreatography and endoscopic sphincterotomy versus conservative treatment for acute pancreatitis due to gallstones. *Lancet* 1988;**2**:979–83.
11 May GR, Shaffner EH. Should elective endoscopic sphincterotomy replace cholecystectomy for the treatment of high risk patients with gall stone pancreatitis. *J Clin Gastroenterol* 1991;13:125–8.
12 Foutch PG. Endoscopic management of large common duct stones. *Am J Gastroenterol* 1991;**86**:1561–5.
13 Leung JWC, Chung SCS, Mok SD, Li AKC. Endoscopic removal of large common bile duct stones in recurrent pyogenic cholangitis. *Gastrointest Endosc* 1988;**34**: 238–41.
14 Chung SCS, Leung JWC, Leong HT, Li AKC. Mechanical lithotripsy of large common bile duct stones using a basket. *Br J Surg* 1991;78:1448–50.
15 Leung JWC, Chung SCS. Electrohydraulic lithotripsy with peroral choledochoscopy. *Br Med J* 1989;**299**: 595–8.
16 Cotton PB, Forbes A, Leung JWC, Dineen L. Endoscopic stenting for long term management of large bile duct stones; a 2–5 year follow-up. *Gastrointest Endosc* 1987;33:401–12.
17 Dowsett JF, Vaira D, Hatfield ARW *et al.* Endoscopic biliary therapy using the combined percutaneous and endoscopic technique. *Gastroenterology* 1989;**96**: 1180–6.
18 Cotton PB. Precut papillotomy—a risky technique for experts only. *Gastrointest Endosc* 1989;35:578–9.
19 Leung JWC, Banez VP, Chung SCS. Precut (needle knife) papillotomy for impacted common bile duct stone at the ampulla. *Am J Gastroenterol* 1990;85: 991–3.
20 Leung JWC, Venezuela RR, Banez VP, Chung SCS, Lau JWY, Li AKC. Endoscopic management of intrahepatic stones. *Gastrointest Endosc* 1991;**37**:256. (Abstract).
21 Bonnel DH, Liguory CE, Comud FE, Lefebvre JF. Common bile duct and intrahepatic stones: results of transhepatic electrohydraulic lithotripsy in 50 patients. *Radiology* 1991;**180**:345–8.
22 Soehendra N. Access to the cystic duct: a new endoscopic therapy for gall bladder diseases. *Endoscopy* 1991;23:36–7.
23 Neoptolemos JP, Carr-Locke DL, Fossard DP. Prospective randomised study of pre-operative endoscopic sphincterotomy versus surgery alone for common bile duct stones. *Br Med J* 1987;**294**:470–4.
24 Hunter JG. Laparoscopic transcystic common bile duct exploration. *Am J Surg* 1992;**163**:53–6.
25 Jacobs M, Verdeja J-C, Goldstein HS. Laparoscopic choledocholithotomy. *J Laparoendosc Surg* 1991;1: 79–82.
26 Cotton PB, Baillie J, Pappas TN, Meyers WS. Laparoscopic cholecystectomy and the biliary endoscopist. *Gastrointest Endosc* 1991;37:94–7.

Chapter 18
The radiological approach to common bile duct stones

H.J. Burhenne & A.F. Watkinson

Introduction

Radiology of the biliary tract began almost immediately after Roentgen's discovery of the X-ray. The first radiographs of gallstones were published in 1896 [1]. In addition to diagnosis, radiologists have developed techniques for the treatment of bile duct stones in the last 2 decades. Removal of bile duct stones is accomplished under fluoroscopic control and is called 'interventional radiology'. This term was coined by Margulis in 1967 [2] to describe the 'growing body of manipulative procedures performed by a physician skillful in radiologic techniques and experienced in the clinical problems'. The beginning of interventional radiology of the biliary tract occurred probably as early as 1921 when two surgeons in Germany, Burckhardt and Müller, reported on percutaneous puncture of the gallbladder, both in cadavers and *in vivo*. They succeeded 'by injection of a shadowing-producing fluid to visualize the gallstones and bile ducts' [3]. They also raised the possibility of dissolving gallstones by injection of chemicals. We can assume that Dr Pribram in Berlin knew about the work of his surgical colleagues when he used ether in 1923 for the attempted treatment of gallstones impacted in the common duct [4]. Part of the success of instillation of fluids in the bile duct for stone passage probably is the result of increased fluid pressure alone. Catheter irrigation through the T-tube tract under fluoroscopic control has been used with good success for the treatment of retained small common duct stones [5].

The radiological interventional approach to bile duct stones is usually indicated when surgical or endoscopic techniques have failed or in patients with a high operative risk.

Imaging of bile duct stones

Advances in imaging modalities of the biliary tract in recent decades have resulted in significant changes in the ability of the radiologist to make a precise diagnosis. Ultrasound, computed tomography (CT), magnetic resonance imaging (MRI), and the development of new radionuclides have played a major role in our ability to diagnose bile duct stones. The oldest radiological imaging technique is the plain radiograph of the abdomen (Fig. 18.1 (a)). This simple and inexpensive examination is sometimes neglected in today's era of high technology imaging. The plain film examination requires no special preparation of the patient, and the results are known immediately. Plain film detection of gallstones depends on their calcium content. Gallstones can even be detected today by this radiographic technique in Egyptian mummies. With progress, however, have come the expensive problems of application of multiple imaging techniques and the need to reduce the incidence of false positive studies.

Ultrasound is a sensitive, non-ionizing and inexpensive method (Fig. 18.2) for investigating calculous gallbladder disease [6], with sensitivities, specificities and accuracies greater than 95% for detecting gallbladder stones. However, its accuracy in choledocholithiasis diagnosis is less, particularly for stones in the distal common duct, with sensitivities reported from 20–75% [7, 8]. The plain radiograph of the abdomen can show gallstones in 10–15% of patients [9], depending on the calcium concentration.

Fig. 18.1 (a) Plain radiograph of the right-upper quadrant shows clips and staples from previous surgery. A calcified common duct stone is detected in the last intercostal space 2 cm to the right of T12–L1 interspace. (b) Computed tomography in the same patient shows a markedly dilated distal common duct. The common duct stone is seen to better advantage. (c) Endoscopic retrograde pancreatico-cholangiography shows the pancreatic duct filled. The stone is seen to lie in a choledochal cyst.

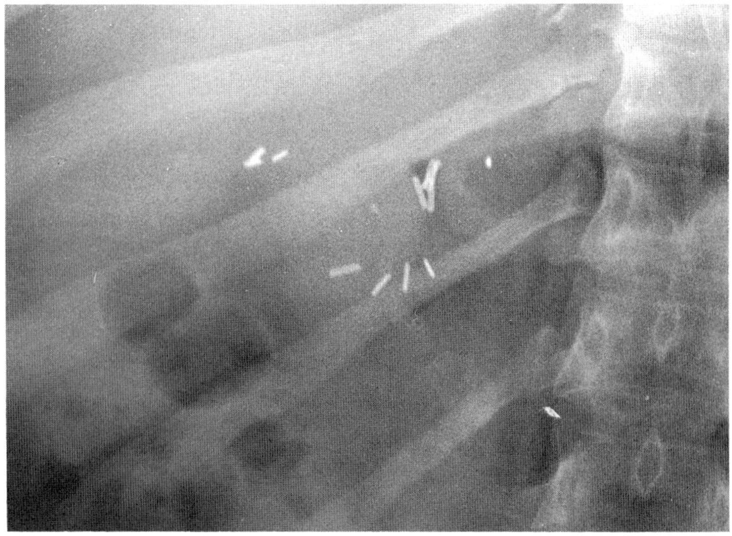

(a)

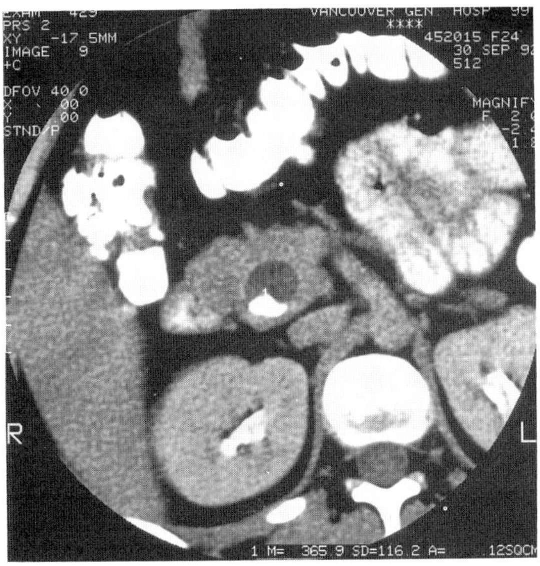

(b)

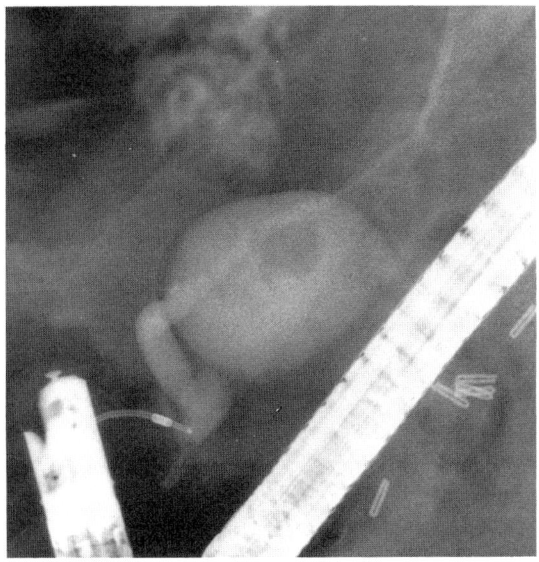

(c)

CT is more sensitive than the plain film (see Fig. 18.1(b)) with accuracies of 89.8%, specificities of 100% and sensitivities of 79.1% being quoted [10]. Early studies, however, to quantitate stone composition and aid differentiation of cholesterol from pigment stones to guide therapeutic dissolution have met with variable success [11–14].

MRI demonstrates stones well, although these are typically of low signal intensity on both T1- and T2-weighted sequences regardless of stone composition, and no correlation has been found between MRI appearances and gallstone composition [15].

Oral cholecystography (OC) has been replaced in the last decade by ultrasound as the modality of choice for investigating gallbladder disease; however, in some instances it is still indicated. It may help to further evaluate patients in which there is a high clinical suspicion of gallstones in which the ultrasound is negative. In addition, it has been used for evaluation of patients for

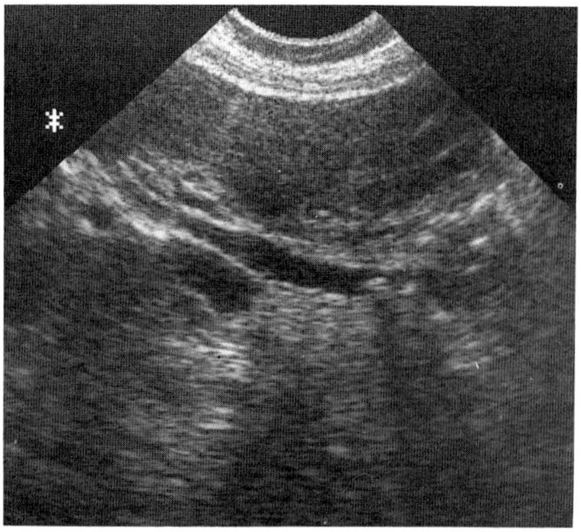

Fig. 18.2 At least two common duct stones seen on ultrasonography.

chemolitholysis, giving information on the size and number of gallstones, as well as the patency of the cystic duct. However, recent studies have achieved comparable results for assessment of cystic duct patency using ultrasonography pre- and post-fatty meals [16].

Intravenous cholangiography is rarely performed now, following published studies of unacceptable contrast reactions [17]. However, some centres are now re-evaluating this cost-effective method of identifying common duct anatomy and the presence of stones pre-operatively in patients going for laparoscopic cholecystectomy [18–20] (Fig. 18.3).

Endoscopic retrograde cholangiopancreatography (ERCP) is the preferred method of cholangiography when choledochal stone disease is suspected on clinical grounds (see Fig. 18.1(c)), with sensitivities varying from 66.7% in non-jaundiced patients to 80.6% in jaundiced patients [7]. If this technique is unsuccessful or non-diagnostic, a percutaneous transhepatic cholangiogram (PTC) helps to define the presence of either obstructing or non-obstructing choledochal calculi, although this may be difficult in the non-obstructed system.

T-tube cholangiography, post-cholecystectomy and common duct exploration, remains an important imaging modality to detect the presence of residual choledochal calculi. Meticulous attention to technical detail is important, utilizing dilute contrast media and excluding air bubbles from the examination tract.

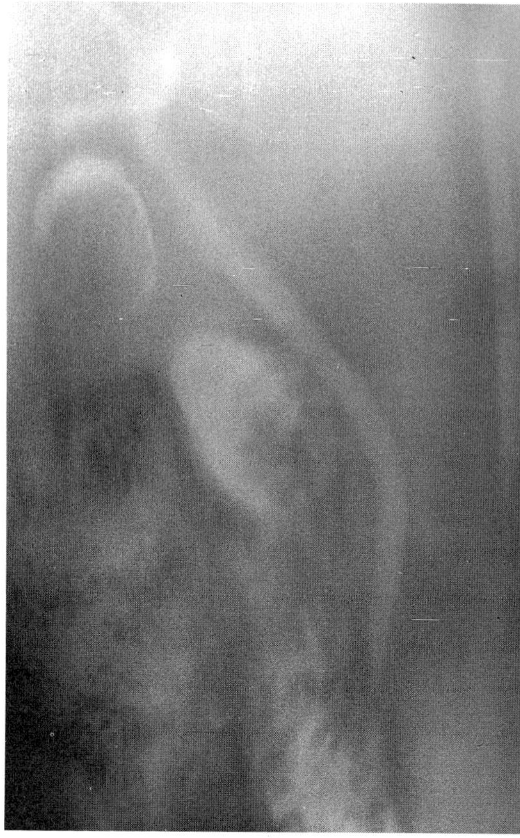

Fig. 18.3 Intravenous cholangiography obtained before laparoscopic cholecystectomy shows a normal common duct. A large gallstone is present in Morison's pouch.

Nuclear imaging, utilizing O-methylimmunodiacetic acid compound (HIDA), or its derivatives, is extremely sensitive in confirming acute cholecystitis with an occluded cystic duct [21]. This is invariably due to a gallstone, although its role in defining biliary calculi further is extremely limited.

Stone extraction via postoperative tract

Retained stones in the common bile duct, as demonstrated on T-tube cholangiography after cholecystectomy, remain a persistent problem.

The use of routine operative cholangiography in open cholecystectomy still yields a false-negative rate of 5% after common duct exploration [22]. Some surgeons advocate performing only selective cholangiography during laparoscopic cholecystectomy [23]. However, 2–12% [24, 25] of patients undergoing cholecystectomy have undetected common bile duct stones. This is in agreement with our experience with patients having no history of jaundice or cholangitis, normal liver function tests, and normal ultrasound having unsuspected bile duct calculi. The radiological interventional technique of percutaneous removal through a T-tube tract, is currently the method of choice for removal of retained calculi, with a success rate in excess of 90% [26]. This success rate has been established with the use of the postoperative sinus tract [27], utilizing a Dormia ureteral stone basket [28] and the addition of a steerable catheter [29].

The procedure can be performed on an outpatient basis on an ambulatory patient requiring no premedication. A pulse oximeter and electrocardiography monitor are routinely used in our institution. If there is a previous history of postoperative infection or pancreatitis, the patient should have an intravenous line established, receive pre-instrumentation antibiotics (ceftizoxine 1 g just prior to the procedure, with three subsequent doses), and be admitted for 24 hours post-procedure for observation.

The T-tube tract should be established over a 5-week period postoperatively (Fig. 18.4). Cholangiography is then performed to visualize the

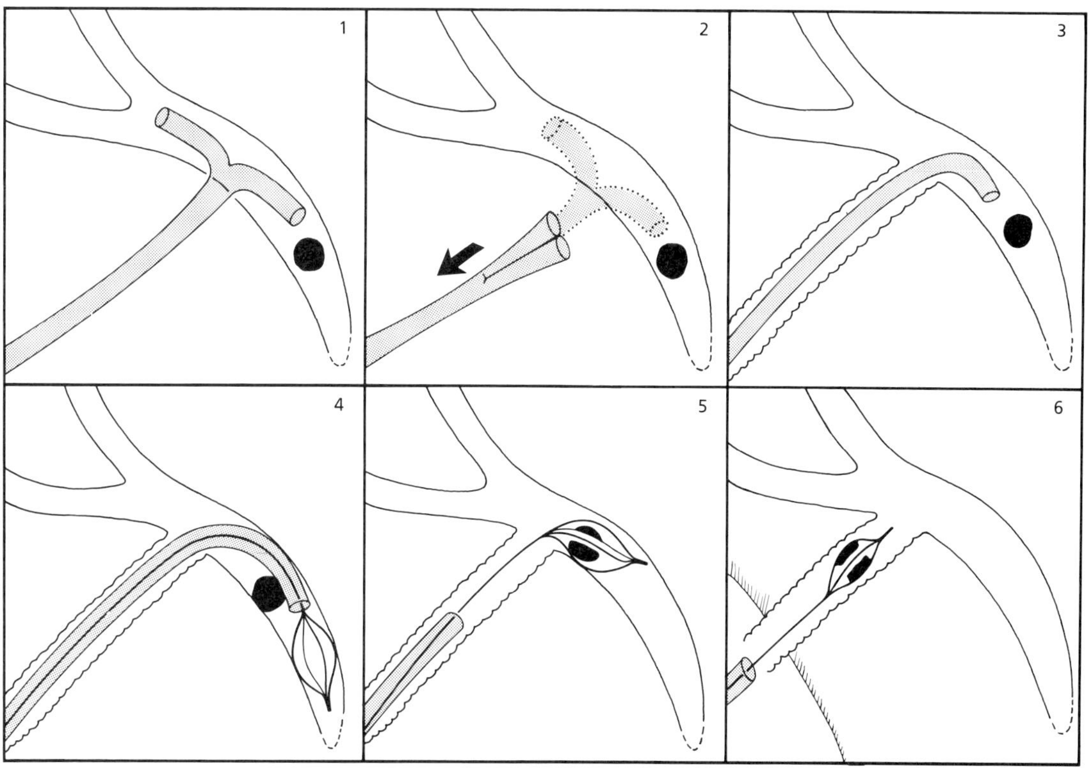

Fig. 18.4 Technical steps for retained common duct stone extraction: (1) Repeat T-tube cholangiogram is obtained on the day of stone extraction 4–5 weeks after choledochotomy. (2) After the location of the retained stone has been ascertained, the T-tube is withdrawn. (3) Using the sinus tract of the T-tube, the steerable catheter is guided into the bile duct, and its moveable tip is advanced beyond the retained stone. (4) The basket is inserted through the steerable catheter, the catheter partially withdrawn, and the basket opened. (5) The open basket is withdrawn in order to engage the stone. The basket is only retracted, never advanced, outside the enclosure of the steerable catheter. (6) The stone is extracted through the drain tract. From Burhenne 1973 [30].

intra- and extrahepatic biliary tree and demonstrate any retained calculi. The T-tube is withdrawn and a 12 F steerable catheter manipulated under fluoroscopy along the tract into the common bile duct and advanced to a position just beyond the retained calculus. The stone basket is then manœuvred through the steerable catheter lumen beyond the retained calculus such that it opens fully when the steerable catheter is partially withdrawn. In one movement, once the basket has engaged the calculus, the steerable catheter and basket are withdrawn together (Fig. 18.5). The basket is only closed and engaged by traction with the tip of the steerable catheter when the stone is too large (>8 mm) to move along the tract and needs fragmenting. This is often easy as large impacted stones are usually relatively soft. This technique of stone extraction was first described in 1972 [29] with success rates in excess of 90% [30–32]. Smaller stones and fragments less than 3 mm usually pass spontaneously or can be pushed with the aid of catheters into the duodenum [33].

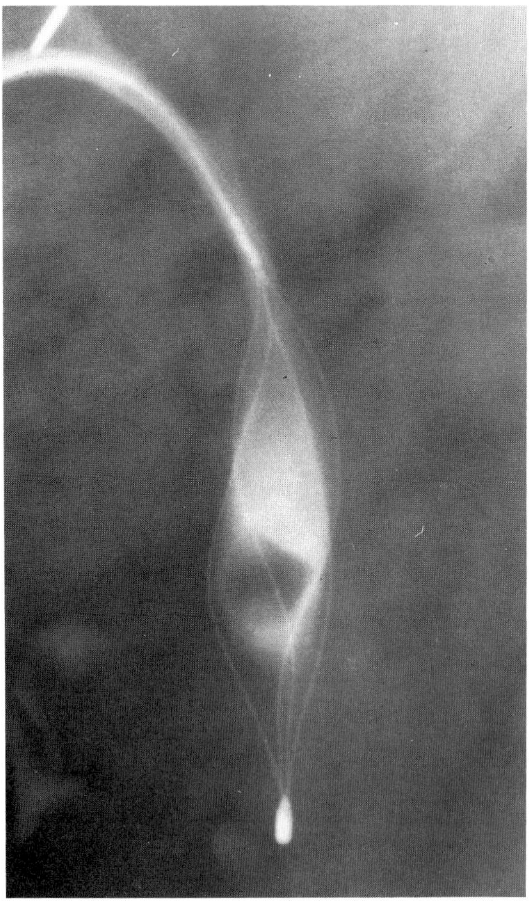

Fig. 18.5 The stone has been engaged in the basket and is withdrawn under fluoroscopic control through the sinus tract.

Forceps, as described by Mazzariello in 1973 [34], have been used with good success; however, we personally only recommend their usage if all other methods have failed. For impacted stones, the use of smaller steerable catheters (8 F), hydrophilic guidewires and a Fogarty vascular balloon may assist passage beyond the stone and its subsequent disimpaction. For impacted stones in the distal common bile duct, we have tried, with variable success, suction applied through the catheter, a strong contrast injection just distal to the stone A morbidity of 5% with no deaths has been reported in 612 patients having percutaneous extraction in the USA [35], although a review of 26 British hospitals demonstrated a morbidity of 9.2% including pancreatitis, fever and tract perforation, and one death from acute pancreatitis [36]. However, with a surgical mortality for re-exploration for retained stones approaching 3%, these results are extremely good [37]. Another technique for small retained common duct stones is a saline washout after intravenous medication to relax the sphincter of Oddi [38]. If no T-tube access is available, endoscopic sphincterotomy and stone removal is the method of choice. It is more expensive, has a lower success rate, and a higher complication rate than the interventional radiological technique. Cotton concluded that it appears reasonable to favour a primary percutaneous radiological approach if the size and position of the T-tube are appropriate and that the convenience of having the T-tube weighed against the potential risk of sphincterotomy [39].

Intrahepatic bile duct stones

Duct stones within the liver which have been displaced from the gallbladder and extrahepatic bile ducts, can be located within the hepatic duct, and can form proximal to the intrahepatic bile duct strictures, particularly when associated with recurrent pyogenic cholangitis. Faceted stones in the bile ducts in an intrahepatic location are usually displaced from the gallbladder or common duct. This displacement can also be noticed during cholangiography injection. Retained stones appearing in the extrahepatic bile ducts after cholecystectomy may have been in an intrahepatic location during operative cholangiography and, for that reason, were overlooked.

If there is access through a postoperative drainage tract, such as a T-tube tract, a steerable catheter can be moved to an intrahepatic location for stone removal. The difficulty here lies in the fact that stone baskets may not move alongside an impacted stone proximally to it (Fig. 18.6). Suction is then applied through the steerable catheter. Also, waiting for several days with the patient ambulatory will often move the stones distally into the extrahepatic ducts. The success rate for percutaneous non-operative stone removal is lower for intrahepatic than for extrahepatic stones. Strictures below intrahepatic stones will have to be dilated with balloon catheters before stone manipulation can be attempted.

If the stone cannot be mobilized from below, transhepatic puncture into the dilated duct proximal to the stone is sometimes required. This is often successful if there are only one or a few intrahepatic stones present. In so-called oriental cholangitis or recurrent pyogenic cholangitis, intrahepatic stones are usually in multiple segments of the liver and this condition can only be palliated by interventional techniques. Because of recurrence of stones in the liver, prolonged access is then usually required. This can be with the use of a U-tube or, better, after surgical choledochojejunostomy with formation of a Hutson loop at the time of surgery. This ensures easy access to the remaining biliary tree percutaneously through the jejunum (Fig. 18.7). The jejunostomy access can also be used for dilating possible strictures at a choledochojejunostomy. Repeated access is provided to the intrahepatic segments using either

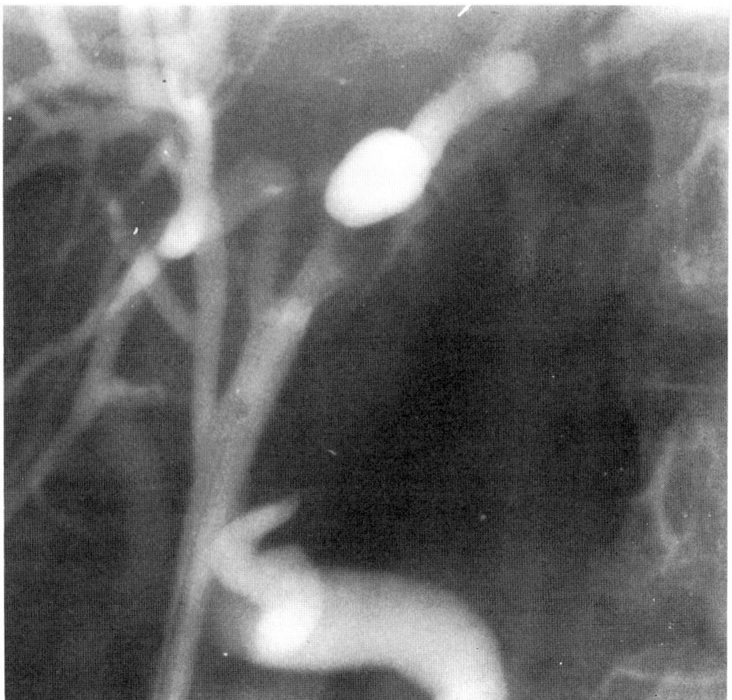

Fig. 18.6 Utilizing a postoperative T-tube tract, the steerable catheter is moved close to the impacted stone in the left hepatic radicle. A Fogarty balloon is inflated with contrast distal to the stone and the stone is moved into the extrahepatic ducts for basket engagement.

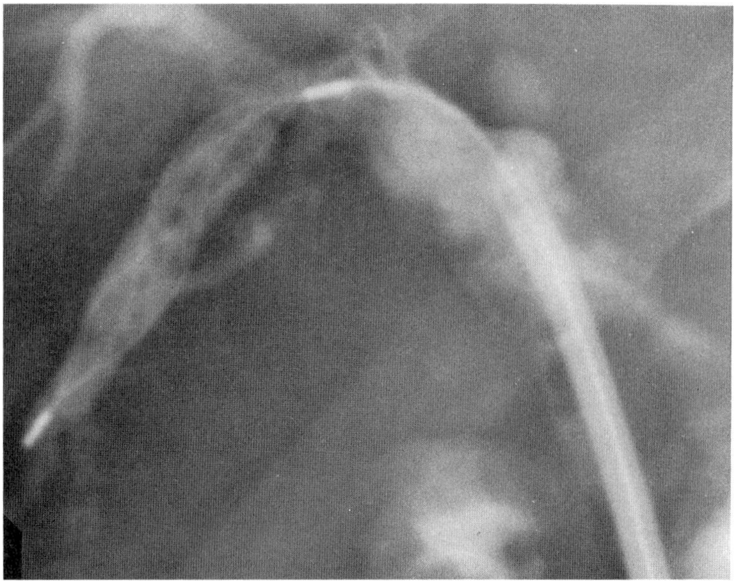

Fig. 18.7 Patient with recurrent pyogenic cholangitis and multiple stones in one right hepatic radicle. The steerable catheter was advanced through a jejunostomy access and a hepatojejunostomy. The basket is placed in the hepatic radicle for palliative stone extraction.

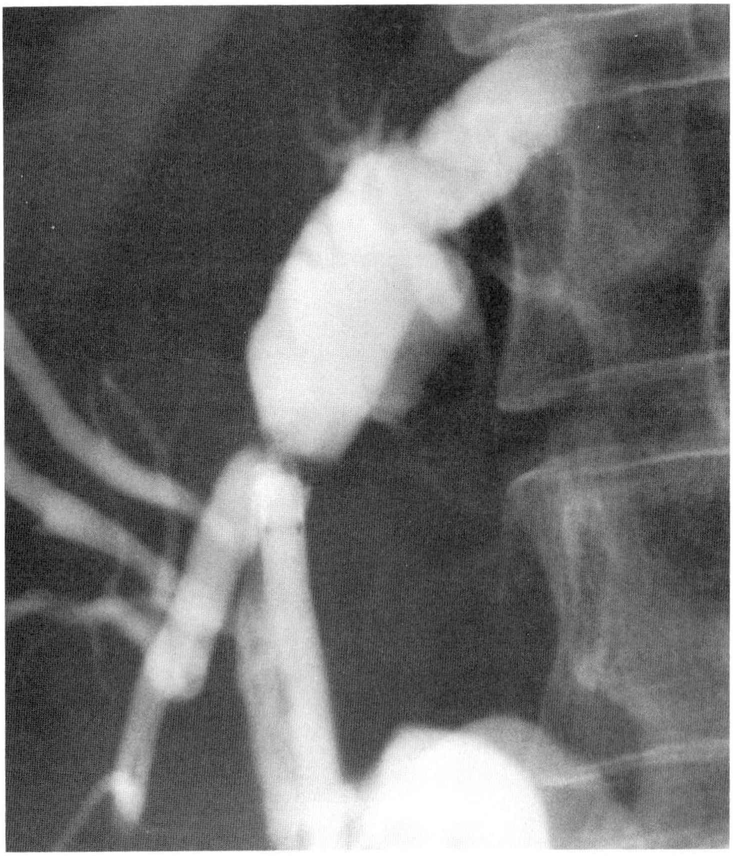

(a)

Fig. 18.8 (a) Stricture in main left hepatic radicle with stones proximally to it.

fibreoptic endoscopes or radiological techniques with a side-to-side or end-to-side biliary-enteric anastomosis; the enteric end being brought out as a cutaneous stoma [40].

Bile duct stricture dilatation

Dilatation of strictures of the bile ducts, both intrahepatic and extrahepatic, is now commonly accomplished as a radiological interventional procedure. It was first reported in 1975 [41]. Even malignant strictures are readily dilated in one setting to accommodate a 14 F catheter for internal biliary drainage [42]. Interventional dilatation of benign bile duct strictures is required if biliary stones are retained proximally to such strictures resulting from cholangitis or previous surgery (Fig. 18.8). It has been suggested that indwelling splint catheters must remain within previous strictures for a period of 8–24 months for the scar to mature and stabilize [43]. Lasting patency following stent removal has been reported in 73% of patients with biliary–enteric anastomosis, and in 88% of patients with primary ductal strictures, for an overall success rate of 78%. However, no definite conclusions can be drawn about the utility of long-term internal–external stenting after stricture dilatation [44]. Balloon dilation can be performed through a choledochojejuno-cutaneous fistula, or through a stomatized jejunal limb [45]. Interventional stricture dilatation is part of the palliative treatment of stone removal in patients with recurrent pyogenic cholangitis in the Orient.

Percutaneous transhepatic approach

Percutaneous transhepatic cholangiography, the

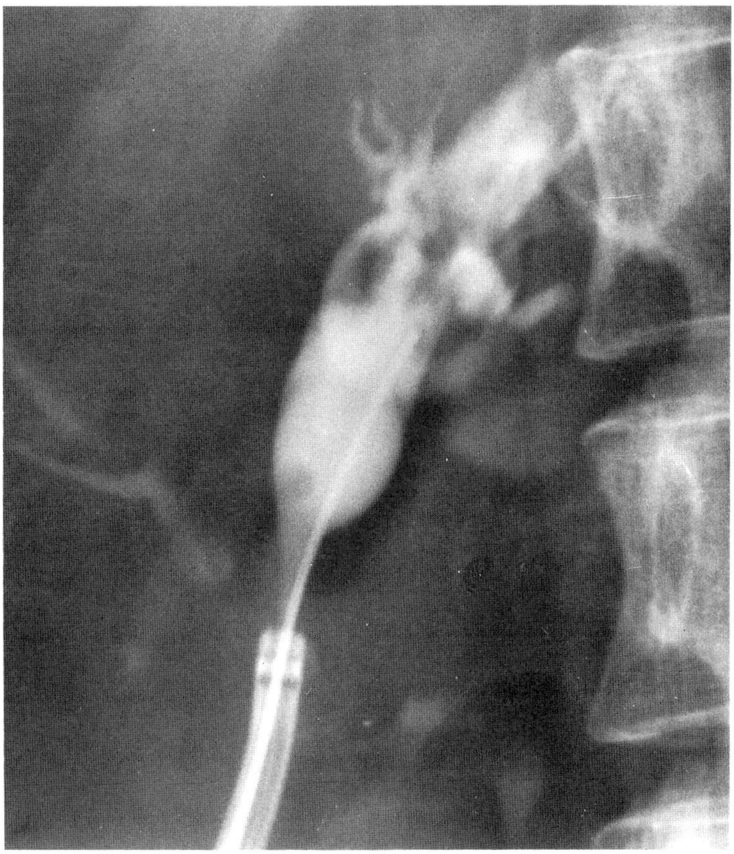

(b)

Fig. 18.8 (b) The stricture has been dilated with balloon technique and stone removal is now possible with a basket through the previous stricture.

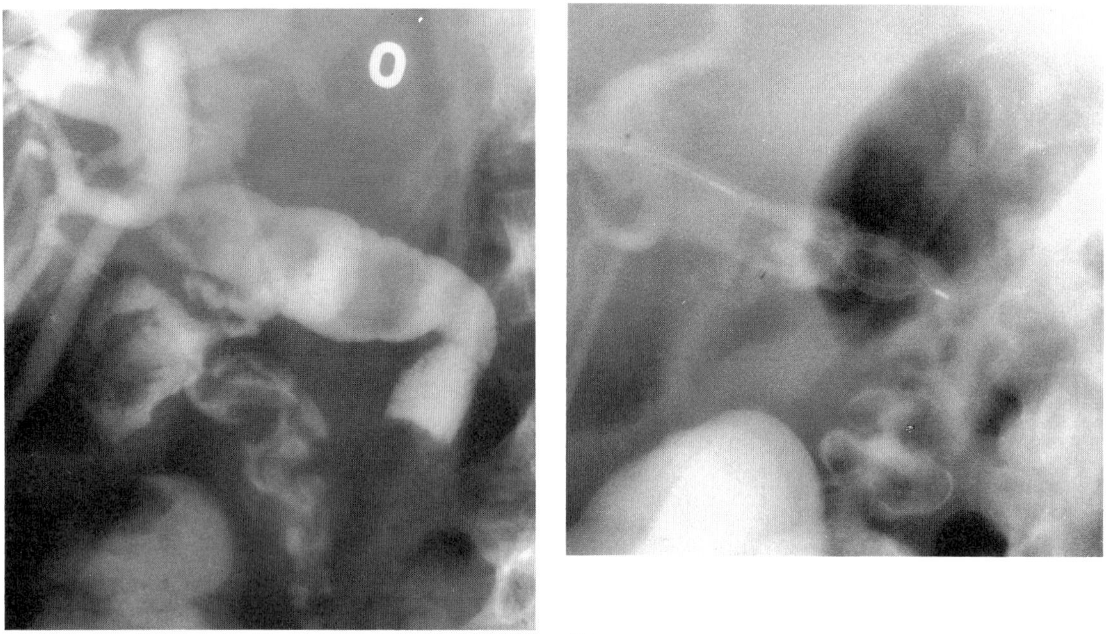

(a) (b)

Fig. 18.9 (a) Patient with multiple common duct stones underwent percutaneous transhepatic puncture because of failed retrograde endoscopic approach. (b) Basket advanced transhepatically engaged common duct stones in sequence and was closed in the duct to fragment these stones.

technical prerequisite for interventional transhepatic procedures, was described in 1937 [46]. In patients with a previously removed gallbladder in which the endoscopic approach to a common duct stone has failed and extra-corporeal shockwave lithotripsy is unavailable, the transhepatic approach described in 1979 [47] can be utilized. Initial diagnostic percutaneous transhepatic cholangiography is performed to confirm and locate the common duct calculus. An intravenous line is established, prophylactic antibiotics are given, and a pulse oximeter and ECG monitor are positioned appropriately. The transhepatic tract is then dilated to 8.3 F and a steerable 8 F Burhenne catheter and stone basket is used to entrap the stone. If the stone is too large to remove, Dotter [47] originally suggested dilatation of the transhepatic tract to a calibre sufficient to allow extraction of the intact stone. After 2–3 days of an indwelling 8.3 F catheter, dilatation and substitution for a larger equivalent can be performed and the calculus can then be removed with a larger basket. However, more recent studies [48–51] suggest that dilatation of the ampulla of Vater or bilio-enteric anastomosis in the instance of a choledochojejunostomy, with a balloon catheter over a guidewire is preferable. The calculus can then be pushed into the duodenum with a soft occlusion balloon (Medi-Tech Inc.) over a guidewire. If the calculus is too large to be pushed or withdrawn, then crushing into multiple fragments with a basket or lithotripsy is our procedure of choice (Fig. 18.9). The fragments can then be removed by the basket technique or may pass into the duodenum spontaneously. Forced injections of saline may assist their passage, or the tip of the catheter may be advanced to push the residual fragments into the duodenum. The drainage catheter should be left *in situ* and follow-up cholangiography performed after 24 hours. If there are no residual fragments at that time, this can then be withdrawn over a guidewire.

Cystic duct stones

Radiological interventional instrumentation via

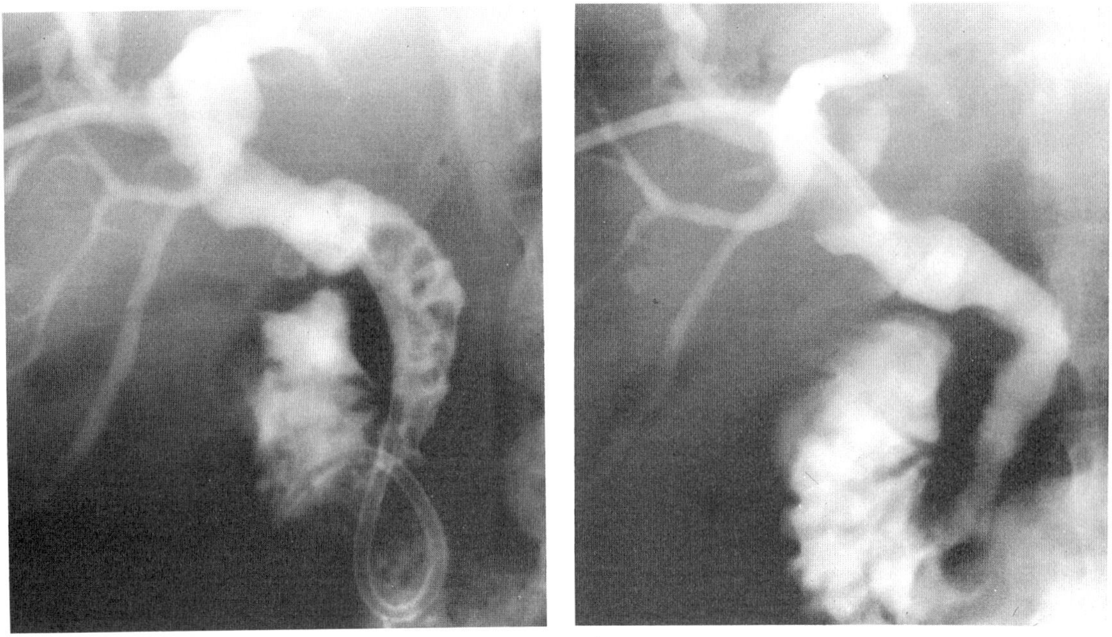

(c) (d)

Fig. 18.9 (*Continued*) (c) Note multiple fragments after transhepatic approach. A transhepatic loop catheter is left in place for further transhepatic procedures if required and in order to permit interventional dilatation of the ampullary segment. (d) Note that all fragments have passed and the steerable catheter is now withdrawn.

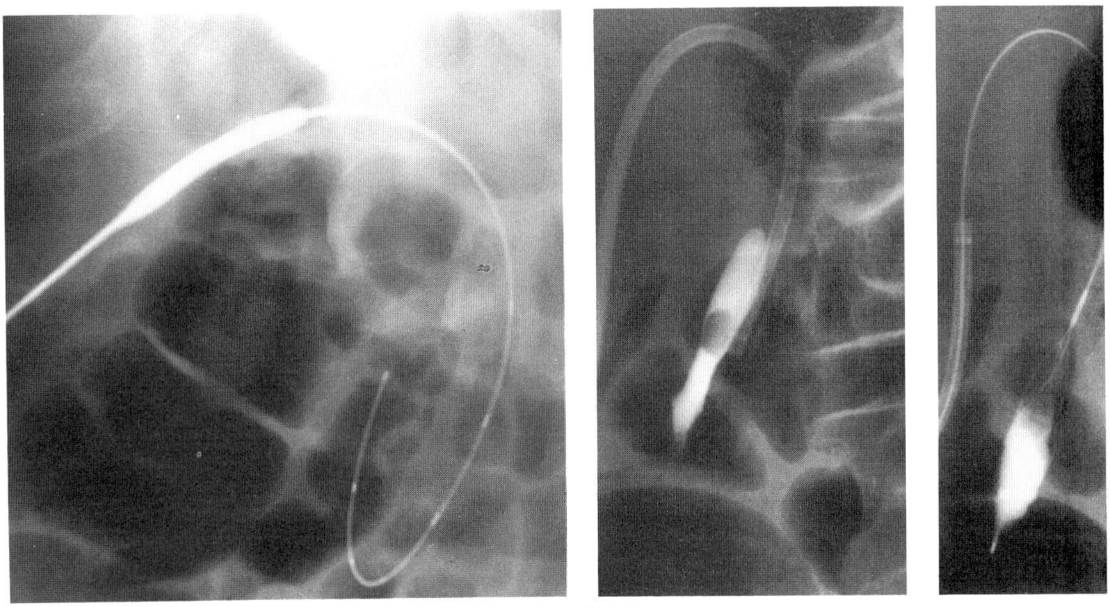

(a) (b)

Fig. 18.10 (a) A guidewire has been advanced from a cholecystostomy through the cystic duct into the common duct. An angiographic balloon catheter is utilized to dilate the cystic duct. (b) The steerable catheter is advanced through the cystic duct into the common duct and selective cholangiography now shows the common duct stone. The stone is engaged in the basket and withdrawn.

a cholecystostomy and removal of an impacted stone in the neck of the gallbladder was described as early as 1974 [52]. This technique can be extended for interventional removal of common bile duct stones after instrumentation and dilatation of the cystic duct (Fig. 18.10) with the use of J-shaped guidewires and balloon catheters [53]. Since the introduction of the Terumo wire with hydrophilic coating, it is now technically easier to cross the cystic duct from the gallbladder into the common duct. Mazzariello reported transcystic duct removal of common duct stones as early as 1976 with success in 20 out of 28 cases [54].

Cholecystostomy under local anaesthesia is performed in our institution in high-risk patients when cholecystectomy is not advisable as the first step (Fig. 18.11). This permits not only removal of stones from the gallbladder but subsequent catheterization of the common duct via the cystic duct with steerable catheter over a guidewire, followed by a basket through the steerable catheter. Balloon dilatation of the cystic duct may be required during the procedure in order to place a large enough catheter in the common bile duct. Dependent on the size of the common duct stones, they may be withdrawn intact in a basket, pushed through the ampulla in the duodenum, or fragmented by closure of the basket and removed in small pieces. If repeated treatment sessions are required, a biliary drainage catheter is left positioned across the cystic duct.

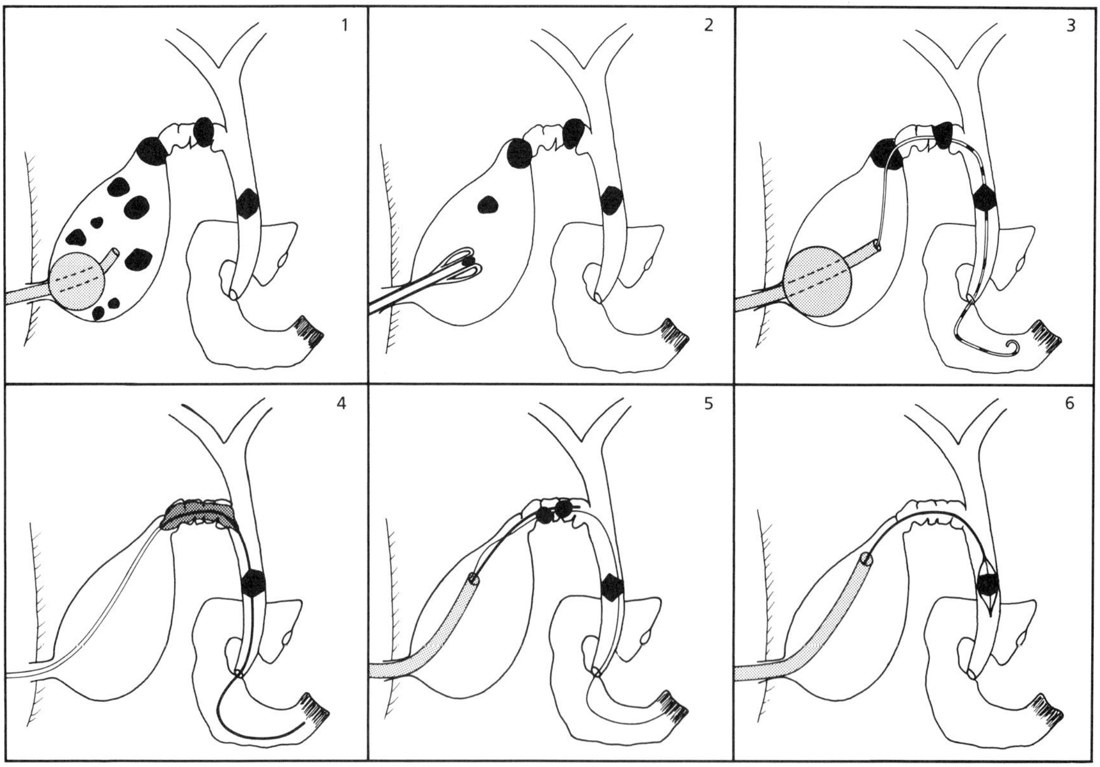

Fig. 18.11(a) Cholecystostomy intervention for cholelithiasis. Mini-cholecystostomy is accomplished under local anaesthesia and the gallbladder fundus is sutured to the abdominal wall. Stones are removed from the gallbladder with the Mazzariello forceps under fluoroscopic control. Drainage catheter with side holes is placed through the cystic and common ducts into the duodenum, followed by removal of cystic duct stones and common duct stones. From Burhenne and Stoller 1985 [71].

Stones impacted in the cystic duct make passage with interventional instrumentation difficult alongside the stone. The success rate for common duct stone removal via the cystic duct is higher than for interventional radiological cystic duct stone removal. We often have to resort to lithotripsy of cystic duct stones if instrumentation is not successful.

Obstructing and impacted cystic duct stones are the usual cause of cholecystitis. Radiological intervention for cystic duct stone removal is not required after percutaneous cholecystostomy if cholecystectomy is planned as a second procedure. If the gallbladder is left in place, however, cystic duct stone removal is required in order to prevent recurrent cholecystitis.

Combined endoscopic and transhepatic approach

Endoscopic removal of common duct stones following sphincterotomy was first reported in 1974 [55]. This usually provides excellent results [56]; however, in less than 10% of patients, it is not possible to cannulate the papilla of Vater, either due to technical difficulty or stenosis [57]. In

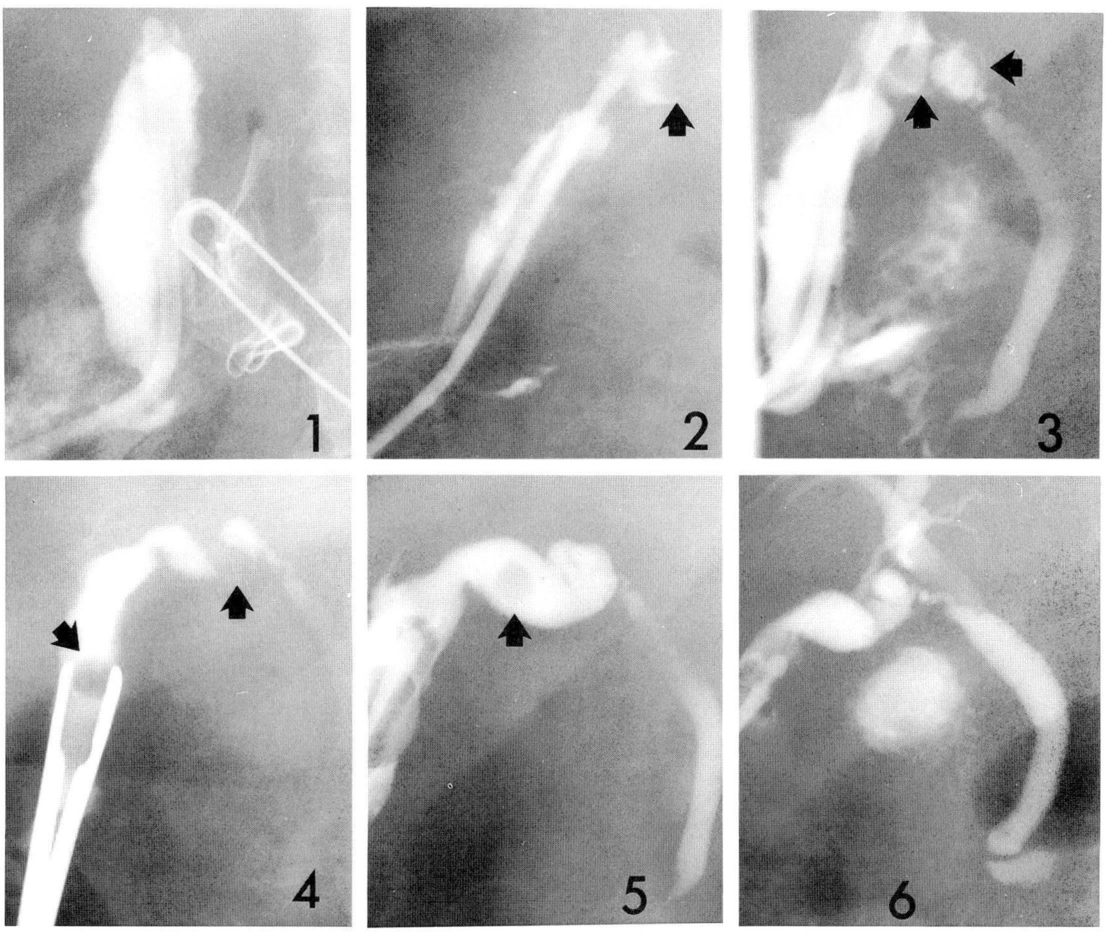

Fig. 18.11(b) Sequence of radiographs following mini-cholecystostomy demonstrating successful cystic duct stone removal.

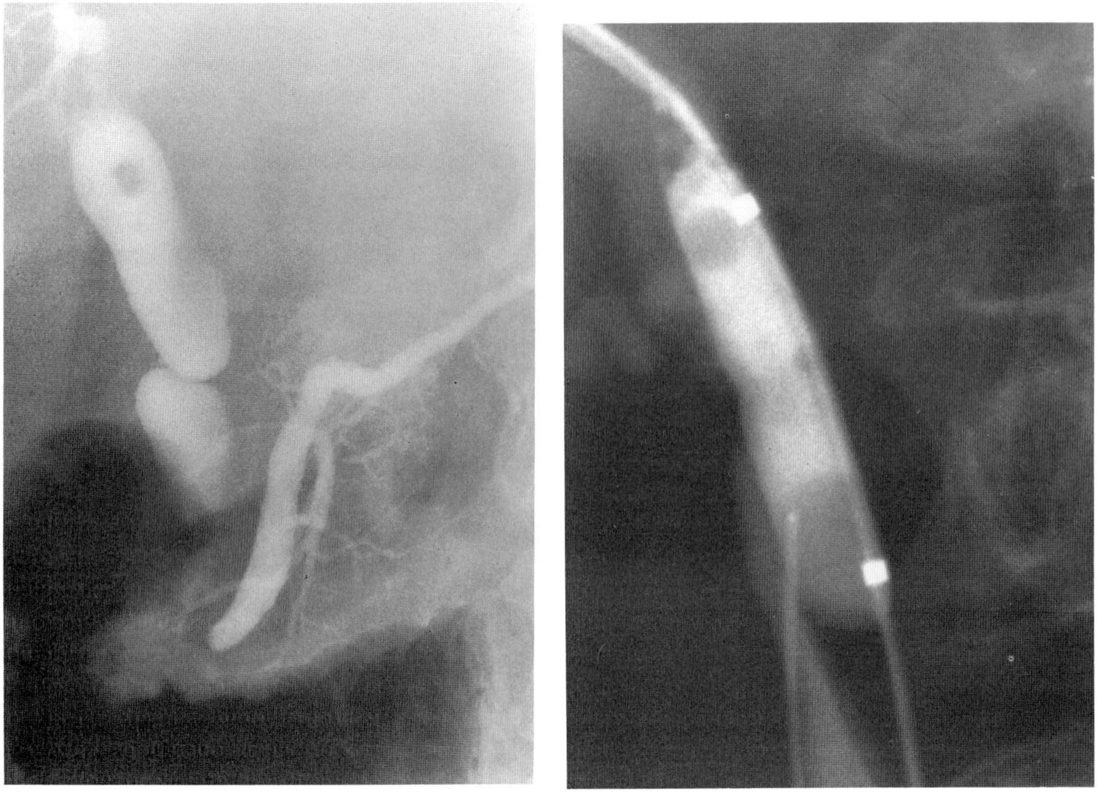

(a) (b)

Fig. 18.12 (a) Endoscopic retrograde approach was unsuccessful in this patient with complications of cholecystectomy. The percutaneous transhepatic cholangiogram shows a postoperative stricture in the common duct with a stone retained above it. The pancreatic duct is filling due to spasm at the ampulla of Vater. (b) Percutaneous transhepatic instrumentation gave good dilatation of the common duct stricture. The guidewire was advanced into the duodenum, grasped by endoscopic means, and the sphincterotomy wire was advanced into the ampullary portion of the duct for sphincterotomy. This permitted intact passage of the retained stone.

the combined approach (Fig. 18.12) access to the biliary tree is first obtained via the transhepatic route and a 5 F Cobra catheter and 0.038 in Teflon-coated exchange guidewire (Cook, Bloomington, USA) are manipulated through the papilla into the fourth part of the duodenum. If the papilla is tight or difficult to negotiate, a Terumo guidewire may be required. The catheter is then firmly taped to the skin at the entry site and the patient is turned over into the standard endoscopy position. After sedation has been given (10 mg intravenous diazemuls), the endoscope is inserted orally and manipulated into the second part of the duodenum. The 5 F Cobra catheter and guidewire are then withdrawn at the skin until the tip can be visualized and grasped by the endoscopic operator (Fig. 18.13). The guidewire can then be withdrawn up the endoscope such that a sphinc-terotomy can be performed in the usual manner with endoscopic access over the guidewire to the common bile duct for basket or balloon removal of calculi. The 5 F catheter, once withdrawn at the skin entry site, cannot be re-advanced due to bacterial contamination. Caution should be exercised on guidewire manipulation into the endoscope as tension, in association with catheter withdrawal, can have a 'cheese-wire' effect at the papilla with uncontrolled sphincterotomy and possible duodenal perforation.

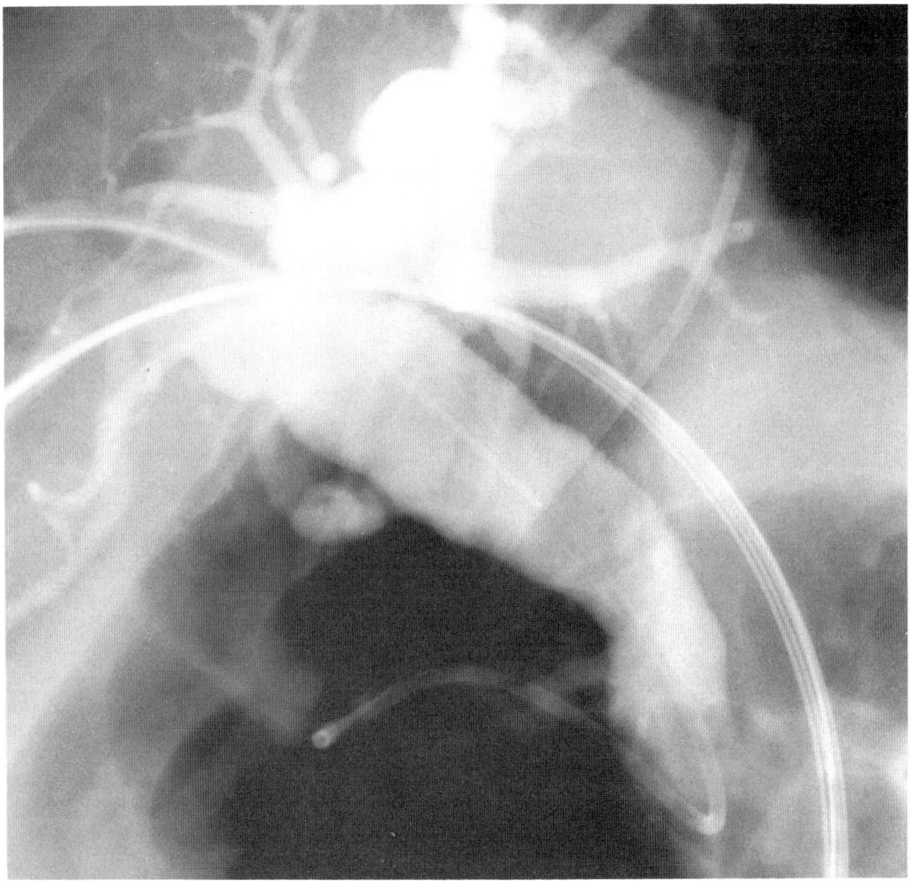

Fig. 18.13 Large common duct stone seen on transhepatic cholangiography in patient with previous cholecystectomy. Retrograde endoscopic approach failed. A catheter and guidewire was advanced via the transhepatic route into the duodenum. The patient is then turned over into the standard endoscopy position and the endoscope is manipulated into the duodenum and the tip of the guidewire is grasped by the endoscopic operator. The guidewire is then withdrawn up the endoscope, permitting sphincterotomy catheter placement in the usual manner.

Adjuvant lithotripsy

Bile duct stones may not be accessible via a postoperative tract or by endoscopic means. We evaluated the role of biliary extracorporeal shock-wave lithotripsy in treating 70 symptomatic patients with bile duct stones in whom endoscopic or percutaneous radiologic attempts at basket extraction failed. The overall successful treatment rate was 83% [58]. Lithotripsy was used as early as 1987 in the treatment of retained cystic duct stones after cholecystectomy [59] (Fig. 18.14). Sauerbruch and Stern reported even slightly better results in 1989 with fragmentation of bile duct stones by shock waves [60]. The usual cause for failure of radiological or endoscopic bile duct stone extraction is the presence of a very large stone which does not permit movement of instruments alongside. Intracorporeal lithotripsy with electrohydraulic shockwaves, a technique which preceded extracorporeal shock-wave development, can also be applied in these cases, either through the T-tube tract as originally reported [61] or via the endoscope. The equipment for intracorporeal lithotripsy costs only a fraction of the expensive machinery for extracorporeal treat-

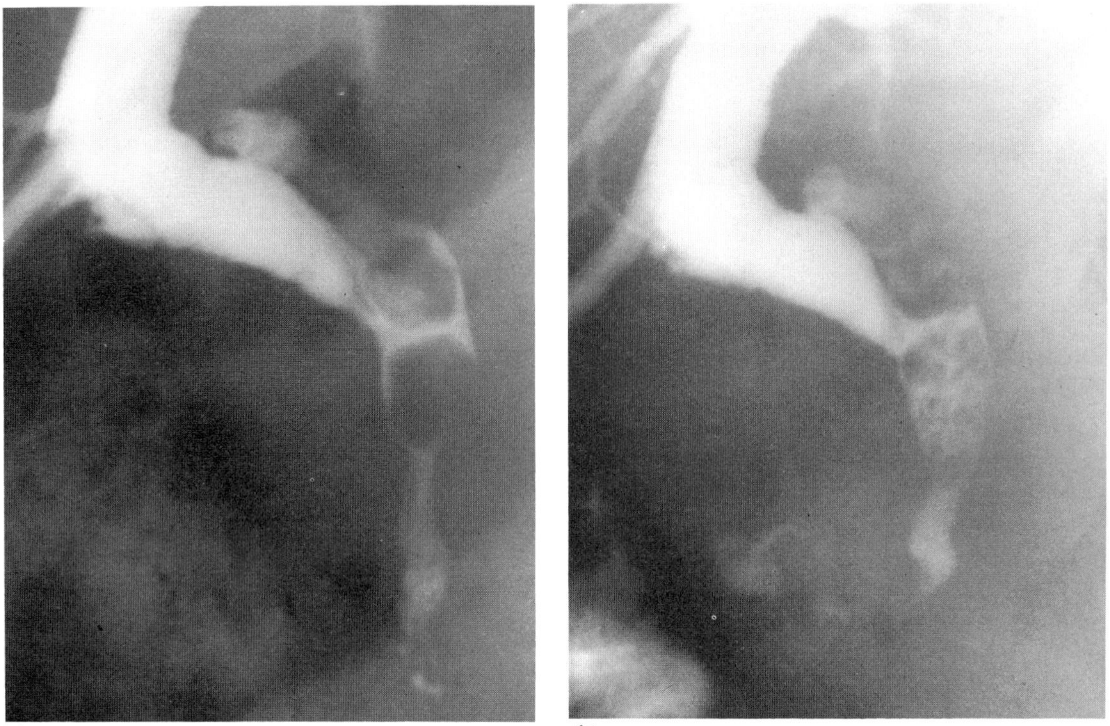

(a) (b)

Fig. 18.14 (a) Two retained stones impacted in a low-inserting cystic duct after cholecystectomy. Manipulation of the retained stones via the T-tube tract was not possible. (b) Extensive fragmentation of the two cystic duct stones is now seen after extracorporeal lithotripsy. The fragments could now be mobilized via the T-tube tract with a steerable catheter and passed spontaneously into the duodenum.

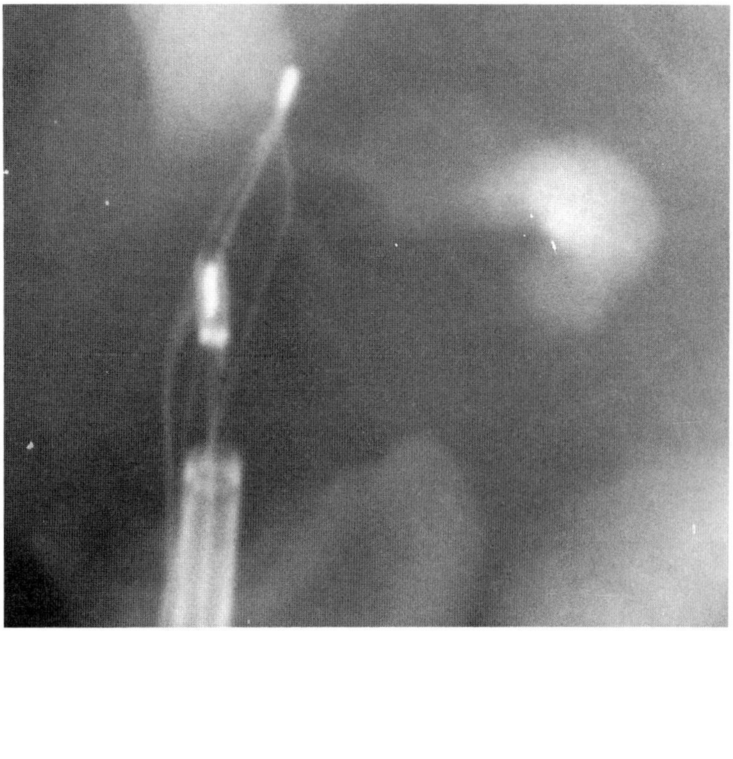

Fig. 18.15 Spot film obtained during intracorporeal lithotripsy of retained common duct stone. The stone has been engaged in the basket and the small platinum electrode was advanced through a steerable catheter against the bile duct stones. Using electrohydraulic shockwaves, the stone was fragmented and the fragments were successfully extracted through the T-tube tract.

ment (Fig. 18.15). Extracorporeal shock-wave lithotripsy can also be employed in the treatment of impacted stones in bile duct diverticula [62].

Stone dissolution

Contact dissolution of gallstones was first described by Walker [63] in 1891 who 1 month after surgical cholecystostomy in a 27-year-old woman, dissolved an impacted cystic duct stone with equal parts of ether and glycerin.

Percutaneous contact dissolution has been shown to be effective in clearing cholesterol gallstones from the gallbladder with minimal complications and undesirable side-effects [64]. More than 400 patients throughout the world have been treated with chemolitholysis using methyl tert-butyl ether (MTBE) [65]. However, with the advent of laparoscopic cholecystectomy, the current role of this technique is limited to those patients who refuse conventional or laparoscopic surgery, and those patients who are not candidates for surgical procedures. Several substances have been used for contact dissolution, including ether [63, 66], chloroform [67], heparin [68], and bile salt solutions [69, 70]. However, due to flammability, toxic side-effects and long dissolution times, none of these are currently in use.

The radiologist and gastroenterologist work together in MTBE stone dissolution techniques.

References

1 Shehadi WH. History of radiology of the biliary tract. *App Radio* 1977;**6**:141–68.
2 Margulis AR. Interventional diagnostic radiology: a new subspeciality. *Am J Roentgenol* 1967;**99**:761.
3 Burckhardt H, Müller W. Experiments of gallbladder puncture. *Deutsche Zeitschrift für Chirurgie* 1921;**162**: 168–178.
4 Pribram BOC. Ether treatment of gallstones impacted in the common duct. *Lancet* 1939;**1**:1311–14.
5 Lamis PA, Letton HJ, Wilson JP. Retained common duct stones: New nonoperative technique for treatment. *Surgery* 1969;**66**:291–6.
6 Cooperberg PL, Burhenne HJ. Real-time ultrasonography: diagnostic technique of choice in calculous gallbladder disease. *N Engl J Med* 1980;**302**:1277–9.
7 Pasanen P, Partenen K, Pikkarainen P, Alhava E, Pirinen A, Jantuinen E. Ultrasonography, CT and ERCP in the diagnosis of choledochal stones. *Acta Radiol* 1992;**33**:53–6.
8 Dong B, Chen M. Improved sonographic visualization of choledocholithiasis. *J Clin Ultrasound* 1987;**15**:185–90.
9 Berk RN. Radiology of the gallbladder and bile ducts. *Surg Clin North Am* 1973;**53**:973.
10 Donner MW, Weiner S. Diagnostic evaluation of abdominal calcifications in acute abdominal disorders. *Radiol Clin North Am* 1964;**2**:145–9.
11 Barakos JA, Ralls PW, Lapin SA *et al.* Cholelithiasis: evaluation with CT. *Radiology* 1987;**162**:415–18.
12 Hickman MS, Schwesinger WH, Bora JD, Kurtin WE. Computed tomographic analysis of gallstones. *Arch Surg* 1986;**121**:289–91.
13 Baron RL, Rohrmann CAJ, Lee SP, Shuman WP, Feefey SA. CT evaluation of gallstones. *In vitro* correlation with chemical analysis. *AJR* 1988;**151**:1123–8.
14 Brakel K, Lametis JS, Nijs HGT, Terpstra OT, Steen G, Blijenberg BC. Predicting gallstone composition with CT. *In vivo* and *in vitro* analysis. *Radiology* 1990;**174**: 337–41.
15 Baron RL, Kuyper SA, Lee SP, Rohrmann CA Jr, Shuman WP, Nelson JA. *In vitro* dissolution of gallstones with MTBE: Correlation with characteristics at CT and MR imaging. *Radiology* 1989;**173**:117–21.
16 McGrath FP, Gibney RG, Burhenne HJ. The value of sonography in determining cystic duct patency. *Clin Radiol* 1992;**46**:34–7.
17 Ansell G. Adverse reactions to contrast agents. Scope of problem. *Invest Radiol* 1970;**5**:374–84.
18 Dubois F, Icard P, Berthelot G, Levard H. Coelioscopic cholecystectomy. *Ann Surg* 1990;**1**:60–2.
19 Joyce WP, Keane R, Burke GJ *et al.* Identification of bile duct stones in patients undergoing laparoscopic cholecystectomy. *Br J Surg* 1991;**78**:1174–6.
20 Burhenne HJ, Watkinson AF. Intravenous cholangiography pre-laparoscopic cholecystectomy. Proceedings of the International Biliary Society Meeting, Chicago, December 1992.
21 Weissman HS, Badia J, Sugarman LA, Kluger L, Rosenblatt R, Freeman LM. Spectrum of 99-mTc IDA cholescintigraphic patterns in actue cholecystitis. *Radiology* 1981;**138**:167–75.
22 Longmire WP Jr The treatment of retained gallstones. *West J Med* 1979;**130**:422–36.
23 Yip AWC, Ny WS, Chow WC, Choi TK, Lam KH. Plea for selective operative cholangiography. *J R Coll Surg Edin* 1991;**36**:21–4.
24 Pagne TJ, Stahlgren LH. Indications and accuracy of operative cholangiography. *Arch Surg* 1980;**115**: 1214–15.
25 Schulenberg CAR. Operative cholangiography: 1 000 cases. *Surgery* 1969;**65**:723–30.
26 Classen M, Ossenberg FW. Nonsurgical removal of common bile duct stones. *Gut* 1977;**18**:760–9.
27 Mondet A. Técnica de la extracción incruenta de los calculos en la litiasis residual del colédoco. *Bol Soc Chir Buenos Aires* 1962;**46**:278.

28 Lagrave G, Plessis JL, Pougeard-Dulimbert G *et al.* Litiase billiare résiduelle: extraction à la sonde de Dormia par de drain de Kehr. *Mem Acad Chir (Paris)* 1969;**95**:431–8.
29 Burhenne HJ. Extraktion von Residual Steinen der Gallenwege ohne Reoperation. *Fortschr Röntgenstr* 1972;**117**:425–8.
30 Burhenne HJ. Nonoperative retained biliary tract stone extraction: a new roentgenologic technique. *Am J Roentgenol* 1973;**117**:388–99.
31 Burhenne HJ. Percutaneous extraction of retained biliary tract stones: 661 patients. *Am J Roentgenol* 1980;**134**:888–98.
32 Garrow DG. The removal of biliary tract stones: report of 105 cases. *Br J Radiol* 1977;**50**:777–84.
33 Fennessy JJ, You KD. A method for the expulsion of stones retained in the common bile duct. *Am J Roentgenol* 1970;**110**:256–9.
34 Mazzariello R. Review of 220 cases of residual biliary tract calculi treated without operation: an eight year study. *Surgery* 1973;**73**:299.
35 Burhenne HJ. Complications of nonoperative extraction of retained biliary tract stones. *Am J Surg* 1976;**131**:260–2.
36 Mason R. Percutaneous extraction of retained gallstones via the T tube tract. British experience in 131 cases. *Clin Radiol* 1980;**31**:497.
37 Smith HW. Problems of retained and recurrent common bile duct stones. *Surgery* 1969;**66**:291.
38 Tritapepe R, de Padova C, de Padova F. Noninvasive treatment for retained common bile duct stones in patients with a T-tube *in situ*. Saline washout after intravenous Ceruletide. *Br J Surg* 1988;**75**:144.
39 Cotton PB. Retained bile duct stones: T-tube in place, percutaneous or endoscopic management? *Am J Gastroenterol* 1990;**85**:1075–8.
40 Hutson DG, Russell E, Shiff E, Levi JJ, Jeffers L, Zeppa R. Balloon dilatation of biliary strictures through a choledochojejunocutaneous fistula. *Ann Surg* 1984; **199**:637–9.
41 Burhenne HJ. Dilatation of biliary tract strictures. *Radiologica Clinica* 1975;**44**:153–9.
42 Burhenne HJ, Morris DC. Biliary stricture dilatation: use of the Grüntzig balloon catheter. *Can Assoc Radiol J* 1980;**31**:196–7.
43 Warren KW, Whitcomb FF Jr. Diagnosis and treatment of benign biliary stricture. *Hospital Practice* 1971;**6**: 62.
44 Mueller PR, van Sonnenberg E, Ferrucci JT Jr *et al.* Biliary stricture dilatation: multicenter review of clinical management in 73 patients. *Radiology* 1986;**160**:17–22.
45 Russell E. Dilatation of biliary stricture through a stomatized jejunal limb. *Acta Radiologica Diagnostica* 1985;**26**:283.
46 Huard P, Do-Xuan-Hop. La ponction transhépatique des canaux biliares. *Bull Soc Med Chir de l'Indochine* 1937;**15**:1090–1100.
47 Dotter CT, Bilbao MK, Katon RM. Percutaneous transhepatic gallstone removal via a needle tract. *Radiology* 1979;**133**:242–3.
48 Clouse ME, Stokes KR, Lee RGL *et al.* Bile duct stones: percutaneous transhepatic removal. *Radiology* 1986;**160**:525–9.
49 Meranze SG, Stein EJ, Burke DR *et al.* Removal of retained common bile duct stones with angiographic occlusion balloons. *AJR* 1986;**146**:383–5.
50 Centola CAP, Jander HP, Stuffer A *et al.* Balloon dilatation of the papilla of Vater to allow biliary stone passage. *AJR* 1981;**136**:613–14.
51 Berkman WA, Bishop AF, Palagallo GL *et al.* Transhepatic balloon dilatation of the distal common bile duct and ampulla of Vater for removal of calculi. *Radiology* 1988;**167**:453–5.
52 Burhenne HJ. Nonoperative roentgenologic instrumentation techniques of the postoperative biliary tract. *Am J Surg* 1974;**128**:111–7.
53 Burhenne HJ. Biliary tract. In: Margulis AR, Burhenne HJ, eds. *Alimentary Tract Radiology*, 3rd edn. St Louis: Mosby, 1983:2318–38.
54 Mazzariello RM. Residual biliary duct stones: Nonoperative treatment of 570 patients. Surgery Annual 8. New York: Appleton-Century-Crofts, 1976:113–14.
55 Classen M, Demling L. Endoskopische Sphincterotomoie der Papilla Vateri und Steinextraktion aus Demductus Choledochus. *Dtsch Med Wochenscht* 1974;**99**:496–7.
56 Cotton PB. Nonoperative removal of bile duct stones by duodenoscopic sphincterotomy. *J Surg* 1980;**67**:1–5.
57 Mason RR, Cotton PB. Combined duodenoscopic and transhepatic approach to stenosis of the papilla of Vater. *Br J Radiol* 1981;**54**:678–9.
58 Lee SH, Fache JS, Burhenne HJ. The value of extracorporeal shockwave lithotripsy in management of bile duct stones. *Am J Roentgenol* 1990;**155**:775–9.
59 Becker CD, Fache JS, Gibney RG, Stoller JL, Burhenne HJ. *Am J Roentgenol* 1987;**148**:1121–2.
60 Sauerbruch T, Stern M. Fragmentation of bile duct stones by extracorporeal shockwaves. *Gastroenterology* 1989;**96**:146–52.
61 Burhenne HJ. Electrohydrolytic fragmentation of retained common duct stones. *Radiology* 1975;**117**:721.
62 Lee SH, Gibney RG, Burhenne HJ. Biliary extracorporeal shockwave lithotripsy in the treatment of an impacted stone in bile duct diverticulum. *Gastrointest Radiol* 1990;**15**:317–19.
63 Walker JW. The removal of gallstones by ether solution. *Lancet* 1989;**1**:874–5.
64 Hofmann AF, Schteingart CD, van Sonnenberg E *et al.* Contact dissolution of cholesterol gallstones with organic solvents. *Gastroenterol Clin North Am* 1991;**20**:183–99.
65 Thistle JL, May GR, Bender CE *et al.* Dissolution of cholesterol gallbladder stones by methyl tert-butyl ether administered by percutaneous transhepatic catheter. *N Engl J Med* 1989;**320**:633–9.

66 Pribram BO. New methods in gallstone surgery. *Surg Gynecol Obstet* 1935;60:55–9.
67 Best PR, Rasmussen JA, Wilson CE. An evaluation of solutions for fragmentation and dissolution of gallstones and their effect on liver and ductal tissue. *Ann Surg* 1953;138:570.
68 Gardner B. Experience with the use of intracholedochal heparinized saline for the treatment of retained common duct stones. *Ann Surg* 1973;177:240–4.
69 Way LW, Motson RW. Part III: Dissolution of retained common duct stones. *Adv Surg* 1976:10:99–119.
70 Landsford C, Mehta S, Kern F. The treatment of retained stones in the common bile duct with sodium cholate infusion. *Gut* 1974;15:48–51.
71 Burhenne HJ, Stoller JL. Mini-cholecystostomy and radiologic stone extraction in high risk cholelithiasis patients. *Am J Surg* 1985;149:632–5.

Chapter 19
Extracorporeal shock wave lithotripsy for common bile duct stones

T. Sauerbruch

The morbidity and mortality of surgical management of gallstones depends on their anatomical location in the biliary tree. Mortality following choledochotomy is nearly five times that of cholecystectomy (between 2% and 4% compared with 0.5%) [1]. The introduction of endoscopic sphincterotomy in 1974 was thus a major advance [2, 3]. The mortality and morbidity are lower than in open surgery. However, in 10–20% of the patients, endoscopic extraction of the calculi is unsuccessful. Using mechanical lithotripsy, contact dissolution, extracorporeal [4] and intracorporeal shock wave lithotripsy, it is now possible to remove bile duct stones without open surgery in the vast majority of patients [1]. It is the purpose of the present chapter to review the technique and the efficacy of extracorporeal shock wave lithotripsy (ESWL) for stones in the biliary tree. The evaluation is based on rather large prospective, although uncontrolled, trials published within the past few years.

Composition of bile duct stones

Around 80% of gallbladder stones are cholesterol stones [5] (on average 70–80% cholesterol). By contrast, bile duct stones are more heterogeneous. These stones may be divided into stones primarily formed in the biliary tree (so-called brown pigment stones), or stones which moved from the gallbladder into the bile ducts (mainly cholesterol stones). Futhermore, there are so-called mixed stones (i.e., stones with a cholesterol core) that have primarily been formed in the gallbladder, and a pigment shell grown in the bile duct (Fig. 19.1). About one-third of all bile duct stones in the western world are cholesterol stones, the rest are pigment or mixed stones [5, 6]. Cholesterol stones are amenable to solvents. Brown pigment stones in the bile ducts, however, are not. They are mainly composed of calcium bilirubinate, calcium carbonate, cholesterol, and fatty acids [6, 7].

In vitro fragmentation of gallstones by ESWL

In the extracorporeal systems, shock waves are generated electrohydraulically, electromagnetically or piezoelectrically [8]. Disintegration of the stones is not only achieved by the direct effects of the shock waves, but also by secondary cavitation phenomena [9, 10].

A stone positioned into the focal area of a shock wave lithotripter is exposed to several hundred and up to several thousand shock waves. Each shock wave creates a rapidly increasing positive pressure ranging between 500 and 1 000 bars which is then followed by a much lower negative pressure causing tensile forces. If the shock wave hits a stone with an acoustic impedance dissimilar to the surrounding medium, part of the pressure wave is transmitted through the stone, part is reflected at the front surface of the stone and part is reflected at the back surface of the stone. This results in pressure and tensile forces which stress the stone material to an extent that it will split. It is believed that in addition microjets, caused by collapsing cavitation bubbles (a phenomenon designed as cavitation) in the surrounding fluid and in the fluid which entered the stone along the split lines, induce considerable further damage to the stone [10]. As far as we know, the chemical composition of stones is not a major determinant

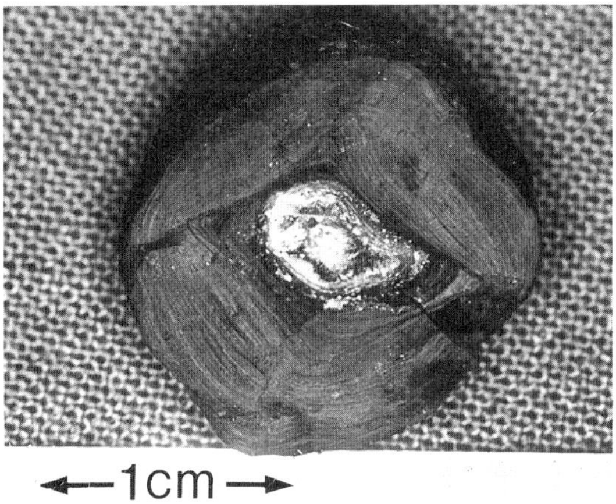

Fig. 19.1 Brown pigment bile duct stone formed arround a cholesterol stone core. The latter probably stems from the gallbladder.

of the disintegration process [9]. The crystalline structure of the stone may be more important. Pure crystalline cholesterol stones are easily crushed by shock-waves. There are some anecdotal reports suggesting that gallstones with a higher content of inorganic calcium salts are more difficult to disintegrate than uncalcified pure cholesterol stones [9].

The surrounding medium of the stone is a further factor influencing stone disintegration. The higher the difference in the acoustic impedance between the stone and the surrounding bile, the higher the pressure built up at the surface borders. From this standpoint, a fluid with a low acoustic impedance and enough potential for generation of cavitation should be ideal for lithotripsy [9]. If probes are placed into the biliary tree, it should be possible to adapt the medium surrounding of the stone to these requirements. However, this has not been studied systematically.

Experience in humans

Extracorporeal shock wave lithotripsy of bile duct stones should be taken into consideration if endoscopic sphincterotomy and attempts of mechanical lithotripsy have failed [11, 12]. Most centres observe the following selection criteria:

1 bile duct stones not extractable endoscopically or percutaneously according to the experience of the individual investigator;

2 successful positioning of the calculi into the focal area of the lithotripter;

3 focal axis of the shock waves avoiding lung, gas-filled bowel loops, vascular aneurysms, calcified vessels or large bone areas;

4 no severe deterioration of coagulation parameters.

To date, most patients have been treated by lithotripter machines with X-ray capability. Radiological monitoring and positioning of the stones is more reliable than ultrasound. Even in experienced hands, adequate detection of unselected bile duct stones succeeds in only half of the patients. On the other hand, intrahepatic stones can be localized to a similar degree with either ultrasound or X-ray. Most investigators use machines fitted with an integrated X-ray system for extrahepatic bile duct stones [12], although reports exist of successful ultrasound stone location [13]. By contrast, machines with an ultrasound monitoring system are often appropriate for intrahepatic stones of the biliary tree.

We prefer shock wave entry from the rear to reduce attenuation of the wave energy by gas-filled bowel loops in the shock wave path (Fig. 19.2). However, clinical practice has shown that a large percentage of patients may also be treated with the shock waves entering from the ventral side.

Since the majority of common bile duct stones are radiolucent, direct injection of the contrast medium is required for visualization of the stones during treatment when using X-ray. This is effected by nasobiliary tubes, T-tubes or a transhepatically placed catheter (Figs 19.3 and 19.4).

When using first generation lithotripters with a large focal dimension and a rather small aperture, lithotripsy may cause sufficient discomfort to warrant anaesthesia. When using the first generation machines, more than half of the patients received general anaesthesia, whereas patients

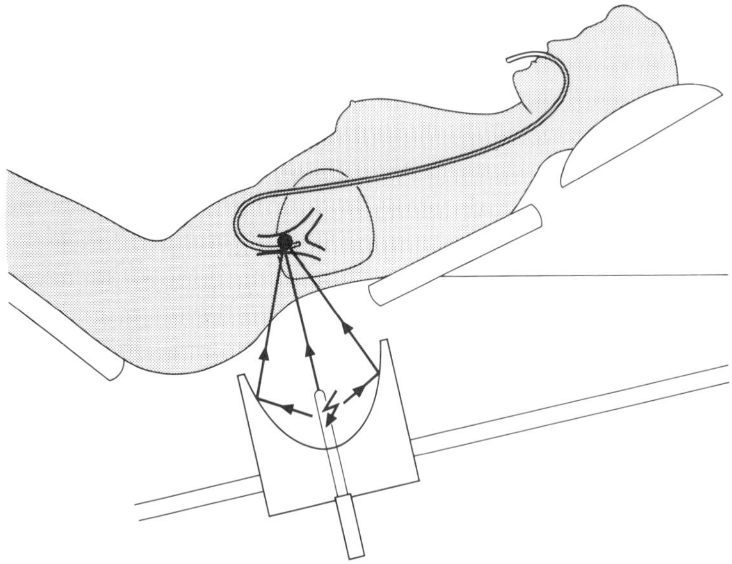

Fig. 19.2 Schematic illustration of Dornier lithotripter HM3 and positioning of the patient for treatment of bile duct stones. The shock waves are generated by underwater spark discharge at the first focus in an ellipsoidal reflector. The stone is positioned at the second (remote) focus. The shock waves are introduced into the body by using a water-bath into which the patient is partially immersed. The bile ducts and the stone are visualized after instillation of contrast medium via a nasobiliary tube employing fluoroscopy. The system also allows positioning and targeting of the stone. After Paumgartner & Sauerbruch [26].

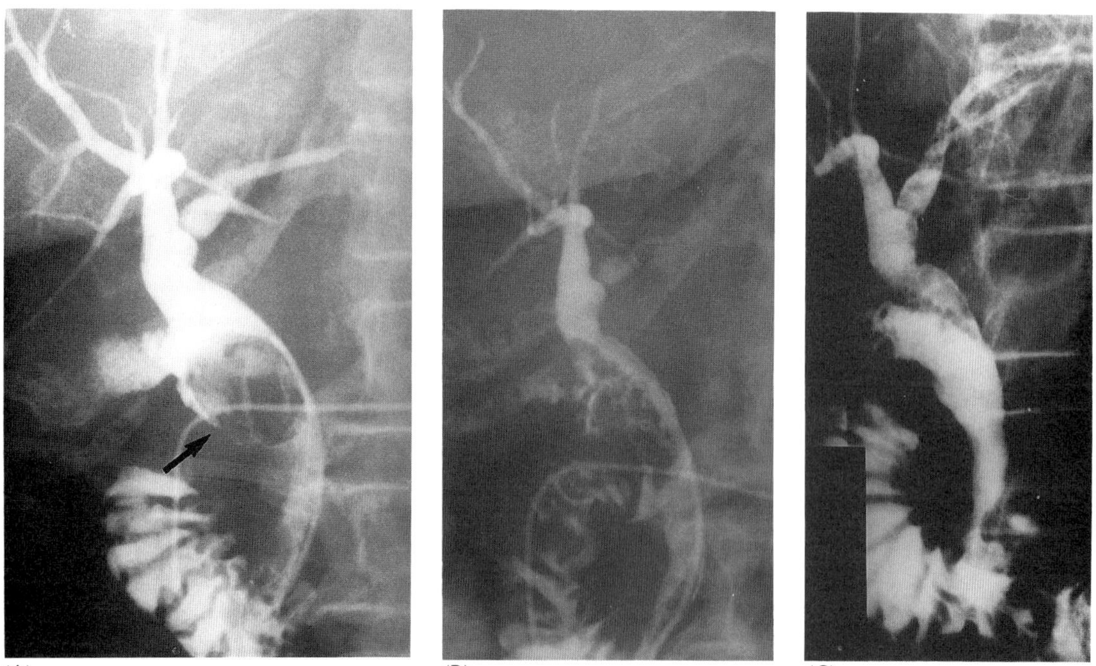

(A) (B) (C)

Fig. 19.3 Common bile duct with a large stone (→), visualized via a nasobiliary tube before (A), immediately after ESWL (B) and after extraction of the fragments. There is now aerobilia in the bile duct (C).

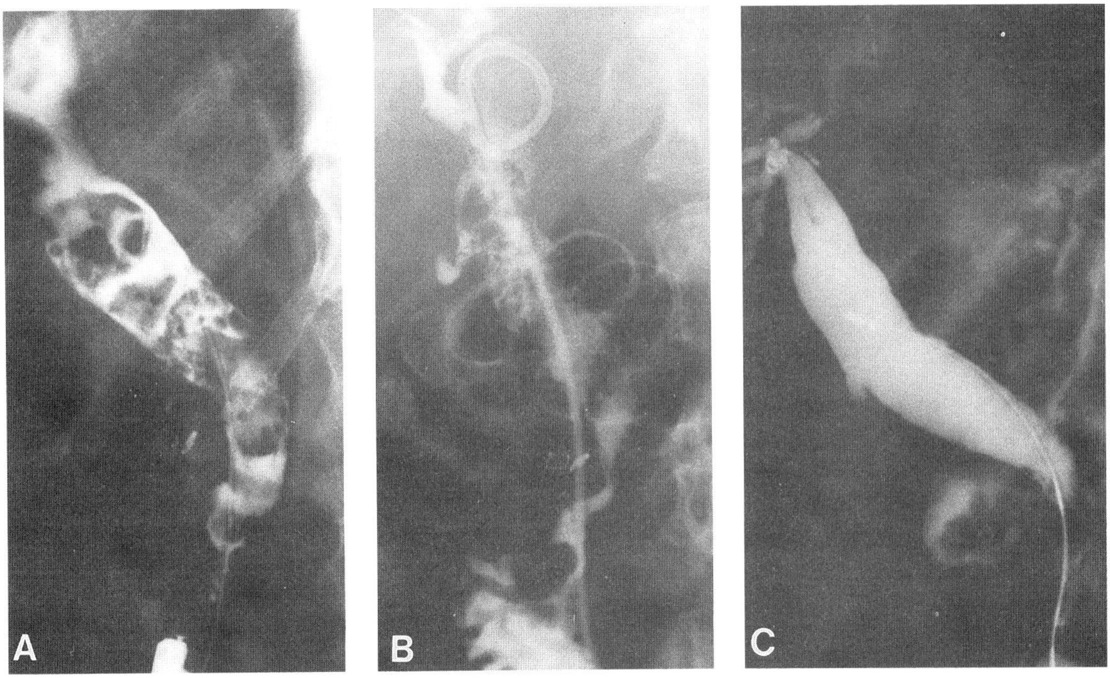

Fig. 19.4 Common bile duct with several large stones before (A), immediately after ESWL (B) and after extraction of the fragments (C). Visualization of the biliary tree is effected by a nasobiliary tube.

treated with other lithotripters frequently received only intravenous sedative analgesia.

Normally the patients receive 1 000–2 000 electrocardiographic (ECG)-triggered shocks and this takes on average 40–60 minutes. About one-third of the patients in the different trials required repeated sessions (Table 19.1).

Adverse effects

Serious adverse effects are rare. The most important complication following ESWL of bile duct stones is septic disease, possibly caused by the introduction of micro-organisms into the blood stream during treatment. This complication occurred in 2–7% of the patients in a larger series [12]. Antibiotic prophylaxis may be expected to reduce biliary-related sepsis after ESWL. Haemobilia and macrohaematuria directly attributable to shock wave tissue damage (occurring in about 5–10% of the patients) are of no clinical relevance. The earlier trials found cardiac arrhythmia a problem during ESWL, but this was not a major problem in more recent trials. Haematoma of the tissue adjacent to the shock wave focus has been observed in about 1% of the patients [11] and there is an anecdotal report of portal venous thrombosis following ESWL.

Efficacy

Disintegration of the stones is achieved in 80–90% of the patients (see Table 19.1). The fragments, however, are rather coarse requiring additional procedures such as endoscopic extraction in up to 90% of the patients. This leads to an overall clearance rate of about 90% of all patients with stones primarily not amenable to routine endoscopic or transhepatic procedures (Fig. 19.5). Success rates observed in patients under general anaesthesia are probably higher than in those treated with intravenous analgesics only.

Table 19.1 ESWL of bile duct stones primarily not amenable to routine endoscopic measures (fully published series with more than 15 patients)

Author	Device	No. of patients	Repeated sessions (%)	General anaesthesia (%)	Monitoring	Success rate (complete clearance of stones) (%)	Hospital mortality
Sauerbruch *et al.* [14]	EH	113	16	78	X-ray	86	1.8
Wenzel *et al.* [15]	EH	55	27	48	X-ray	92	0
Bland *et al.* [16]	EH	42	36	32	X-ray	74	0
Ihse *et al.* [17]	EH	15	13	0	X-ray	67	0
Eckhauser *et al.* [18]	EH	16	19	100	X-ray	94	0
Sauerbruch *et al.* [12]	EH	103	33	75	X-ray	88	1
Lee *et al.* [19]	EH, EM	70	Most	0	X-ray	61	0
den Toom *et al.* [20]	EH, EM	62	53	23	X-ray	79	0
Schulz *et al.* [21]	EM	65	32	0	X-ray	69	0
Ginestal-Cruz *et al.* [22]	EM	30	47	0	X-ray	80	7
Staritz *et al.* [23]	EM	33	?	0	X-ray	64	0
Ponchon *et al.* [24]	EH	19	16	0	Ultrasound	53	0
Weiss *et al.* [25]	PE	32	25	0	Ultrasound	75	0
Weber *et al.* [13]	PE	19	47	0	Ultrasound	79	0

EH: Electrohydraulic device (mostly HM3 – Dornier); EM: Electromagnetic device (mostly Lithostar – Siemens); PE: Piezoelectric device (mostly Wolf).

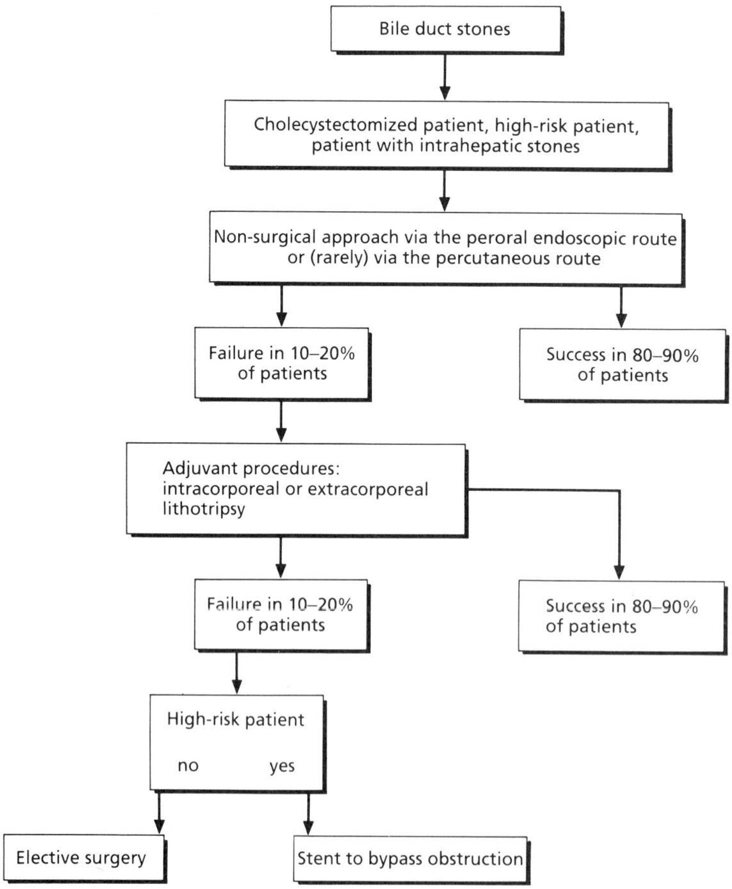

Fig. 19.5 Algorithm for the treatment of bile duct stones. From Sauerbruch & Neubrand [27].

Conclusion

Extracorporeal lithotripsy of gallstones was introduced in 1985 [4] for the treatment of bile duct stones primarily not amenable to routine endoscopic measures. Since that time its value has been confirmed in a number of fully published trials (see Table 19.1). Adverse effects are rare and mostly minor. Therefore, it should be used after failure of mechanical lithotripsy if a lithotripter with radiographic devices is available at the institution.

References

1 Sauerbruch T. Non-surgical management of bile duct stones refractory to routine endoscopic measures. *Baillière's Clin Gastroenterol* 1992;**6**:799–817.

2 Classen M, Demling L. Endoskopische Sphinkterotomie der Papilla Vateri und Steinextraktion aus dem Ductus choledochus. *Dtsch Med Wochenschr* 1974;**99**: 496–7.

3 Kawai K, Akasake Y, Murakami K *et al.* Endoscopic sphincterotomy of the ampulla of Vater. *Gastrointest Endosc* 1974;**20**:148–51.

4 Sauerbruch T, Delius M, Paumgartner G *et al.* Fragmentation of gallstones by extracorporeal shock waves. *N Engl J Med* 1986;**314**:818–22.

5 Sauerbruch T, Stellaard F, Soehendra N, Paumgartner G. Cholesteringehalt von Gallengangssteinen. *Dtsch Med Wochenschr* 1983;**108**:1099–1102.

6 Wosiewitz U, Schenk J, Sabinski F, Schmack B. Investigation of common bile duct stones. *Digestion* 1983;**26**:43–52.

7 Neoptolemos JP, Hofmann AF, Moossa AR. Chemical treatment of stones in the biliary tree. *Br J Surg* 1986;**73**:515–24.

8 Sauerbruch T, Holl J, Sackmann M, Paumgartner G. The role of extracorporeal lithotripsy (ESWL) in the treatment of gallstones. *Endoscopy* 1988;**20**:305–8.

9 Sauerbruch T, Neubrand M, Lobentanzer H. *In vitro* fragmentation of gallstones. In: Paumgartner G, Sauerbruch T, Sackmann M, Burhenne HJ, eds. *Lithotripsy and Related Techniques for Gallstone Treatment.* St Louis: Mosby Year Book, 1991:7–13.

10 Sass W, Bräunlich M, Hayler M *et al.* Analysis of shock wave destruction of stones by high-speed films and microscopy. In: Paumgartner G, Sauerbruch T, Sackmann M, Burhenne HJ, eds. *Lithotripsy and Related Techniques for Gallstone Treatment.* St Louis: Mosby Year Book, 1991:17–26.

11 Sauerbruch T. Extracorporeal shock wave lithotripsy of bile duct stones. In: Paumgartner G, Sauerbruch T, Sackmann M, Burhenne HJ, eds. *Lithotripsy and Related Techniques for Gallstone Treatment.* St Louis: Mosby Year Book, 1991:247–51.

12 Sauerbruch T, Holl J, Sackmann M, Paumgartner G. Fragmentation of bile duct stones by extracorporeal shock wave lithotripsy: a five-year experience. *Hepatology* 1992;**15**:208–14.

13 Weber J, Adamek HE, Riemann JF. Extracorporeal piezoelectric lithotripsy for complicated bile duct stones. *Am J Gastroenterol* 1991;**86**:196–200.

14 Sauerbruch T, Stern M, and the Study Group for Shockwave Lithotripsy of Bile Duct Stones. Fragmentation of bile duct stones by extracorporeal shock waves: a new approach to biliary calculi after failure of routine endoscopic measures. *Gastroenterology* 1989;**96**:146–52.

15 Wenzel H, Greiner L, Jakobeit Ch, Lazica M, Thüroff J. Extrakorporale Stoßwellenlithotripsie von Gallengangssteinen. *Dtsch Med Wochenschr* 1989;**114**:738–43.

16 Bland KI, Jones RS, Maher JW *et al.* Extracorporeal shock-wave lithotripsy of bile duct calculi: an interim report of the Dornier U.S. bile duct lithotripsy prospective study. *Ann Surg* 1989;**209**:743–53.

17 Ihse I, Borch K, Carlsson P, Lindström E, Tiselius HG. Extracorporeal shock-wave lithotripsy of bile-duct stones: initial Swedish experience. *Act Chir Scand* 1990;**156**:87–90.

18 Eckhauser FE, Raper StE, Knol JA *et al.* Extracorporeal lithotripsy—an important adjunct in the nonoperative management of retained or recurrent bile duct stones. *Arch Surg* 1991;**126**:829–35.

19 Lee SH, Fache JS, Burhenne HJ. The value of extracorporeal shock-wave lithotripsy in the management of bile duct stones. *Am J Rœntgenol* 1990;**155**:775–9.

20 den Toom R, Nijs HGT, van Blankenstein M, Laméris JS, Schröder FH, Terpstra OT. Extracorporeal shock wave treatment of common bile duct stones: experience with two different lithotriptors at a single institution. *Br J Surg* 1991;**78**:809–13.

21 Schulz HJ, Brien G, Kunz B *et al.* Extrakorporale Stoßwellenlithotripsie (ESWL) der Choledocholithiasis. *Z Klin Med* 1989;**44**:2349–50.

22 Ginestal-Cruz A, Grima N, Duarte V, Tavora I, Pinto Correia J. Extracorporeal shock wave lithotripsy for large common bile duct stones: an extension of the endoscopic approach. *J Lithotripsy Stone Dis* 1989;**1**: 272–81.

23 Staritz M, Rambow A, Grosse A *et al.* Electromagnetically generated extracorporeal shockwaves for fragmentation of extra- and intrahepatic bile duct stones: indications, success and problems during a 15 months clinical experience. *Gut* 1990;**31**:222–5.

24 Ponchon T, Martin X, Barkun A, Mestas JL, Chavaillon A, Boustière Ch. Extracorporeal lithotripsy of bile duct stones using ultrasonography for stone localization. *Gastroenterology* 1990;**98**:726–32.

25 Weiss W, Türk C, Brownstone E *et al.* Klinische Relevanz der extrakorporalen Stoßwellenlithotripsie (ESWL) bei Choledocholithiasis. *Wien Klin Wochenschr* 1989;**101**:629–31.

26 Paumgartner G, Sauerbruch T. Extracorporeal shock wave lithotripsy of gallstones. In: Zakim D, Boyer ThD, eds. *Hepatology. A Textbook of Liver Disease*, 2nd edn. Philadelphia: Saunders 1990:1561–8.

27 Sauerbruch T, Neubrand M. Nonsurgical management of gallstones. In: Boyer JL, Ockner RK, eds. *Progress in Liver Diseases*. Philadelphia: Saunders, 1992:193–218.

Chapter 20
Peroral cholangioscopic lithotripsy by using electrohydraulic shock waves

H. Saisho, T. Tsuyuguchi, T. Yamaguchi, H. Yugi & M. Ohto

Endoscopic papillotomy (EPT) has been the treatment of choice for common bile duct stones for over a decade. When the stones are too large to pass through the incised papilla, mechanical lithotripsy (ML) may be used to crush them into fragments. Success rates of between 72–94% [1–5] (77% in our own experience) have been reported for this technique. However, mechanical lithotripsy may sometimes be time-consuming and frustrating when the stone is not trapped properly in the basket. Recently, electrohydraulic and laser lithotripsy techniques have been introduced for fragmenting large biliary stones [6, 7]. Although these elaborate techniques may overcome the limitations of ML, the high energies required must be carefully controlled to avoid accidental bile duct injuries.

With the recent advent of thin endoscopes, electrohydraulic lithotripsy has become feasible under direct vision during peroral cholangioscopy; this is called peroral cholangioscope electrohydraulic lithotripsy (POCS-EHL) [8, 9]. In this chapter we will describe our techniques of POCS-EHL and discuss the clinical results of the procedure in patients with difficult extra- and intrahepatic biliary stones.

Patients and methods

Patients

From 1987 to 1990, EPT for bile duct stones was performed in 302 patients. Thirty-five patients (11.6%) were subjected to peroral cholangioscope lithotripsy because of failure of mechanical lithotripsy. These included 19 patients with common duct stones and 16 patients with intrahepatic stones (16 males and 19 females). The age range was from 37–84 years (Table 20.1).

Instrumentation and procedure

We used a mother–baby scope system of a TJF M-20 duodenoscope and a Type J or CHF B-20 cholangioscope (Olympus Optical Co., Tokyo) (Table 20.2). The cholangioscope (i.e., the baby scope) has a 1.7 mm (in inner diameter) channel available for passing small instruments. Through this, 3 F guage electrodes were passed and the shock waves were generated by an electrohydraulic generator (SD-1 Stone Disintegrator, Northgate Research, USA) (Figs 20.1 and 20.2).

EPT was performed initially in all patients. The preparation of the patient was similar to that for EPT. Additionally, just before the procedure, 5–10 mg of diazepam was administered intravenously depending on the patient's general condition.

Following EPT, a 0.89 mm guide wire was inserted into the common bile duct. The cholangioscope was then introduced into the common bile duct over the guide wire. The wire was withdrawn and irrigation performed by manual injection of saline through the instrument channel of the baby scope to obtain a clear endoscopic view. A 3-port stop cock connector was attached to the inlet of the instrument channel to provide irrigation during lithotripsy.

The flexible cholangioscope was readily advanced to the hepatic bifurcation. While further insertion depended on the anatomy, we frequently achieved access to the liver segment containing the stone.

Table 20.1 Patients' characteristics ($n = 35$)

COMMON BILE DUCT STONES	
Patients	19
Male/Female	9/10
Age (median)	50–84 (72) years
Previous cholecystectomy	8
Characteristics of stones	
Number	
single	4
two	9
>two	6
Size (maximum)	
<20 mm	5
20–25	8
>25	6
Location or situation	
Confluence	3
Column formation	5
Prepapillary impaction	2
Lodged elsewhere	5
Floating	4
INTRAHEPATIC STONES	
Patients	16
Male/Female	7/9
Age (median)	37–77 (56.5)
Previous cholecystectomy and/or choledocholithotomy	11
Biliary stricture	
Hilar	5
Intrahepatic	2
Stone distribution	
Extrahepatic stones combined	8
Both lobe	10
Left lobe	4
Right lobe	2

When the stone was visualized the electrode was inserted and 5–10 mm of its firing chamber projected from the tip of the scope. Under endoscopic control the tip of the electrode was manœuvred close to the stone surface. The generator electrohydraulic (SD-1) was set to an output voltage of 55–70 V and a double-shot firing made. The unit was activated by a foot switch.

The results of stone fragmentation and removal were assessed on radiological and endoscopic findings.

Table 20.2 Specifications of the mother–baby scope system Mother scope (Olympus TJF type M20)

Optical system	Side view	
	View field	80°
	Focus fixed	5–60 mm
Distal end	Outer diameter	14.8 mm
Bending part	Bending angle	Up 120°, Down 90°
		Right 110°, Left 90°
Flexible part	Outer diameter	13 mm
Working length		1 215 mm
Total length		1 550 mm
Working channel	Inner diameter	5.5 mm
Baby scope (Olympus CHF type B20)		
Optical system	Straight view	
	View field	100°
	Focus fixed	3–50 mm
Distal end	Outer diameter	4.1 mm
Bending part	Bending angle	Up 160°
		Down 100°
Flexible part	Outer diameter	4.5 mm
Working length		1 870 mm
Total length		2 190 mm
Working channel	Inner diameter	1.7 mm

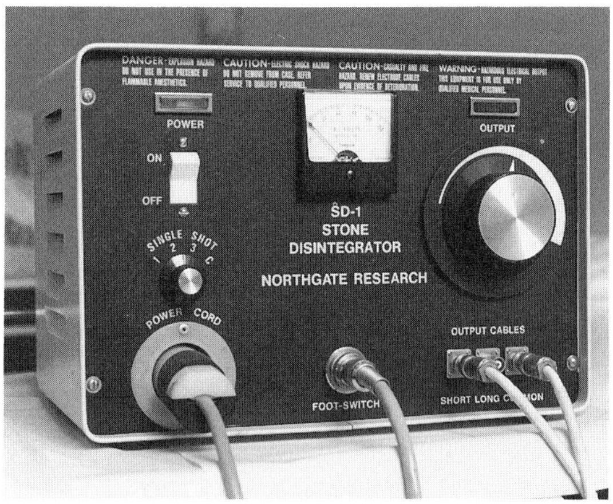

Fig. 20.1 The front view of the stone disintegrator (SD-1, Northgate Research Co.).

Results

Common bile duct stones

Nineteen patients had single or multiple common

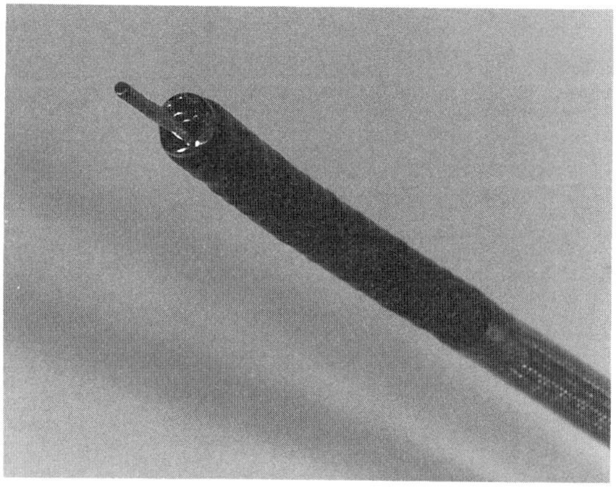

Fig. 20.2 3 F electrode projected from the distal end of the baby scope.

bile duct stones, whose size ranged from 11 × 12 mm to 45 × 56 mm with a mean of 19 × 23 mm. Stones were tightly compacted in the duct in 15 of the 19 patients, including column stones in five, confluent stones in three and stones lodged elsewhere in seven patients.

Acceptable stone fragmentation was achieved in a single session in 11 patients. Repeated lithotripsy was necessary for firm or large stones. Moreover, when a stone was impacted in the terminal common bile duct, positioning of the electrode could be difficult. Thus, two sessions were necessary in four patients, and more than two in the remaining four patients. However, POCS-EHL was eventually successful in all patients (Table 20.3).

After successful stone disintegration, the fragments were allowed to pass spontaneously or were removed by a basket with or without mechanical lithotripsy. Nasobiliary drainage was used to avoid cholangitis during treatment and no serious

Table 20.3 Results of POCS-EHL in the patients with common bile duct stones (n = 19)

Success in stone fragmentation	19*
Success in stone clearance	19
Complications	0

* Treatment sessions (mean) 1–10 (2.2) attempts/patient.

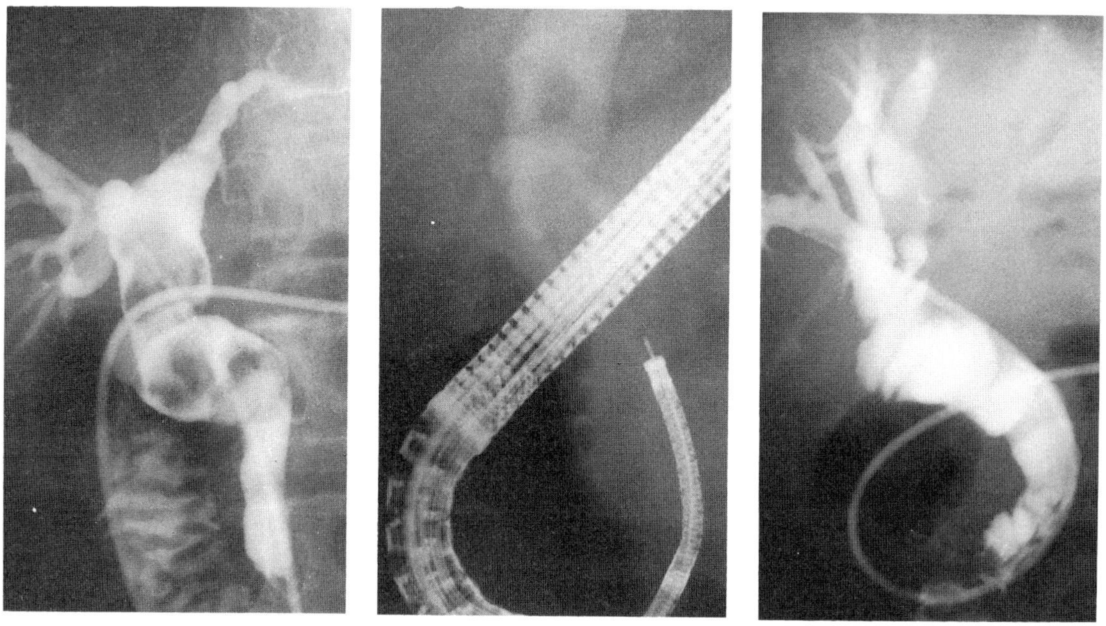

Fig. 20.3 Successful peroral cholangioscopic electrohydraulic lithotripsy (POCS-EHL) in a patient with common bile duct stones. (a) A pre-operative cholangiogram by a N–B tube showing three large stones conformed in the upper segment of the common bile duct. (b) An X-ray film during the procedure of POCS-EHL with a mother–baby scope (TJF-M20:CHF-B20). (c) The successful stone removal proven on the postoperative cholangiogram.

complications occurred in our patients. Stone clearance was achieved in all these patients (Fig. 20.3).

Intrahepatic stones

The baby scope was introduced in the right or left hepatic duct. Peroral endoscopy was generally restricted to the second order branches of the superior segments in both the lobes. The inferior branches, such as the posterior inferior branch in the right lobe and the lateral inferior branch in the left lobe, were usually inaccessible.

A biliary stricture was often associated with intrahepatic stones, and in fact, blocked endoscopic access in seven of the 16 patients. Five of these patients had post-cholecystectomy stricture

Table 20.4 Results of the endoscopic treatment in the patients with intrahepatic stones ($n = 16$)

Patients with accessible stones		14
POCS-EHL attempted		11*
Success in stone fragmentation	11	
Success in stone clearance		
Complete	7	
Fairly complete (>80%)	2	
Partial	2	
Complications	1 (transient bleeding)	
Other POCS applications attempted		3
Success in stone clearance		
Complete	3	

* Treatment sessions (mean) 1–9 (3.6) attempts/patient.

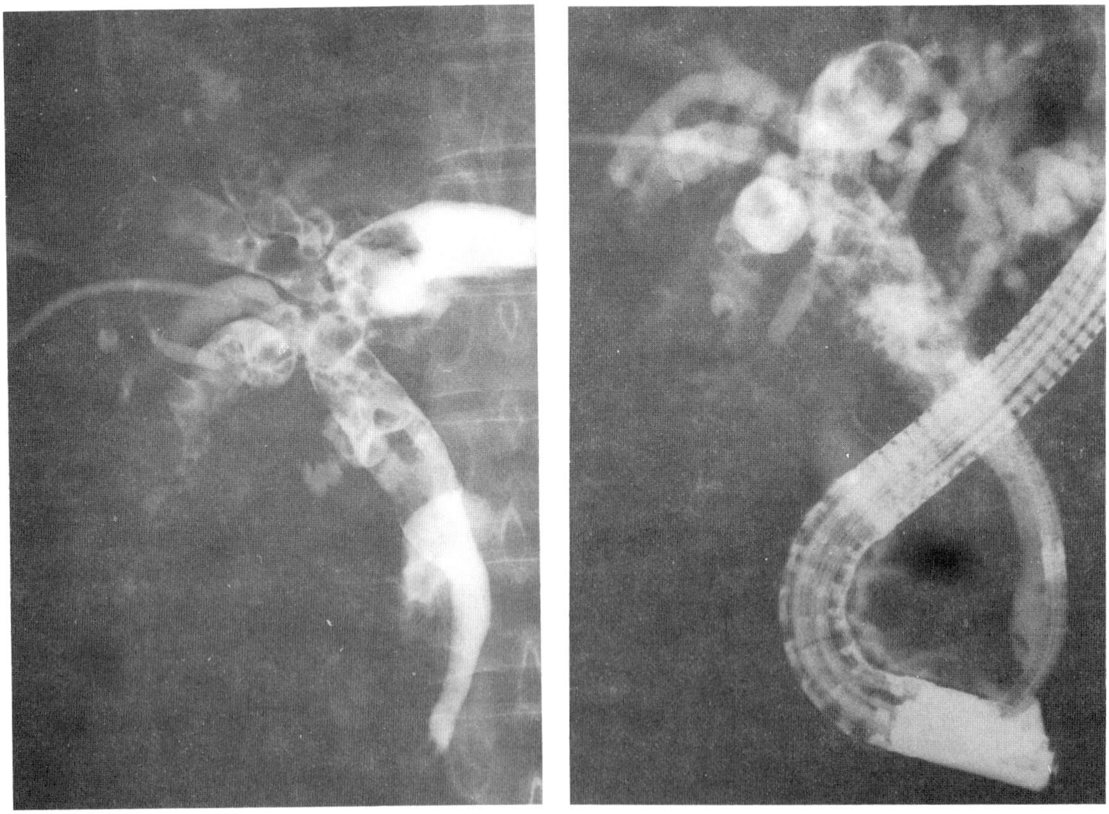

Fig. 20.4 Successful POCS-EHL in a patient with intra- and extrahepatic duct stones. (a) A pre-operative cholangiogram by a PTC tube showing a lot of stones broadly distributed in the intrahepatic bile ducts and in the upper segment of the common bile duct. (b) A cholangiogram during the successful stone fragmentation by POCS-EHL.

at the hepatic hilum, while another two had primary short strictures in the left hepatic duct and in the left lateral segment duct respectively. Dilatation with a balloon catheter was attempted successfully in the five patients with post-cholecystectomy stricture. Thus, the leading stone was located under endoscopic vision in 14 of 16 patients. Unsuccessful dilatation of the stricture accounted for the two failures. In two patients, stones were removed under endoscopic control using a basket and a Nd:YAG laser was attempted in one patient. Therefore, POCS-EHL was performed in 11 patients (Table 20.4).

In several patients the leading stones were successfully fragmented by POCS-EHL, allowing the proximal stones to move distally. When reasonably small, these migrated into the common bile duct.

The mean number of treatment sessions was 3.6 per patient. Except for one episode of transient bleeding there were no significant complications.

Finally, complete clearance of the stones was achieved in 10 of the patients (Fig. 20.4). Fairly complete (>80%) or partial (80% or less) removal was obtained in 4 patients, where retained stones were mostly found in the inferior subsegmental branches.

Discussion

Over the last 2 decades, various innovations in biliary lithotripsy have become available in combination with endoscopy. These include mechanical lithotripsy (ML), intracorporeal electrohydraulic or laser lithotripsy, and extracorporeal shock wave lithotripsy (ESWL). Mechanical

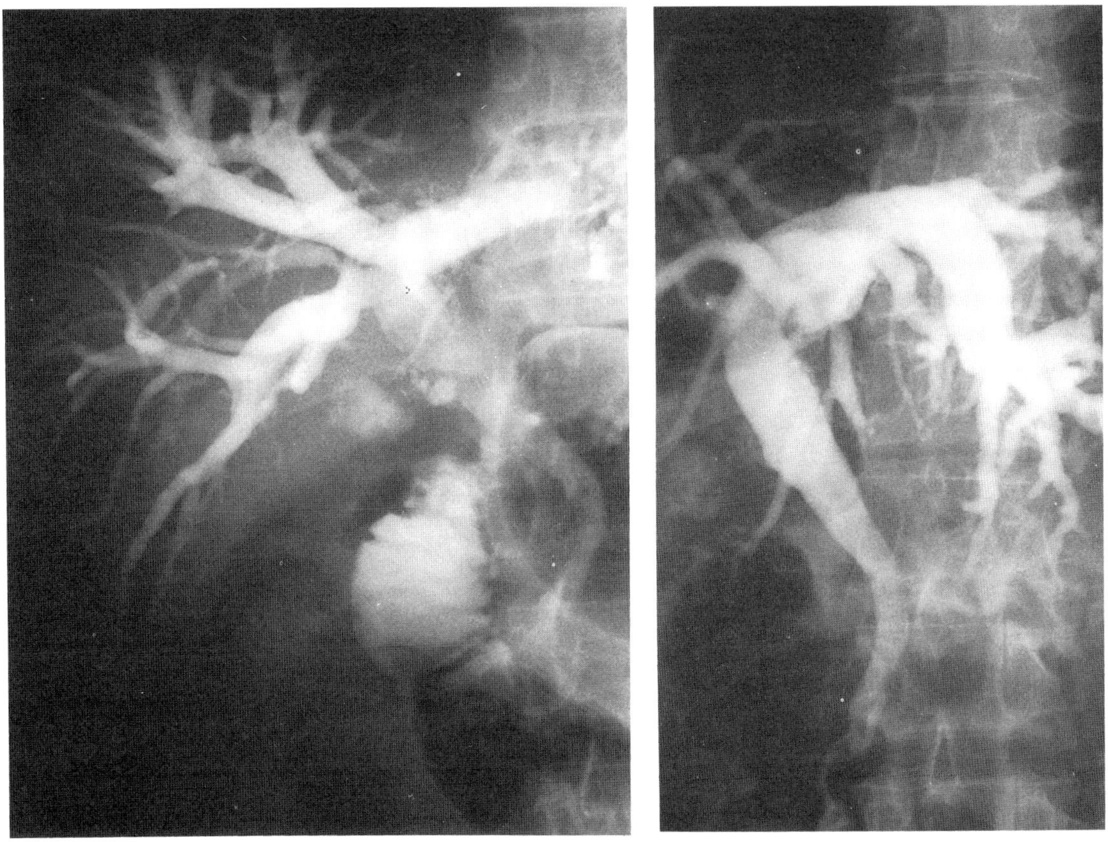

Fig. 20.4 (*Continued*) (c) and (d) The postoperative cholangiograms showing a complete clearance of the stones.

lithotripsy is limited by the location and size of the stones [3, 4] while the laser system is much more expensive compared with the electro-hydraulic generator. ESWL is also dependent on the location, number and consistency of the stones [10–15].

In 1975, Burhenne first used electrohydraulic lithotripsy (EHL) via a percutaneous route and under fluroscopic control for the treatment of a biliary stone [16]. In the 1980s, the procedure was successfully attempted with percutaneous cholangioscopy [17–23].

In 1977 Koch *et al.* performed biliary lithotripsy via a duodenoscope and under fluoroscopic control using a specially designed lithotripsy probe with a Dormia basket [24]. They attempted the procedure in three patients and obtained one successful stone removal. Several other authors have described lithotripsy probes, which were similarly integrated with a basket or a balloon and used under fluoroscopic control [25–28]. However, with the development of the mother–baby scope system, the electrode has been applied under direct vision via peroral cholangioscopy [8, 9, 29].

Close cooperation between the two endoscopists is required to perform mother–baby cholangioscopy; one controls the mother scope, while the other manœuvres the cholangioscope. Nevertheless, the retrograde access to bile duct stones has several advantages compared with the percutaneous route. Firstly, once an adequate papillotomy has been established the peroral access route is permanent. This may be useful if another treatment for retained or recurring stones is required at a later date. Secondly, the stone fragments can easily pass through the incised papilla, and the complications and discomfort associated with the percutaneous route are avoided completely. The intubation of the papilla with the baby scope (CHF-B20), even if it is flexible, may be difficult and we found use of a guide wire very helpful in this situation, especially when the papilla was not widely opened.

An impacted stone at the distal end of the common bile duct may pose a challenge when using the retrograde approach and additional manœuvres may be required. Sometimes, the stone may be forced back into the duct by pushing with the tip of the scope or the mother scope may be advanced distally to facilitate manipulation of the baby scope.

In our experience, post-cholecystectomy strictures at the hepatic hilum were easily dilated with a balloon dilator so that the proximal stones could be treated. Thus, the presence of a biliary stricture is not always a serious contraindication to the use of retrograde lithotripsy.

In the case of large stones, accumulation of fragments generated during lithotripsy obscured the endoscopic view. Repeated sessions were required in eight (42%) of 19 patients with common bile duct stones (2–4 sessions) and in nine (82%) of 11 patients with intrahepatic stones (2–9 sessions).

In experimental studies of electro-hydraulic shock wave lithotripsy, perforation of the duct wall occurred when the electrode tip came into direct contact with the mucosal surface [24, 26, 30]. It is important, therefore, to centre the electrode in the duct space to avoid contact with the wall. Endoscopic guidance is obviously superior to fluroscopic guidance in this regard. However, accurate control of the probe may not be easy in a small and tortuous duct. We experienced transient bleeding in a single patient with intrahepatic stones. Otherwise, there were no serious adverse effects attributable to electro-hydraulic lithotripsy in our study.

Laser lithotripsy may be a more promising and less hazardous technique than electro-hydraulic lithotripsy [31–34]. Ultrathin laser fibres may allow miniaturization of the endoscopic system, thus simplifying the procedure. However, the high cost of laser systems still precludes its routine use.

In conclusion, peroral cholangioscopic electro-hydraulic lithotripsy is a safe, efficacious and low-cost alternative to other surgical and non-surgical interventions in the managment of difficult biliary stones, when endoscopic access to the papilla is possible. It is especially indicated in patients with common bile duct stones, where bile duct clearance can often be frequently accomplished in one or two treatment sessions.

References

1 Runge D, Gebhardt J, Burmeister W, Wurbs D. Mechanische Lithotripsie von Gallengangssteinen. *Dtsch Med Wochenschr* 1985;110:1981–3.
2 Siegel JH, Pullano W, Ramsey WH. Lithotripsy–to crush or to explode: State of the art. *Gastrointest Endosc* 1986;**32**:172. (Abstract).
3 Schneider MU, Matek W, Bauer R, Domschke W. Mechanical Lithotripsy of bile duct stones in 209 patients–effect of technical advances. *Endoscopy* 1988;**20**:248–53.
4 Siegel JH, Ben-Zvi JS, Pullano WE. Mechanical lithotripsy of common duct stones. *Gastrointest Endosc* 1990;**36**:351–6.
5 Show MJ, Dorsher PJ, Vennes JA. A new mechnical lithotripter for the treatment of large common bile duct stones. *Am J Gastroenterol* 1990;**85**:796–8.
6 Classen M, Hagemuller F, Knyrim K, Frimberger E. Giant bile duct stones–Non-surgical treatment. *Endoscopy* 1988;**20**:21–6.
7 Slivka A, Carr-Locke DL. Therapeutic biliary endoscopy. *Endoscopy* 1992;**24**:100–19.
8 Ponchon T, Chavaillon A, Ayela P, Lambert R. Retrograde biliary ultrathin endoscopy enhances biopsy of stenoses and lithotripsy. *Gastrointest Endosc* 1989; **35**;292–7.
9 Leung JWC, Chung SSC. Electrohydraulic lithotripsy with peroral choledochoscopy. *Br Med J* 1989;**299**: 595–8.
10 Sauerbruch T, Stern M, The study group for shock-wave lithotripsy of bile duct stones. Fragmentation of bile duct stones by extracorporeal shock waves: a new approach to biliary calculi after failure of routine endoscopic measures. *Gastroenterology* 1989;**96**:146–52.
11 Wenzel H, Greiner L, Jakobeit Ch *et al.* ExtraKorporale Stosswellenlithotripsie von Gallengangssteinen. *Dtsch Med Wochenschr* 1989;**114**:738–43.
12 Moodey FG, Amerson JR, Berci G *et al.* Lithotripsy for bile duct stones. *Am J Surg* 1989;**158**:241–7.
13 Bland KI, Jones RS, Maher JW *et al.* Extracorporeal shock-wave lithotripsy of bile duct calculi. *Ann Surg* 1989;**209**:743–55.
14 Ponchon T, Martin X, Barkun A *et al.* Extracorporeal lithotripsy of bile duct stones using ultrasonography for stone localization. *Gastroenterology* 1990;**98**:726–32.
15 Lee SH, Fache JS, Burhenne HJ. The value of extracorporeal shock-wave lithotripsy in the management of bile duct stones. *AJR* 1990;**155**:775–9.
16 Burhenne HJ. Electrohydrolytic fragmentation of retained common duct stones. *Radiology* 1975;**117**: 721–2.
17 Ebbs SR, Beckly DE, Hammonds JC, Teasdale C. Percutaneous electrohydraulic lithotripsy of retained bile duct calculus. *Br Med J* 1986;**292**:94.
18 Hwang MH, Lee HH, Lin J *et al.* Transcholecystic endoscopic choledocholithotripsy: successful management of retained common bile duct stone. *Endoscopy* 1987;**19**:24–7.
19 Liguory CL, Bonnel D, Canard JM *et al.* Intracorporeal electrohydraulic shock wave lithotripsy of common bile duct stones: preliminary results in 7 cases. *Endoscopy* 1987;**19**:237–40.
20 Ponchon T, Valette PJ, Chavaillon A. Percutaneous electrohydraulic lithotripsy under endoscopic control. *Gastrointest Endosc* 1987;**33**:307–9.
21 Mo L-R, Hwang M-H, Yueh S-K, Yueh S-K *et al.* Percutaneous transhepatic choledochoscopic electrohydraulic lithotripsy (PTCS-EHL) of common bile duct stones. *Gastrointest Endosc* 1988;**34**:122–5.
22 Picus D, Weyman PJ, Marx MV. Role of percutaneous intracorporeal electrohydraulic lithotripsy in the treatment of biliary tract calculi. *Radiology* 1989;**170**:989–93.
23 Bonnel DH, Liguory CE, Cornud FE, Lefebvre J-F. Common bile duct and intrahepatic stones: results of transhepatic electrohydraulic lithotripsy in 50 patients. *Radiology* 1991;**180**:345–8.
24 Koch H, Stolte M, Walz V. Endoscopic lithotripsy in the common bile duct. *Endoscopy* 1977;**9**:95–8.
25 Frimberger E, Kuhner W, Weingart J, Ottenjann R. Eine neue Methode der elektrohydraulischen cholelithotripsie (Lithoklasie). *Dtsch Med Wochenschr* 1982; 107:213–15.
26 Nakajima M, Fujimoto S, Imaoka W *et al.* Endoscopic electrohydraulic lithotripsy (EEL) of biliary tract stones. *Gastroenterol Endosc* 1982;**24**:1391–1400 (in Japanese).
27 Tanaka M, Yoshimoto H, Ikeda S, Itoh H. Endoscopic electrohydraulic lithotripsy for choledocholithiasis: dog experiments and preliminary clinical experience. *Gastroenterol Endosc* 1982;**24**:1544–51.
28 Siegel JH, Ben-Zvi JS, Pullano WE. Endoscopic electrohydraulic lithotripsy. *Gastrointest Endosc* 1990;**36**:134–6.
29 Riemann JF, Kohler B, Weber J, Schlauch D. Intraductal shockwave lithotripsy in complicated common bile duct stones. *Clin Investig* 1992;**70**:148–51.
30 Harrison J, Morris DL, Haynes J *el al.* Electrohydraulic lithotripsy of gall stones–*in vitro* and animal studies. *Gut* 1987;**28**:267–71.
31 Ell Ch, Lux G, Hochberger J *et al.* Laserlithotripsy of common bile duct stones. *Gut* 1988;**29**:746–51.
32 Cotton PB, Kozarek RA, Schapiro RH *et al.* Endoscopic laser lithotripsy of large bile duct stones. *Gastroenterology* 1990;**99**:1128–33.
33 Ponchon T, Gagnon P, Valette P-J *et al.* Pulsed dye laser lithotripsy of bile duct stones. *Gastroenterology* 1991;**100**:1730–6.
34 Neuhaus H, Hoffmann W, Zillinger C, Classen M. Laser lithotripsy of difficult bile duct stones under direct visual control. *Gut* 1993;**34**:415–21.

Chapter 21
Cholecystectomy and colon cancer

A.D. Spigelman

Introduction

Colorectal cancer is the second most frequent cause of death in the western world [1]. Numerous studies have investigated a possible relationship between cholecystectomy for gallstones and the subsequent risk of cancer of the large bowel. The implications of such a relationship, were it to be valid, are several. Firstly, a strong relationship would target a group of patients at high-risk for colorectal cancer for screening, thereby facilitating earlier treatment with an anticipated improvement in survival. Secondly, it would imply a common aetiology for gallstones and colorectal cancer that might be a fruitful path for basic research into the causation of colorectal cancer. Thirdly, if the performance of a cholecystectomy *per se*, rather than the presence of gallstones correlates with colorectal cancer, then enthusiasm for removal of the gallbladder might be tempered. The pendulum would swing away from cholecystectomy back to conservation of the gallbladder [2]. In this chapter I will focus on the relationship between cholecystectomy and colorectal cancer and summarize some of the key work which has directly addressed the proposed gallstone–cholecystectomy–colorectal cancer link.

Why should cholecystectomy predispose to colorectal cancer?

The relationship between bile acids and colon cancer has been the subject of much investigation for the following reasons:

1 bile acids stimulate the proliferation of colonic epithelial cells [3];
2 abnormal bile acid profiles have been identified in patients who have colonic adenomas (premalignant polyps) or who have colonic cancer [4, 5];
3 cholecystectomy may change the composition of [6] and enhance the circulation of the bile acid pool [7, 8];
4 an increase in secondary bile acids has been found to occur after cholecystectomy [6].

However, many of these findings have not been confirmed in studies conducted by other groups. Nevertheless, the reported increase in secondary bile acids after cholecystectomy may inhibit the activity of hepatic enzyme systems which act to detoxify environmental carcinogens [9]. Such carcinogens may then be excreted into bile and thence into the lumen of the intestinal tract. Bile salts themselves can be converted to methylcholanthrene, which is a potent carcinogen [3]. It is also of interest that patients with familial adenomatous polyposis, who inevitably develop colon cancer unless the colon is removed, also have abnormal bile acid profiles [10]. Moreover, bile acid profiles change after colectomy, and it has been suggested that this altered profile mediates a reduction in rectal cell proliferation, which is accompanied by the regression of rectal polyps in patients with polyposis [11]. Abnormalities in bile acid metabolism have also been advanced as an explanation for an excess of large bowel adenomas and cancers in patients, 10 or more years after truncal vagotomy for benign peptic ulcer disease [12].

Cholecystectomy and colorectal cancer

Animal studies

A number of investigators have studied the

effects of known large bowel carcinogens (dimethylhydrazine or its metabolite methylazoxymethanol) in animals with and without cholecystectomy. Werner *et al.* [13] found colonic tumours in 18 of 19 mice (95%) treated with dimethylhydrazine and cholecystectomy compared with 15 of 19 mice (79%) given the carcinogen alone. This study is often cited in support of the cholecystectomy–colon cancer link because the colon-cancer yield was significantly greater in the carcinogen plus cholecystectomy group (13 mice (68%)) compared with 3 mice (16%) in the carcinogen-alone group. However, premalignant adenomas were found in 12 (63%) of the carcinogen-alone group compared with 5 (26%) in the carcinogen plus cholecystectomy group. Therefore, one can conclude that cholecystectomy perhaps hastens the adenoma–carcinoma sequence in this experimental model. The study of Schattenkerk *et al.* [14] purports to demonstrate a lack of effect of cholecystectomy on the frequency of carcinogen-induced colon cancer in mice. There was certainly no difference in the number of mice with colon tumours between groups given carcinogen and cholecystectomy (17 out of 31 mice (55%)) or carcinogen and a sham operation (15 out of 32 mice (47%)). However, the total number of cancers was greater in the cholecystectomy group. That is, 30 colorectal cancers were found in the 31 cholecystectomized mice compared with 21 such cancers in the 32 sham-operated mice [14]. These findings again suggest that cholecystectomy hastens the adenoma–carcinoma sequence. Narisawa *et al.* [15] found an increase in the percentage of mice who had large bowel cancer after cholecystectomy plus carcinogen (31%) compared with mice who had carcinogen alone (20%), although this difference was not statistically significant. Faecal bile acids were measured in this study, and in the cholecystectomy group the level of primary bile acids was found to be significantly increased, with an unchanged level of secondary bile acids. Because the primary bile acids are weaker promoters of cancer than are their secondary counterparts, the authors used this finding to explain the lack of statistical significance in the increase in colon cancer observed in the cholecystectomy group. As in the study of Werner *et al.* [13], the performance of a cholecystectomy in the absence of exogenous carcinogen did not lead to colon cancer. The human situation is more likely to equate with the cholecystectomy plus exogenous carcinogen exposure scenario, as humans are exposed to a myriad of carcinogens in everyday life [16].

In contrast to the murine studies, hamsters given carcinogen plus cholecystectomy were found to have a significantly greater number of large bowel neoplasms compared with hamsters given carcinogen alone. However, the difference was mainly in the yield of precancerous adenomas rather than in frank cancer [17]. In keeping with the mouse experiments reported above, Hickman *et al.* [18] found no difference in large bowel cancer yield between mice given carcinogen and cholecystectomy or sham operation. However, indices of cell proliferation (a likely marker of cancer risk) [19] were found to be significantly increased in mice who had not received carcinogen but who had undergone cholecsystectomy over the levels seen in non-carcinogen sham-operated animals.

Human studies

Bandettini *et al.* [20], used the mitotic index as a means of measuring cell proliferation in the colon of a small number of patients with gallstones (before and shortly after surgery), or who had undergone cholecystectomy several years earlier, and in healthy controls. Whereas the mitotic index results for control and pre-cholecystectomy patients were similar, the index for patients who had undergone cholecystectomy many years before was significantly higher than that for controls. The mitotic index was seen to rise significantly within 6 months of cholecystectomy.

Epidemiological studies

Cholecystectomy and colorectal cancer

For every study that shows an increased risk for colorectal cancer in the presence of a history of cholecystectomy there is another which fails to demonstrate such a link. Mannes *et al.* [21] demonstrated a significantly increased risk for colorectal adenomatous polyps and cancers in 78 patients who were 10 or more years post-cholecystectomy over an otherwise matched group of patients who were less than 10 years after cholecystectomy. In a study of 72 patients, Llamas *et al.* [22] failed to demonstrate an overall association between previous cholecystectomy and colorectal adenomas, but did find an excess risk for women who had undergone cholecystectomy over those who had not had this operation. Cholecystectomy was particularly associated with right-sided colonic adenomas. Neugut *et al.* [23, 24], in two separate studies, were unable to confirm an association between colorectal adenomas in women and cholecystectomy.

Vernick *et al.* [25] demonstrated a positive relationship between cholecystectomy and right-sided colon cancer in a retrospective study of 706 cases. These authors conceded that this finding may have been influenced by two areas of bias, namely the possibility of misdiagnosis leading to cholecystectomy while symptoms were due to right-sided colon cancer and the possibility that information about gallbladder disease might be more readily entered into the notes of patients presenting with right-sided abdominal pain. Turnbull *et al.* [26] found an excess risk for colorectal cancer in females who had undergone cholecystectomy in a case control study involving 305 large bowel cancer patients and matched controls. This association was attributed to an excess of rectal cancer in the test group, the overall relative risk (the increased risk relative to the normal population) being 2.7. Turunen and Kivilaakso [27], in a retrospective autopsy study, also found an increased risk for colorectal cancer in cholecystectomy patients, but here the risk was greatest for right-sided colon cancer. No association was found between the incidence of unoperated gallstones and colorectal cancer in this study. Linos *et al.* [28] found a significant excess of colon cancer in 1221 post-cholecystectomy females. In this retrospective study the relative risk for colon cancer in females was 1.7 (95% confidence intervals 1.1–2.5), rising to 2.1 for females with right-sided colon cancer. A similar relative risk was obtained by Vernick and Kuller [29] in a smaller case control study. A higher relative risk for colon cancer (4.39) was found for patients who had undergone cholecystectomy in an Asian population [30]. Several other studies have also shown a statistically significant association between right-sided colon cancer and a history of a prior cholecystectomy [31–33]. One study showed a significantly increased risk for colon cancer in males only [34]. These studies suggest that prospective screening of the large bowel should be undertaken in patients with a past history of cholecystectomy. When such a study was performed, 12 asymptomatic patients were found to have colorectal neoplasia (4 patients with cancer; 8 with adenomas) [35]. Only 3 patients in a control group of post-mortem patients were found to have tumours (all adenomas).

Other studies [36–45] have failed to show a significantly increased risk for colon cancer in post-cholecystectomy patients. Subgroup analysis according to sex, site of tumour, or length of time after cholecystectomy also did not demonstrate that cholecystectomy led to an excess risk. The largest of these studies involved over 16 000 patients [39, 43].

Gallstones and colorectal cancer

Some studies [46, 47] have failed to confirm the abnormalities in biliary bile acid composition following cholecystectomy observed by others [6, 48, 49]. If a link exists between the gallbladder and colon cancer, then perhaps this association is based on the presence of gallstones rather than the performance of a cholecystectomy. Thus, lithogenic bile might be carcinogenic in the colon, perhaps as a result of bacterial degradation [50, 51]. One study that conflicts with this hypothesis has demonstrated that 13 patients with gallstones had higher secondary bile acid levels in their bile than did eight control patients [52]. However, the 10 patients with colon cancer had similar levels of these bile acids in their bile to the control group (i.e., lower than the level found in the gallstone group of patients). Deficiencies of this study included the small number of patients studied and the lack of information on the age distribution of these patients (age can influence bile acid metabolism) [53].

Epidemiological studies that have tested for an association between gallstones and colon cancer have produced differing results. Both conditions are very common in most countries where these studies have been undertaken, and this feature would make it difficult for all but the strongest of associations to be easily discernible. Doouss and Castleden [54] did not show a relationship between the two disorders. Linos *et al.* [55] showed an apparent link, but concluded that this was due to bias arising from the probability that patients undergoing follow-up for colon cancer would be more likely to have gallstones detected than others. Perhaps confirming this source of bias, the excess risk for colon cancer was indeed found to be confined to patients with asymptomatic gallstones. In a large study from Sweden, gallstone disease was found to be significantly associated with the risk for gastrointestinal cancer, although nearly half of the discussion in this paper is devoted to addressing three potential sources of bias [56]. Allende *et al.* [57] found significantly higher rates of colorectal cancer in female patients who had had a cholecystectomy or who had gallstones. A Danish study showed a significantly higher prevalence of gallstone disease in colorectal cancer patients than in controls, although the 95% confidence intervals were only just above unity, suggesting only a weakly significant relationship [58]. Finally, a large case-control study demonstrated a statistically significant increased risk for both colon cancer and rectal cancer in patients with a history of cholelithiasis [59].

Conclusion

From the studies reviewed in this chapter, it can be seen that the link between gallbladder disease, cholecystectomy and colorectal cancer is, if it exists at all, most likely to be a weak one. Until such times as a large definitive prospective study is done, it seems prudent to screen those patients who are 10 or more years post-cholecystectomy, although the evidence for such a policy is not convincing. At best it might be said that the case for a relationship between gallstones, cholecystectomy and colorectal cancer is unproven. In the light of our present knowledge, cholecystectomy is not contraindicated on the grounds of its colorectal carcinogenic potential.

References

1 Ron E, Lubin F. Epidemiology of colorectal cancer and its relevance to screening. *Front Gastrointest Res* 1986;10:1–34.
2 Walsh TN, Russell RCG. Cholecystectomy and gallbladder conservation. *Br J Surg* 1992;**79**:4–5.
3 Nair PP. Role of bile acids and neutral sterols in carcinogenesis. *Am J Clin Nutr* 1988;**48**:768–74.
4 Moorehead RJ, Campbell GR, Donaldson JD, McKelvey STD. Relationship between duodenal bile acids and colorectal neoplasia. *Gut* 1987;**28**:1454–9.
5 Imray CHE, Radley S, Davis A *et al.* Faecal unconjugated bile acids in patients with colorectal cancer or polyps. *Gut* 1992;**33**:1239–45.
6 Pomare EW, Heaton KW. The effect of cholecystectomy on bile acid metabolism. *Gut* 1973;**14**:753–62.
7 Moorehead RJ, McKelvey STD. Cholecystectomy and colorectal cancer. *Br J Surg* 1989;**76**:250–3.
8 McMichael AJ, Potter JD. Host factors in carcinogenesis: certain bile-acid metabolic profiles that selectively increase the risk of proximal colon cancer. *J Natl Cancer Inst* 1985;**75**:185–91.
9 Hayes JD, Mantle TJ. Inhibition of hepatic and extrahepatic glutathione-*S*-transferases by primary and secondary bile acids. *Biochem J* 1986;**233**:407–15.
10 Spigelman AD, Owen RW, Hill MJ, Phillips RKS, Biliary bile acid profiles in familial adenomatous polyposis. *Br J Surg* 1991;**78**:321–5.
11 Cats A, Kleibeuker JH, Kuipers F *et al.* Changes in rectal cell proliferation and intestinal bile acids after subtotal colectomy in familial adenomatous polyposis. *Cancer Res* 1992;**52**:3552–7.
12 Mullan FJ, Wilson HK, Majury CW *et al.* Bile acids and the increased risk of colorectal tumours after truncal vagotomy. *Br J Surg* 1990;**77**:1085–90.
13 Werner B, deHeer K, Mitschke H. Cholecystectomy and carcinoma of the colon: an experimental study. *Z Krebsforsch* 1977;**88**:223–30.
14 Schattenkerk ME, Li AKC, Jeppsson BW *et al.* Cholecystectomy has no influence on frequency of chemically induced colonic cancer in mice. *Br J Cancer* 1980;**42**:791–3.
15 Narisawa T, Sano M, Sato M, Takahashi T, Tanida N, Shimoyama T. The correlation between cholecystectomy and fecal bile acids, and large bowel cancer induced with 1,2-dimethylhydrazine in mice. *Dis Colon Rectum* 1985;**28**:27–30.
16 Beach AC, Gupta RC. Human biomonitoring and the

^{32}P-postlabeling assay. *Carcinogenesis* 1992;13:1053–74.

17 Kuniyasu T, Tanaka T, Shima H, Sugie S, Mori H, Takahashi M. Enhancing effect of cholecystectomy on colon carcinogenesis induced by methylazoxymethanol acetate in hamsters. *Dis Colon Rectum* 1986;**29**:492–4.

18 Hickman MS, Salinas HC, Schwesinger WH. Does cholecystectomy affect colonic tumorigenesis? *Arch Surg* 1987;**122**:334–6.

19 Cohen SM, Ellwein LB. Cell proliferation in carcinogenesis. *Science* 1990;**249**:1007–11.

20 Bandettini L, Filipponi F, Romagnoli P. Increase in mitotic index of colonic mucosa after cholecystectomy. *Cancer* 1986;**58**:685–7.

21 Mannes AG, Weinzierl M, Stellard F, Thieme C, Wiebecke B, Paumgartner G. Adenomas of the large intestine after cholecystectomy. *Gut* 1984;**25**:863–6.

22 Llamas KJ, Torlach LG, Ward M, Bain C. Cholecystectomy and adenomatous polyps of the large bowel. *Gut* 1986;**27**:1181–5.

23 Neugut AI, Johnsen CM, Forde KA, Treat MR, Nims C, Murray D. Cholecystectomy and adenomatous polyps of the colon in women. *Cancer* 1988;**61**:618–21.

24 Neugut AI, Murray TI, Garbowski GC. Cholecystectomy as a risk factor for colorectal adenomatous polyps and carcinoma. *Cancer* 1991;**68**:1644–7.

25 Vernick LJ, Kuller LH, Lohsoonthorn P, Rycheck RR, Redmond CK. Relationship between cholecystectomy and ascending colon cancer. *Cancer* 1980;**45**:392–5.

26 Turnbull PRG, Smith AH, Isbister WH. Cholecystectomy and cancer of the large bowel. *Br J Surg* 1981;**68**:551–3.

27 Turunen MJ, Kivilaakso EO. Increased risk of colorectal cancer after cholecystectomy. *Ann Surg* 1981; **194**:639–41.

28 Linos DA, Beard CM, O'Fallon WM, Dockerty MB, Beart RW, Kurland LT. Cholecystectomy and carcinoma of the colon. *Lancet* 1981;ii:379–81.

29 Vernick LJ, Kuller LH. Cholecystectomy and right sided colon cancer: an epidemiological study. *Lancet* 1981;ii:381–3.

30 Lee HP, Gourley L, Duffy SW, Esteve J, Lee J, Day NE. Colorectal cancer and diet in an Asian population: a case-control study among Singapore Chinese. *Int J Cancer* 1989;**43**:1007–1116.

31 Alley PG, Lee SP. The increased risk of proximal colonic cancer after cholecystectomy. *Dis Colon Rectum* 1983;**26**:522–4.

32 Mamianetto A, Cinto RO, Altolaguirre D, Bosicio OA, Heidenreich A, Salomon M. Relative risk of colorectal cancer after cholecystectomy. A multicentre case-control study. *Int J Colorect Dis* 1988;3:215–18.

33 Soltero E, Cruz NI, Nazario CM, Lopez RE, Alonso A, Rios CF. Cholecystectomy and right colon cancer in Puerto Rico. *Cancer* 1990:**66**:2249–52.

34 Nielsen GP, Theodors A, Tulinius H, Sigvaldason H. Cholecystectomy and colorectal carcinoma: a total-population historical prospective study. *Am J Gastroent* 1991;**86**:1486–9.

35 Moorehead RJ, Wilson HK, Mills JOM, McKelvey STD. Cholecystectomy and the development of colorectal neoplasia: a prospective study. *Ann Roy Coll Surg Eng* 1989;**71**:37–9.

36 Weiss NS, Daling JR, Chow WH. Cholecystectomy and the incidence of cancer of the large bowel. *Cancer* 1982;**49**:1713–15.

37 Narisawa T, Sano M, Sato M, Takahashi T, Arakawa H. Relationship between cholecystectomy and colonic cancer in low-risk Japanese population. A preliminary study. *Dis Colon Rectum* 1983;**26**:512–15.

38 Abrams JS, Anton JR, Dreyfuss DC. The absence of a relationship between cholecystectomy and the subsequent occurrence of cancer of the proximal colon. *Dis Colon Rectum* 1983;**26**:141–4.

39 Adami HO, Meirik O, Gustavsson S, Nyren O, Krusemo UB. Colorectal cancer after cholecystectomy: absence of risk increase within 11–14 years. *Gastroenterology* 1983;**85**:859–65.

40 Blanco D, Ross RK, Paganini-Hill A, Henderson BE. Cholecystectomy and colonic cancer. *Dis Colon Rectum* 1984;**27**:290–2.

41 Spitz MR, Russell NC, Guinee VF, Newell GR. Questionable relationship between cholecystectomy and colon cancer. *J Surg Oncol* 1985;**30**:6–9.

42 Kaibara N, Wakatsuki T, Mizusawa K, Sugesawa A, Kimura O, Koga S. Negative correlation between cholecystectomy and the subsequent development of large bowel carcinoma in a low-risk Japanese population. *Dis Colon Rectum* 1986;**29**:644–6.

43 Adami HO, Krusemo UB, Meirik O. Unaltered risk of colorectal cancer within 14–17 years of cholecystectomy: Updating of a population-based cohort study. *Br J Surg* 1987;**74**:675–8.

44 Friedman GD, Goldhaber MK, Quesenberry CP. Cholecystectomy and large bowel cancer. *Lancet* 1987; i:906–8.

45 Kune GA, Kune S, Watson LF. Large bowel cancer after cholecystectomy. *Am J Surg* 1988;**156**:359–62.

46 van der Linden W, Katzenstein B, Nakayama F. The possible carcinogenic effect of cholecystectomy. No postoperative increase in the proportion of secondary bile acids. *Cancer* 1983;**52**:1265–8.

47 Adler RD, Metzger AL, Grundy SM. Biliary lipid secretion before and after cholecystectomy in American Indians with cholesterol gallstones. *Gastroenterology* 1976;**66**:1212–17.

48 Almond HR, Vlachevic ZR, Bell CC, Gregory DH, Swell L. Bile acid pool kinetics and biliary bile acid composition before and after cholecystectomy. *N Eng J Med* 1973;**289**:1213–16.

49 Hepner GW, Hofmann AF, Malagedala JR, Szczepanik PA, Klein PD. Increased bacterial degradation of bile acids in cholecystectomized patients. *Gastroenterology* 1974;**66**:556–64.

50 Hill MJ. Bile, bacteria and bowel cancer. *Gut* 1983;**24**: 871–5.

51 Hill MJ. Bile flow and colon cancer. *Mutagenesis* 1990;238:313–20.
52 Castleden WM, Detchon P, Misso NLA. Biliary bile acids in cholelithiasis and colon cancer. *Gut* 1989;30:860–5.
53 Nagengast FM, van der Werf SDJ, Lamers HLM, Hectors MPC, Buys WCAM, van Tongeren JHM. Influence of age, intestinal transit time, and dietary composition on fecal bile acid profiles in healthy subjects. *Dig Dis Sci* 1988;33:673–8.
54 Doouss TW, Castleden WM. Gallstones and carcinoma of the large bowel. *NZ Med J* 1973;77:162–5.
55 Linos DA, O'Fallon M, Thistle JL, Kurland LT. Cholelithiasis and carcinoma of the colon. *Cancer* 1982;50:1015–19.
56 Lowenfels AB, Domellof L, Lindstrom CG, Bergman F, Monk MA, Sternby NH. Cholelithiasis, cholecystectomy, and cancer: a case-control study in Sweden. *Gastroenterology* 1982;83:672–6.
57 Allende HD, Ona FV, Davis HT. Gallbladder disease: risk factor for colorectal carcinoma? *J Clin Gastroenterol* 1984;6:51–5.
58 Jorgensen T, Rafaelsen S. Gallstones and colorectal cancer–there is a relationship, but it is hardly due to cholecystectomy. *Dis Colon Rectum* 1992;35:24–8.
59 Vecchia CL, D'Avanzo B, Negri E, Franceschi S. History of selected diseases and the risk of colorectal cancer. *Eur J Cancer* 1991;27:582–6.

Chapter 22
Iatrogenic injuries of the bile duct

W.C. Chapman & I.S. Benjamin

Introduction

While accidental injury of the bile duct may occur during the course of a number of operative procedures, such as partial gastrectomy, most such injuries occur during cholecystectomy or common bile duct exploration. These injuries often result in severe morbidity for affected patients which may require lifelong medical attention and necessitate repeated operations and radiological interventions. This can be particularly tragic, since many of the patients are young women in good health prior to their elective cholecystectomy.

Many factors have been suggested which may predispose to iatrogenic bile duct injury including variations in vascular and biliary anatomy and severe inflammation in region of the bile duct from recent cholecystitis [1–3]. However, the most common cause of bile duct injury is a failure of the surgeon to dissect and identify ductal structures adequately before transecting the apparent 'cystic duct'. Thus, some surgeons have suggested that iatrogenic injury of the bile duct, occurring during 'open' or laparoscopic cholecystectomy, should be entirely preventable [4–7].

After the introduction of laparoscopic cholecystectomy in the USA and Europe, some reports suggested that there might be an increased incidence of iatrogenic bile duct injury associated with this new procedure [6, 8]. This has brought about a heightened awareness of the potential for bile duct injuries during cholecystectomy. While the follow-up period is still too short to determine if laparoscopic removal of the gallbladder is inherently associated with a higher rate of bile duct injuries it has been suggested that laparoscopic cholecystectomy be performed only by specialist biliary surgeons [9]. Whether or not this is so, any surgeon performing either laparoscopic or open cholecystectomy should have a thorough understanding of the treatment options for bile duct injury, should this eventuality occur. Repeated attempts at surgical repair or interventional radiological procedures should probably be performed only in tertiary referral centres with a special interest in this problem, since the likelihood of success diminishes with each additional procedure [4–6]. The most likely procedure to succeed is the first one performed after the bile duct injury.

Incidence and contributing factors

The precise incidence of this complication is difficult to determine with certainty, but has been reported to occur in approximately 0.1–0.5% of open cholecystectomies [5, 8, 10, 11]. In an early report following the introduction of laparoscopic cholecystectomy in the USA, Cameron and Gadacz [8] suggested that the incidence of iatrogenic bile duct injury might be up to 10-fold higher when the gallbladder was removed laparoscopically. However, this has not yet been proven in large follow-up reviews.

Johnston has suggested that three factors primarily contribute to iatrogenic injury of the bile duct: 'dangerous pathology, dangerous anatomy, and dangerous surgery' [4]. In the patient with recent acute cholecystitis or pancreatitis, there may be a significant degree of inflammation in the region of the porta hepatis, making dissection and identification of the cystic duct and common duct extremely difficult. In this setting it may be necessary to open the gallbladder to identify the region of the neck of the organ. Occasionally, in difficult cases, it is prudent to leave a portion of the neck of the gallbladder *in situ*, and close this after removing any stones from the gallbladder itself. Another option in particularly severe cases of inflammation is to perform only a cholecystostomy, avoiding dissection in the region of the common bile duct. In this situation, cholecystectomy can be performed at a later date when the acute inflammation has subsided. Performance of cholecystostomy is increasingly rare now, and 'partial cholecystectomy', as described above, has been a safe and effective option in our experience.

An additional, less common, situation in which the pathology may contribute to ductal injury is in the Mirrizzi syndrome [13], in which a stone impacted in the cystic duct or the neck of the gallbladder erodes into the adjacent common hepatic duct. If this situation is not properly identified, a common duct injury may result when the neck of the gallbladder and cystic duct are being dissected.

In the setting of portal hypertension, cholecystectomy becomes particularly hazardous because of the numerous large venous collaterals in the region of the porta [14, 15]. If significant bleeding is encountered during cholecystectomy, then ductal injury may result when the surgeon tries to stop the haemorrhage and is forced to operate in an obscured field. The indications for cholecystectomy in cirrhotic patients must, therefore, be carefully considered, and safe procedures such as partial cholecystectomy adopted in these cases. Severe cirrhosis is a relative contraindication to laparoscopic cholecystectomy.

There are many anatomical variations of the cystic and hepatic ducts with which the surgeon performing cholecystectomy must be familiar [3, 5]. The most common of these are shown in Fig. 22.1, and may contribute to accidental injury to the common duct if not appreciated. In particular, the very short or absent cystic duct, the cystic duct which enters the right hepatic duct, and the cystic duct which passes posterior to the common hepatic duct may all contribute to ductal injury. Sectoral ducts may be ligated in error in cases where there is a low union of right and left hepatic ducts. With careful dissection and operative cholangiography the surgeon can usually identify these anomalies before any ducts are divided.

The most common contributing factor to iatrogenic ductal injury, however, is probably a failure of the surgical technique [3–7, 16, 17]. In several European studies, the majority of ductal injuries occurred when the operation was being performed by junior surgical staff [18] who had only performed between 25 and 100

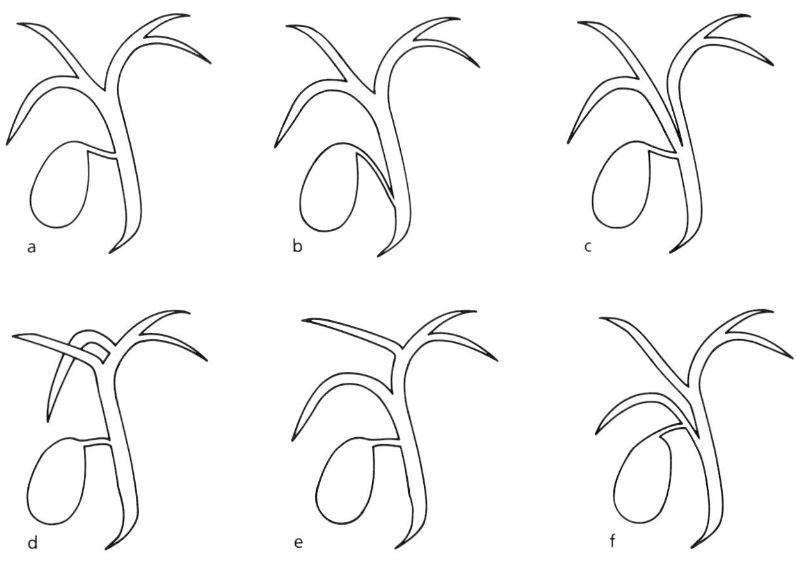

Fig. 22.1 Common anomalies of the bile ducts.

cholecystectomies and were not being supervised by a consultant surgeon [19]. In some training systems, junior surgeons perform the majority of elective cholecystectomies: this was the case in 62% of 1 000 cholecystectomies performed in three UK district hospitals [20]. With this level of experience, the surgeon may have a degree of overconfidence and may not appreciate the extent of anatomical variation possible, and thus injure the bile duct.

While intraoperative cholangiography has traditionally been used primarily to detect common duct calculi, it has also been suggested as an adjunct, which if used routinely, might diminish the incidence of ductal injuries in both open [3, 5, 11, 21, 22] and laparoscopic cholecystectomies [23, 24]. To this point, in Blumgart's report of 78 bile duct injuries [1] it was found that in only 29% of cases had a cholangiogram been performed at the time of the original cholecystectomy. Likewise, in a nationwide review of bile duct injuries in Sweden by Andren-Sandberg *et al.* [19], while 95% of patients did have operative cholangiograms, the surgeon proceeded with the ductal transection (and common duct injury) in 49% of cases without waiting for the cholangiogram films to return from being developed. There has been much debate regarding the need for routine cholangiography and whether this practice would in fact prevent ductal injuries [5, 24–29]. It is likely, however, that this practice would identify patients with ductal anomalies and assist in the immediate identification of injuries when they occurred. If a cholangiogram is performed, we feel that no ductal structure should be transected if there is any doubt regarding the anatomy until the films have been developed and reviewed.

Hermann [11] has noted that many surgeons use a fundus-first technique of gallbladder dissection when there is a significant degree of inflammation in the region of the triangle of Calot, but revert to an initial ductal dissection when the degree of inflammation is less. He suggests that the fundus-first technique is safer and ought to be used in all cases to minimize the risk of ductal injury. Other authors disagree [19], however, and do not feel that this technical point would reduce the number of injured bile ducts. In the series of bile duct injuries from Sweden [19], 48% of the gallbladders were excised starting at the fundus. Thus the fundus-first technique does not completely protect against ductal injury, and its adoption should not lead to a false sense of security in gallbladder dissection.

It remains a frustrating observation that many cases of bile duct injury occur when there is normal biliary anatomy and a minimally inflamed gallbladder. In fact, it is frequently noted by the operating surgeon that the initial cholecystectomy was 'an easy dissection' and he is, therefore, 'very surprised' that a ductal injury was subsequently discovered [5, 6, 18]. Lord Smith has called this a problem of the 'lazy' surgeon [3], particularly when no cholangiogram was performed or was performed but improperly interpreted. In this setting he feels that a failure in the surgical technique or a period of inattention by the operating surgeon makes a significant contribution to the iatrogenic injury.

After the introduction of laparoscopic cholecystectomy into clinical practice in the USA and Europe, some authors suggested that there might be an increased incidence of common duct injuries compared with the traditional open procedure [8]. One reason for this concern was the perceived impairment of visualization when operating via a laparoscope compared with a generous laparotomy incision. In practice, however, the 16-fold magnification provided by the laparoscope can allow excellent visualization of structures in the operative field. However, the standard laparoscopic port placement at the umbilicus, while optimal for imaging of the gallbladder and cystic duct, is not ideal for imaging of the common bile duct, which lies beneath and parallel to the scope. One suggestion [29] to overcome this problem has been the use of a laparoscope with a 30–45° viewing angle, which may improve visualization of the common duct in difficult cases.

With any new invasive procedure, the incidence of complications is generally highest during the early learning phase. Meyers *et al.* [30] in a collective review of 1 518 laparoscopic cholecystectomies performed in the USA suggested that this is the case for laparoscopic bile duct injuries. In this series, there was an overall incidence of common duct injuries of 0.5% for the 59 surgeons who participated in the study. However, the incidence of ductal injury was 2.2% during the first 13 laparoscopic cholecystectomies that any given surgeon performed, but subsequently fell to 0.1% after this point had been passed. This 'learning curve' factor seems to agree with older studies of bile duct injuries occurring during open cholecystectomy in the UK, where 85% of the ductal injuries in one large review [18] occurred when a junior surgical registrar was performing the open cholecystectomy without supervision by a consultant. It is still too early to determine if there will in fact be an increased incidence of ductal injury associated with laparoscopic cholecystectomy once the 'learning curve' period has passed.

Presentation

The majority of bile duct injuries are recognized at the time of cholecystectomy or in the immediate postoperative period. The presence of bile leakage from a drain site or from the wound itself, or the rapid onset of jaundice or a rising bilirubin provides clear evidence that a ductal injury has probably occurred. A small subset of patients with iatrogenic strictures present after a prolonged interval from the time of their original cholecystectomy; we have had a patient present 25 years after the time of her original cholecystectomy with a bile duct stricture. In these cases of late presentation, it is always difficult to determine the exact cause of the original injury, but this most probably involves an ischaemic insult to the duct. Northover *et al.* using resin dye castings, have demonstrated that the blood supply to the common duct arises from two lateral vessels at the 3 o'clock and 9 o'clock positions (with a third retroportal vessel in 32% of cases) [31]. If the duct is mobilized excessively or dissected free of its adjacent tissue, then this vascular supply may be jeopardized without any actual direct trauma to the duct. Because of the slow but marked response of the bile duct to ischaemia, there may be a prolonged interval between the original insult and the manifestations of the bile duct stricture.

Patients who present late after their bile duct injury may suffer recurrent bouts of cholangitis with or without right upper quadrant pain. They may have a normal bilirubin but the alkaline phosphatase is usually elevated. While these episodes may initially resolve with antibiotic treatment alone, most such patients will continue to have repeated attacks and risk the ultimate development of biliary cirrhosis [32, 33]. Additionally, these patients will frequently be found to have biliary sludge and primary intrahepatic calculi associated with stasis and infection, which may cause further obstruction and aggravate the situation. This syndrome of chronic or intermittent incomplete biliary obstruction is potentially most serious, and such patients should be aggressively investigated and considered for biliary bypass, if a stricture is present, to avoid the long-term complications [33, 34].

Evaluation of injury

With the exception of an injury that is detected during the course of a cholecystectomy, the nature of the bile duct injury should be evaluated thoroughly before the patient is taken to the operating theatre—the operating room itself is not the place to sort out these often difficult problems. The surgeon must have a clear understanding of the anatomy of the bile duct injury and have a specific plan for repair before commencing an operative procedure.

In the patient with a recent bile duct injury the initial work-up and evaluation should be directed towards correction of any metabolic deficits and the treatment of any ongoing sepsis. If there is a subdiaphragmatic or subhepatic abscess this should be drained, preferably by percutaneous puncture under computed tomography (CT) or ultrasound guidance [35] and the patient treated with directed antibiotic therapy. These problems should be well under control before any attempt at biliary bypass is undertaken. If an abscess is discovered at the time of exploration for biliary bypass, this may require drainage alone at the initial procedure to avoid creation of an anastomosis in the midst of a contaminated field and the risk of anastomotic breakdown or further stricture formation.

Most patients with a biliary stricture have undergone a previous invasive procedure and almost all will have infected bile. Therefore, these patients should have routine antibiotic prophylaxis before any invasive radiological or operative procedure. We prefer to use a ureidopenicillin and an aminoglycoside for antibiotic prophylaxis, since the most common organisms cultured from bile in these patients are *Enterococcus*, *E. coli*, and *Klebsiella*, which may not be adequately covered with single agent cephalosporin coverage. Routine bile cultures should be obtained at the time of radiological or operative bypass, since subsequent wound and abdominal infections are likely to be caused by the organisms present in the bile at the time of the operative procedure. The operative bile culture should, therefore, be used to direct antibiotic treatment should an infective complication develop in the postoperative period.

Laboratory and non-invasive radiographic studies are usually abnormal in the early period in the patient with a bile duct injury. The majority of patients with a ductal injury will have elevation of the serum alkaline phosphatase, and the serum bilirubin may be elevated if any degree of ductal obstruction is present or if a biliary fistula is incompletely drained. The gamma glutaml transpeptidase (GT) and serum transaminases may also be elevated, especially in cases of severe or prolonged obstruction, and in the presence of severe cholangitis.

Abdominal ultrasonography should probably be performed as the initial radiological study in all patients with a suspected bile duct injury. It may demonstrate dilated extrahepatic and intrahepatic ducts depending on the location and degree of obstruction present, but the ductal size may be normal in the presence of a biliary fistula or in cases of long-standing partial obstruction with biliary fibrosis or cirrhosis. Additionally, ultrasonography will demonstrate undrained fluid collections or abscesses in the perihepatic region. This imaging method may also be helpful in suggesting changes of cirrhosis, splenomegaly, and portal hypertension, which are particularly important considerations in planning an intervention in any such patient.

Biliary isotopic scanning (i.e., HIDA, PRIDA, etc.) may prove helpful in certain circumstances such as demonstrating that a biliary fistula is present, or if there is complete obstruction of the bile duct. If, however, there is only partial obstruction of the bile duct, then this imaging method may not demonstrate any abnormality. Furthermore, it will not provide the anatomical detail necessary to plan the operative bypass procedure. This non-invasive imaging method is probably most useful in the long-term follow-up of patients after biliary enteric anastomosis has been performed [36].

Other non-invasive imaging methods such as CT or magnetic resonance (MR) scanning are not routinely helpful after biliary injury, but may be helpful in certain situations. If the patient has had long standing but unequal biliary obstruction (i.e., total occlusion of one duct with partial occlusion of the opposite duct) or a vascular injury, there may be significant lobar fibrosis and atrophy with consequent hyperplasia of the opposite liver lobe (this more often occurs with right-sided atrophy and left-sided hyperplasia). This may be evident on direct cholangiography, but is often particularly well delineated on CT scanning (Fig. 22.2). Additionally, perihepatic fluid collections and abscesses can also be visualized and percutaneous drains placed if necessary.

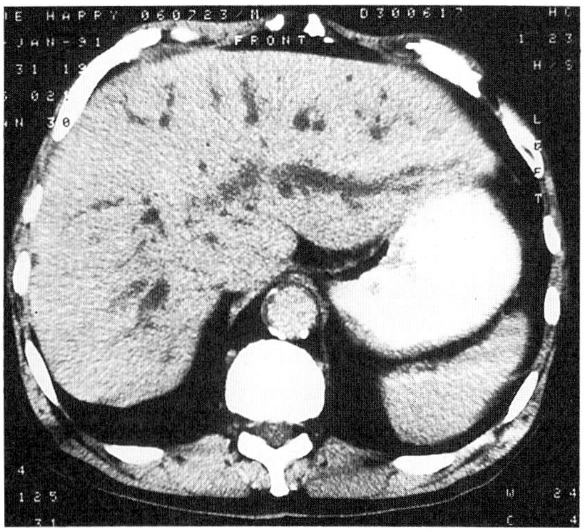

Fig. 22.2 CT scan showing atrophy/hyperplasia complex. Note increased size of left lobe of liver.

In almost all patients with biliary injuries, it is essential to define the proximal ductal anatomy cholangiographically. This can sometimes be performed via a common duct catheter if one was placed at a previous operation. However, in most cases it is necessary to perform either an endoscopic retrograde cholangiogram (ERCP) and/or a percutaneous transhepatic cholangiogram. The importance of the pre-operative definition of the injury cannot be overemphasized in this situation, because it is of critical importance to determine the precise anatomy of the sectoral hepatic ducts in relation to the site of the injury, in order to ensure that all ducts will be drained by the treatment method adopted. Moreover, the level of the injury will have a major impact both on the planned operative procedure and on the long-term prognosis. Cholangiography may additionally demonstrate intraductal gallstones which are frequently present after ductal injury and should be removed at the time of biliary bypass.

Several methods of classification of the biliary injury have been proposed, but the method almost universally adopted is that of Bismuth [21] shown in Fig. 22.3 and outlined below.

Type I. Injury to the lower common duct with at least 2 cm of intact common hepatic duct.

Type II. Injury to the upper common duct less than 2 cm from the level of the hepatic duct confluence.

Type III. Injury at the level of the right and left ductal confluence, with no remaining common hepatic duct stump.

Type IV. Injury involving the left and right hepatic ducts which are separated and non-communicating.

Type V. Injury involving a right-sided sectoral duct with or without injury to the left or common hepatic ducts.

This classification system is helpful in categorizing the type of ductal injury and is useful in planning the operative procedure and in determining the prognosis after repair (see below).

Occasionally, arteriography is helpful in patients with previous ductal injuries but is usually not necessary. Blumgart *et al.* [1] performed arteriography selectively, and found a coexisting vascular injury in over 50% of patients with ductal injuries as well as evidence of portal hypertension in 20%.

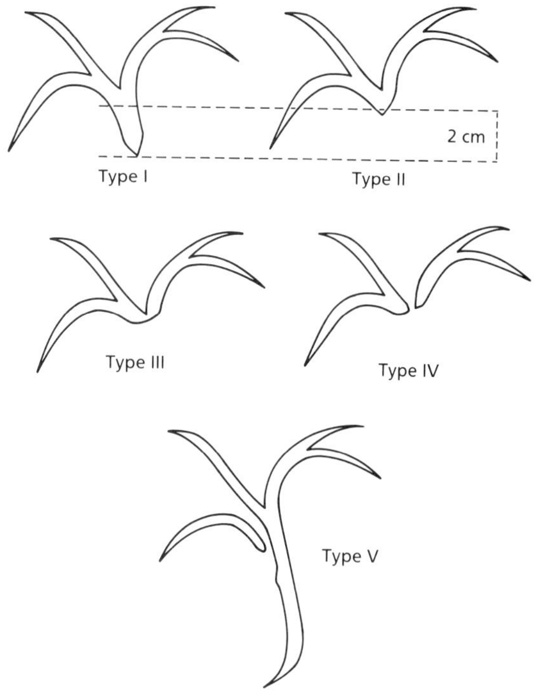

Fig. 22.3 Bismuth classification scheme, modified from drawings by Bismuth [21].

Patients with suspected cirrhosis and portal hypertension (15% in some series) [37, 38] pose a particularly difficult problem, which must be addressed before attempting a biliary procedure. In the past, authors have recommended a portosystemic shunt prior to the biliary bypass [37], but this procedure has a high mortality rate. In such patients it may be helpful to perform upper gastrointestinal endoscopy to assess and treat varices, and because this group has a very high mortality rate when undergoing biliary bypass, alternative, lesser procedures should be carefully considered.

Treatment

The course of action chosen in any patient with a bile duct injury depends in a large part on the nature of the injury and the time at which the injury is discovered. While many bile duct injuries are recognized at the time of the original procedure (usually cholecystectomy), others will not be identified until the postoperative period when either the patient becomes jaundiced, or develops signs of biliary peritonitis, or a bile leak from a drain site, or from the abdominal wound. With the increasing popularity of laparoscopic cholecystectomy, recognition of bile duct injuries may be delayed, since this procedure is frequently performed on an ambulatory basis and patients may not be in the hospital for a long enough period for the signs of this complication to develop. In our experience treating nine laparoscopic cholecystectomy injuries during the last 12 months, two were recognized at the time of operation, two presented before the patient's discharge, and in five cases the patient was readmitted with jaundice or biliary peritonitis.

When a bile duct injury is recognized during cholecystectomy, then a definitive procedure should usually be performed at that time. If a cholangiogram has not been obtained, then this should be performed as an initial step to delineate the injury and to define the remainder of the biliary anatomy. In the case of a laparoscopic cholecystectomy, this will almost always need conversion to an open laparotomy.

The specific method of repair for an injury discovered at the time of cholecystectomy will depend to a large extent on the nature of the injury. If the patient has received only a partial scissor transection, it may be possible to repair this by direct suture closure and T-tube drainage with the tube exiting from a different location (usually lower in the common bile duct) and one limb of the T-tube placed across the site of injury. This might occasionally be a successful method of repair for a complete transection; however, the approximated ends must be under no tension and the least amount of bile duct dissection necessary for the anastomosis should be performed, since this can lead to increased ischaemia of the bile duct and recurrent stricture formation [31, 39].

If there is a greater degree of tissue damage or an associated electrocautery injury, as is often the case, then primary bile duct repair is unlikely to be successful, and a hepaticojejunostomy should instead be considered. Previously, choledochoduodenostomy has been suggested as a treatment option in the patient with a bile duct injury. However, this method of repair has a higher rate of recurrent stricture formation [40], probably because of the constant bathing of the anastomosis with gastric and intestinal contents.

In the majority of patients with a bile duct injury, the procedure most likely to provide the best long-term results is a Roux-en-Y hepaticojejunostomy. For optimal results, the duct to intestinal anastomosis should be a direct mucosa to mucosa sutured anastomosis, which can be performed in the majority of patients [5]. Additionally, any fibrotic tissue at the site of the duct stricture should be excised and the anastomosis performed above this level to healthy, well perfused duct tissue.

The studies by Northover and Terblanche [31, 39, 41] suggest that if the duct was transected in its mid-portion, one explanation for failure of an anastomosis at this level might be the resulting ischaemia of the duct in this region. They reviewed their bile duct bypass results and found that patients who had a 'high' anastomosis (within 2 cm of the bile duct bifurcation in the liver) had a lower incidence of recurrent stricture formation compared with those who had a 'low' anastomosis (greater than 2 cm from the duct bifurcation). Thus, they suggest that even in patients who have a 'low' ductal injury, the likelihood of a successful repair is improved if the duct to intestinal anastomosis is performed at the bifurcation of the left and right ducts. We would caution that anastomoses performed at this level, when unsuccessful, make subsequent procedures which become necessary very difficult. We would instead suggest that the biliary–enteric anastomosis be performed to the upper common hepatic duct (within 2 cm of the bifurcation), if this is intact and without significant scar formation.

Some surgeons in the past have advocated loop hepaticojejunostomy with or without jejunojejunostomy for biliary diversion [42]. This procedure is less satisfactory than Roux-en-Y diversion because of the increased contamination at the anastomotic site [17]. We routinely make the Roux limb of jejunum at least 70 cm in length to prevent reflux of intestinal contents upwards to the level of the anastomosis. We prefer to perform the duct to intestinal anastomosis in an end to side fashion using a single layer of interrupted absorbable monofilament suture as previously described by Voyles *et al.* [43]. We place a small Silastic catheter across the anastomosis which is used for postoperative cholangiography and removed between 1–2 weeks postoperatively if there are no reasons to leave it in place.

In a small subset of patients, recurrent strictures or intrahepatic stones may develop after the biliary bypass has been performed. For this reason, we routinely create an access loop by tacking the distal 10 cm of the Roux limb to the anterior abdominal wall (Fig. 22.4) [44]. We mark the location of this site by placing a 2/0 stainless steel suture circumferentially at the distal end of the Roux limb, fixed flush with the parietal peritoneum. If needed, this limb can be accessed under fluoroscopic guidance at a later date and manipulations carried out with a combination of fluoroscopy and cholangioscopy, as needed. We have performed this access loop in over 75 patients (unpublished series) and have not encountered any complications from this addition to the standard Roux-en-Y hepaticojejunostomy. It adds little time to the operative procedure and we feel should be considered in any patient being treated for a bile duct stricture, particularly if the

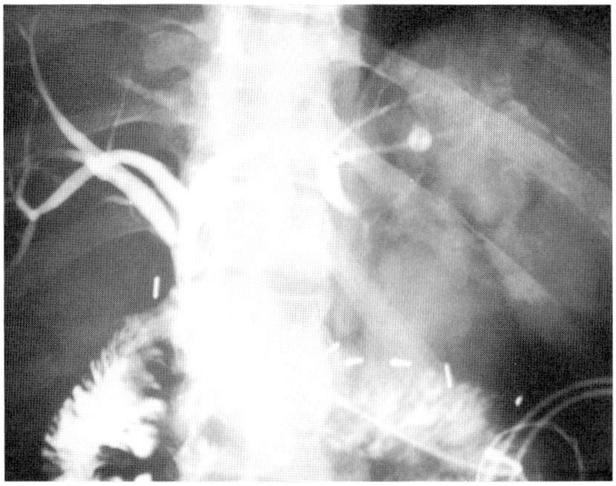

Fig. 22.4 Roux-en-Y hepaticojejunostomy with an access loop fixed to the anterior abdominal wall for radiological access.

repair has been difficult or if there are intrahepatic stones or strictures present.

The majority of patients with iatrogenic bile duct strictures should probably be treated with operative bypass with a Roux loop as their primary procedure. If these patients develop a second or even third recurrent stricture, these often can still be successfully repaired with hepaticojejunostomy [33]. In a recent review of 130 patients treated at the Hammersmith Hospital, London (unpublished data), 81 patients (62%) had undergone at least one previous attempt at bile duct bypass and 14 patients (18.5%) had 2 or more attempts. Eighty-three per cent of the latter group were successfully treated with an operative mucosa to mucosa bypass.

However, in some patients with Bismuth type IV strictures or cirrhosis and portal hypertension, attempts at operative bypass may be particularly hazardous. In this group, consideration should be given to balloon dilatation of the stricture, either by a transhepatic route or via an access loop, if one has been previously created [33, 35, 45]. In several such patients previously bypassed but without an access loop, we have operated solely to mark and tack the Roux loop to the abdominal wall for subsequent radiological dilatation of the bile duct stricture.

In the patient with a recurrent bile duct stricture in whom a repeat attempt at operative bypass has failed or seems unwise, consideration may be given to balloon dilatation [46] and possibly placement of a metal stent across the stricture [49]. The Gianturco self-expanding stents (Fig. 22.5) can be placed either endoscopically or radiologically [47, 48] via a transhepatic approach. These exert a steady continuous pressure at the site of the stricture and over 1–2 months will enlarge the stricture and subsequently maintain continuous outward pressure. The length of the stricture must be shorter than the length of the stent for this method of treatment to be successful and it must be possible to pass a guidewire across the stricture. For strictures that are longer than the Gianturco stent, it may be possible to place the longer Wallstent (Fig. 22.6), although these have less expanding force and are generally used for malignant strictures [49]. Both types of prosthesis

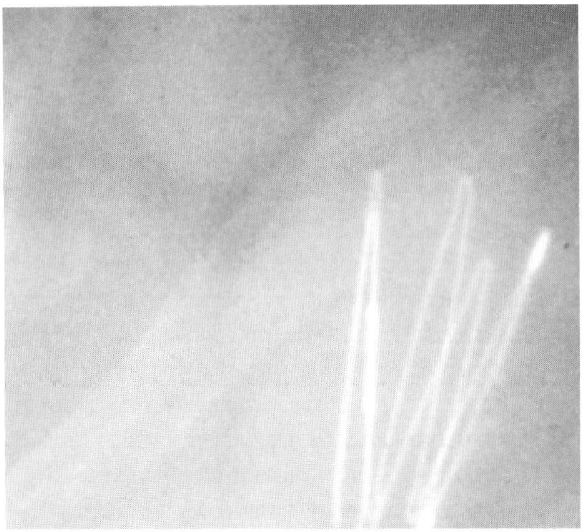

Fig. 22.5 The metal Gianturco stent, used in treatment of benign strictures felt not to be amenable to surgical bypass. The stent is shown fully expanded some days after insertion.

are expensive and have not been used for a long enough period to evaluate their long-term efficacy. Therefore, we recommend their consideration only in patients in whom it is felt that a operative bypass cannot be successfully performed or in whom the operative risk is judged too great.

In the past the mucosal graft technique has been advocated for use in high bile duct strictures where a direct sutured anastomosis was thought to be impossible [3, 18, 50]. However, this procedure is associated with a high rate of recurrent bile duct strictures (22% in Lord Smith's series) [51]. The left hepatic duct almost invariably has a long extra-hepatic course and can usually be isolated by lowering the hilar plate as described originally by Hepp and Couinaud [52]. Once the left duct has been isolated, by following the duct to the right, the right duct can likewise be dissected for a sufficient length for a direct sutured anastomosis in the majority of patients. In Blumgart's series, there were 20 patients who had previously undergone mucosal graft procedures at outside centres because their strictures were thought to be too high in location for a direct sutured bypass. Using the approach to the left duct as described above, a sutured Roux-en-Y hepaticojejunostomy was possible in 19 [1].

Results

In most series of iatrogenic bile duct injuries, approximately 85–90% of patients have undergone successful repair and remain asymptomatic with normal liver enzymes following biliary bypass [1, 2, 40, 42, 53]. In the 10–15% of patients who do develop a recurrent stricture, most can undergo a subsequent successful operative bypass with good long-term results [53]. In assessing these results, patients should probably be followed at least 3–5 years before concluding that their risk of recurrent stricture formation is mini-

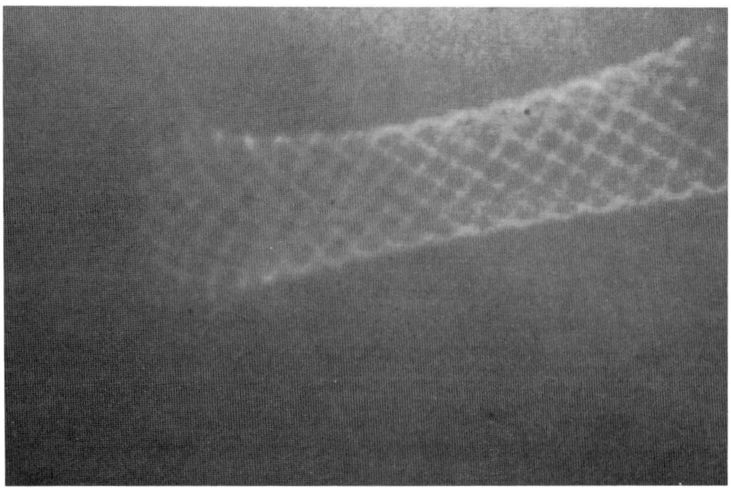

Fig. 22.6 Photograph of expanded Wallstent, used primarily for malignant strictures, but occasionally helpful for long benign strictures.

mal, although in one series 10% of patients with recurrent strictures presented more than 7 years after previous repair of an iatrogenic stricture [33].

Many factors influence the results of ductal repair following iatrogenic injury, including the nature and location of the injury, the time at which the injury is recognized (intraoperatively or postoperatively), coexisting abscess formation or sepsis, the presence of significant parenchymal disease, and the type of repair employed. Pitt *et al.* [40] performed a long-term retrospective study of 138 patients with bile duct injuries who were managed at their institution to determine factors which influenced recurrent stricture formation after bile duct repair. They found that results were significantly improved when a Roux-en-Y loop was employed for a sutured mucosa to mucosa anastomosis (compared with choledochoduodenostomy, simple loop choledochojejunostomy, etc.) and results were increasingly worsened by the number of previous attempts before referral to their centre. Additionally, younger patients (<30 years of age) had a better outcome than did older patients in this series [40]. Our own experience [1, 5] has shown that the higher the level of the injury (i.e., Bismuth type III and IV), the worse the results.

Primary end to end repair, with or without T-tube drainage, has been reported to be associated with a very high incidence of recurrent stricture formation, in some series up to 80% [10, 54]. The true results of this type of repair, however, are very difficult to determine with certainty, since those patients who have a successful repair may never come to further medical attention. It is probably true that this method of repair is associated with a high rate of recurrence unless there is only a clean limited injury with minimal adjacent tissue damage.

The issue of transanastomotic stenting following biliary bypass (and the length of time that this is necessary) has long been a controversial topic. Some surgeons feel that this is unnecessary [2, 5, 33] while other studies have suggested improved results when a transanastomotic tube was left in place for a prolonged period following stricture repair [12, 16, 40]. We prefer to leave a small transanastomotic tube in place after biliary bypass to obtain a postoperative cholangiogram, but do not feel that it is necessary to 'stent' the anastomosis.

The operative mortality rate after biliary–enteric anastomosis in most series is very low, usually below 5%. The greatest risk factor associated with this procedure appears to be the coexistence of cirrhosis and portal hypertension. In Blumgart's series [1], bile duct bypass in this setting was associated with a 36% mortality, while in patients without liver disease and portal hypertension who underwent bile duct bypass procedures the mortality was only 3.2%.

Besides recurrent stricture formation, most complications after biliary bypass are infective. In most series, this has meant a wound infection rate of 5–25% [1, 53], with a small incidence of subdiaphragmatic and subhepatic abscesses. Major complications are unusual and most frequently occur in patients with liver damage and portal hypertension [1].

Conclusions

Iatrogenic injury of the bile duct occurs almost exclusively during the course of cholecystectomy or common bile duct exploration, though more rarely with a variety of other upper abdominal procedures. Sometimes there may be contributing factors such as aberrant anatomy or marked local inflammation which obscures the true location of the common bile duct, but in the majority of cases this injury probably occurs because of inexperience of the operating surgeon or carelessness on his/her part. Thus, most bile duct injuries could be prevented with more care on the part of the operating surgeon and better supervision of the inexperienced surgeon, whether this involves a surgical trainee or an experienced surgeon learning laparoscopic cholecystectomy.

Many bile duct injuries are recognized at the time of cholecystectomy, during the course of the dissection, or in the early postoperative period. Any patient who deviates from the usual postoperative course after cholecystectomy (i.e., prolonged ileus, progressive distension, jaundice, bile drainage from wound or drain tract, etc.) should be monitored very closely and investigated for a bile duct injury. When a bile duct injury is discovered during the course of a cholecystectomy or in the early postoperative period, the repair performed will depend primarily on the injury sustained. Ductal transections with minimal adjacent tissue damage may be successfully treated with end to end repair and T-tube drainage. However, most ductal injuries will require Roux-en-Y hepaticojejunostomy for optimal results, and sometimes this procedure can be difficult since the bile duct is often not dilated.

In the patient who presents at a later time after the bile duct injury, patience is to be encouraged in the investigation and repair. Drainage of abscesses and fistulae with directed antibiotic treatment is critically important during the earliest phases of the management. Unless the patient has an undrained biliary fistula with peritonitis, it is unusual to have to operate urgently after a ductal injury. Instead it is preferable to define the bile duct injury fully by careful cholangiography and treat the patient conservatively during this early phase, if possible. This has the additional advantage of allowing ductal dilatation, making the subsequent bypass procedure easier to perform.

At the time of biliary stricture repair most patients can be treated with a sutured mucosa to mucosa Roux-en-Y hepaticojejunostomy. Even in the presence of scarring in the region of the porta from previous procedures, this can usually be performed using a left duct approach and tracing this to the right-sided ducts. We prefer to perform the duct to enteric anastomosis using interrupted absorbable monofilament suture and we routinely create an access loop in addition by tacking the distal 10 cm of the Roux loop to the anterior abdominal wall.

Eighty-five to 90% of patients with bile duct injuries can be successfully treated using this approach, and reoperation with repeat bypass will be successful in the majority of those who fail this initial bypass attempt. The likelihood of successful bypass decreases, however, with each successive bypass attempt, and repeated interventions should only be performed in specialist centres with a interest in such bile duct strictures.

Partial or complete biliary obstruction causes hepatic fibrosis and ultimately will lead to the development of biliary cirrhosis and portal hypertension. Biliary bypass in the setting of portal hypertension is particularly hazardous with reported operative mortality rates of over 30%. In this group of patients, non-operative measures such as percutaneous or endoscopic dilatation and stent placement may play a greater role, although the long-term place of such treatments has yet to be completely defined.

References

1 Blumgart LH, Kelley CJ, Benjamin IS. Benign bile duct stricture following cholecystectomy: critical factors in management. *Br J Surg* 1984;71:836–43.
2 Bismuth H, Franco D, Corlette MB *et al.* Long term results of Roux-en-Y hepaticojejunostomy. *Surg Gyn Obstet* 1978;146:161–7.
3 Smith R. Injuries of the bile ducts. In: Smith R, Sherlock S, eds. *Surgery of the Gallbladder and Bile Ducts*. London: Butterworth, 1981:361–81.
4 Johnston GW. Iatrogenic bile duct stricture: an avoidable surgical hazard? *Br J Surg* 1986;73:245–7.
5 Blumgart LH. Benign biliary strictures. In: Blumgart LH, ed. *Surgery of the Liver and Biliary Tract*, Vol 1. Edinburgh: Churchill Livingstone, 1988:721–52.
6 Garden OJ. Iatrogenic injury to the bile duct. *Br J Surg* 1991;78:1412–13.
7 Way LW. Bile duct injury during laparoscopic cholecystectomy. *Ann Surg* 1992;215:195.
8 Cameron JL, Gadacz TR. Laparoscopic surgery. *Ann Surg* 1991;213:1–2.
9 Smith R. Injuries to the common bile duct during laparoscopic cholecystectomy (letter). *Br Med J* 1991; 303:1475.
10 Andren-Sandberg A, Johansson S, Bengmark S. Accidental lesions of the bile duct at cholecystectomy: results of treatment. *Ann Surg* 1985;201:452–5.
11 Hermann RE. A plea for a safer technique of cholecystectomy. *Surgery* 1976;76:609–13.
12 Moossa AR, Block GE, Skinner DB. Reconstruction of high biliary tract strictures employing transhepatic intubation. *Surg Clin N Amer* 1976;56:73–81.
13 Mirrizzi PL. Sindrome del conducto hepatico (sindrome hepaticiano). *J Internat Chirurgie* 1948;8:731–4.
14 Aranha GV, Sontag SJ, Greenlee HB. Cholecystectomy in cirrhotic patients: a formidable operation. *Am J Surg* 1982;143:55–60.
15 Schwartz SI. Biliary tract surgery and cirrhosis: a critical combination. *Surgery* 1981;90:577–83.
16 Warren KW, McDonald WM. Facts and fiction regarding strictures of the extrahepatic bile ducts. *Ann Surg* 1964;159:996–1010.
17 Way LW, Bernhoft RA, Thomas MJ. Biliary stricture.

Surg Clin N Amer 1981;**61**:963–72.

18 Smith R. Obstructions of the bile duct. *Br J Surg* 1979;**66**:69–79.

19 Andren-Sandberg A, Alinder G, Bengmark S. Accidental lesions of the common bile duct at cholecystectomy: pre- and perioperative factors of importance. *Ann Surg* 1985;**201**:328–32.

20 Habib NA, Cox S, Salem R *et al.* Biliary surgery in three district general hospitals: factors contributing to mortality. *Br J Clin Pract* 1988;**42**:329–32.

21 Bismuth H. Postoperative strictures of the bile duct. In: Blumgart LH, ed. *The Biliary Tract*. Edinburgh: Churchill Livingstone, 1982:209–18.

22 Moossa AR, Mayer AD, Stabile B. Iatrogenic injury to the bile duct: who, how, where? *Arch Surg* 1990;**125**: 1028–31.

23 Phillips EH, Berci G, Carroll B *et al.* The importance of intraoperative cholangiography during laparoscopic cholecystectomy. *Am Surg* 1990;**56**:792–5.

24 Berci G, Sackier JM, Partlow MP. Routine or selected intraoperative cholangiography during laparoscopic cholecystectomy? *Am J Surg* 1991;**161**:355–60.

25 Scott-Coombes D, Thompson JN. Bile duct stones and laparoscopic cholecystectomy: selective intraoperative cholangiography is the best strategy. *Br Med J* 1991; **303**:1281–2.

26 Cuschieri A, Dubois F, Mouiel J *et al.* The European experience with laparoscopic cholecystectomy. *Am J Surg* 1991;**161**:385–7.

27 Peters JH, Ellison C, Innes JT *et al.* Safety and efficacy of laparoscopic cholecystectomy: a prospective analysis of 100 initial patients. *Ann Surg* 1991;**213**:3–12.

28 Blatner ME, Wittgen CM, Andrus CH *et al.* Cystic duct cholangiography during laparoscopic cholecystectomy. *Arch Surg* 1991;**126**:646–9.

29 Peters JH, Gibbons GD, Innes JT *et al.* Complications of laparoscopic cholecystectomy. *Surgery* 1991;**110**: 769–78.

30 Meyers WC, Branum GD, Farouk M *et al.* A prospective analysis of 1518 laparoscopic cholecystectomies. *NEJM* 1991;**324**:1073–8.

31 Northover JM, Terblanche J. A new look at the arterial supply of the bile duct in man and its surgical implications. *Br J Surg* 1979;**66**:379–84.

32 Lygidakis NJ, Carlet F. Structural and functional biliary changes secondary to extrahepatic biliary obstruction. *Endoscopy* 1989;**21**:321–3.

33 Pellegrini CA, Thomas MJ, Way LW. Recurrent biliary stricture: patterns of recurrence and outcome of surgical therapy. *Am J Surg* 1984;**147**:175–80.

34 Benjamin IS. Biliary tract obstruction. *Surg Gastroenterol* 1983;**2**:105–20.

35 Zuidema GD, Cameron JL, Sitzman JV *et al.* Percutaneous transhepatic management of complex biliary problems. *Ann Surg* 1983;**197**:584–93.

36 Collins PG, Gorey TF. Iatrogenic biliary stricture: presentation and management. *Br J Surg* 1986;**71**:980–2.

37 Sedgwick CE, Poulantzas JK, Kune GA. Management of portal hypertension secondary to bile duct strictures: review of 18 cases with splenorenal shunt. *Ann Surg* 1966;**163**:949–53.

38 Kelly CJ, Benjamin IS, Blumgart LH. Portal hypertension and post-cholecystectomy biliary strictures. *Dig Surg* 1986;**3**:292–6.

39 Terblanche J, Allison HF, Northover JM. An ischemic basis for biliary strictures. *Surgery* 1983;**94**:52–7.

40 Pitt HA, Miyamoto T, Parapatis SK *et al.* Factors influencing outcome in patients with postoperative biliary strictures. *Am J Surg* 1982;**144**:14–21.

41 Terblanche J, Worthley CS, Krige JE. High or low hepaticojejunostomy for bile duct strictures? *Surgery* 1990;**108**:828–34.

42 Braasch JW, Bolton JS, Rossi RL. A technique of biliary tract reconstruction with complete follow-up in 44 consecutive cases. *Ann Surg* 1981;**194**:635–8.

43 Voyles CR, Blumgart LH. A technique for the construction of high biliary–enteric anastomoses. *Surg Gyn Obstet* 1982;**154**:885–7.

44 Krige JE, Bornman PC, Harris-Jones EP *et al.* Modified hepaticojejunostomy for permanent biliary access. *Br J Surg* 1987;**74**:612–13.

45 Vogel SB, Howard RJ, Caridi J *et al.* Evaluation of percutaneous transhepatic balloon dilatation of benign biliary strictures in high-risk patients. *Am J Surg* 1985;**149**:73–9.

46 Mueller PR, van Sonnenberg E, Ferrucci JT *et al.* Biliary stricture dilatation: multicenter review of clinical management in 73 patients. *Radiology* 1986;**160**:17–22.

47 Coons HG. Self-expanding stainless steel biliary stents. *Radiology* 1989;**170**:979–83.

48 Uchida BT, Putnam JS, Rosch J. Modification of Gianturco expandable wire stents. *AJR* 1988;**150**: 1185–7.

49 Roddie ME, Adam A. Metallic stents in biliary disease. *Baillière's Clin Gastro*, 1992;6:341–54.

50 Wexler MJ, Smith R. Jejunal mucosal grafts: a sutureless technic for repair of high bile duct strictures. *Am J Surg* 1975;**129**:204–11.

51 Knight M, Smith R. Benign bile duct stricture following cholecystectomy: critical factors in management. *Br J Surg* 1985;**72**:327.

52 Hepp J, Couinaud C. L'abord et l'utilisation du canal hepatique gauche dans les reparations de la voie biliare principale. *Presse Med* 1956;**64**:947–8.

53 Gernst JF, Broniatowski SB, Vogt D *et al.* Benign biliary strictures: an analytic review. *Surgery* 1986;**99**:409–13.

54 Csendes A, Diaz JC, Burdiles P *et al.* Late results of immediate primary end to end repair in accidental section of the common bile duct. *Surg Gyn Obstet* 1989;**168**:125–30.

Chapter 23
Gallstone pathogenesis and management: prospects for the future

H.A. Pitt

For almost 100 years, open cholecystectomy was essentially the only treatment for gallbladder stones. Similarly, open choledochotomy was once the gold standard for the management of choledocholithiasis. During this same period from the late 19th through the first three-quarters of the 20th century, our knowledge of gallstone pathogenesis was limited and focussed on the gallbladder where most stones form. Over the past 25 years, however, both our understanding of gallstone formation and options for treatment have increased dramatically. During this relatively short period of time, the pendulum has swung toward non-operative therapy and back again to surgery with the introduction of laparoscopic cholecystectomy. This chapter will review the state-of-the-art in the 1990s and what to expect in the 21st century.

Gallbladder stones

The vast majority of gallstones can be classified into three types: cholesterol; black pigment; and brown pigment stones [1]. In Western countries approximately 75% of gallstones are cholesterol, 20% are black pigment and 5% are brown pigment stones [2]. A simple method to differentiate these three types is by the amount of cholesterol they contain (Fig. 23.1). Cholesterol gallstones contain approximately 85% cholesterol by weight whereas black pigment stones contain only 1–2% and brown pigment stones are composed of approximately 10–15% cholesterol. So-called 'mixed' stones, which contain 15–50% cholesterol, are rare, and this term is often misapplied to cholesterol stones most of which also contain some calcium bilirubinate and other calcium salts.

Multiple risk factors have been identified for gallstone formation (Table 23.1). These factors can be subclassified into general and specific factors. Major factors that probably impact on all three types of gallstones include age, gender, diet and genetics. All types of gallstones increase with age. Gallstones are rare in children and in some countries, such as Sweden and Chile, occur in 60% of adults reaching the 8th decade. In some African countries, on the other hand, gallstones are rare, even in elderly adults, suggesting that both diet and genetics are important risk factors. Cholesterol and black pigment stones occur more commonly in women, whereas brown pigment bile duct stones are found more often in men [2].

Pathogenesis

Approximately 25 years ago the focus of research on cholesterol gallstone pathogenesis switched from the gallbladder to the liver. As a result, the importance of the hepatic secretion of cholesterol saturated bile became the goal of most research in the 1970s. During this time, the role of hydroxyl-methyl-glutaryl-coenzyme A (HMG-CoA) reductase, 7 α-hydroxylase, and acyl-coenzyme A cholesterol transferase in cholesterol secretion, conversion to bile salts and cholesterol storage, respectively, were defined. Moreover, the relative increase or decrease in the activity of these hepatic enzymes in patients with gallstones was defined [1].

During the 1980s, some of the focus of research went back to the gallbladder. The importance of gallbladder hypomotility and the fact that this

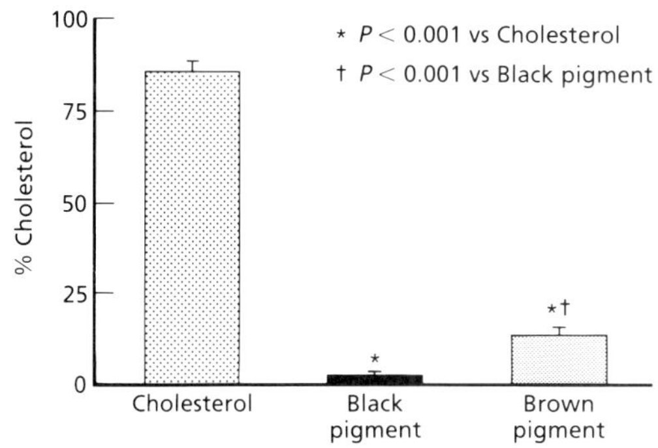

Fig. 23.1 The percent of cholesterol by dry weight in patients with cholesterol ($n = 46$), black pigment ($n = 17$) and brown pigment ($n = 5$) stones. From Kaufman *et al.* [2].

phenomenon precedes gallstone formation were appreciated [3]. In addition, the early increase in mucus secretion by the gallbladder was discovered. In recent years, the importance of nucleation of cholesterol crystals has been the object of much research. Nonmucin glycoproteins including immunoglobulins have emerged as important pro- and antinucleating agents [4]. In the future the relative importance of these nucleating factors should be clarified, and with this knowledge innovative pharmacological manipulations may become available to prevent gallstone formation.

The pace of research in pigment gallstone formation has been somewhat slower. Clearly, the precipitation of calcium with bilirubin is a key factor in both black and brown pigment stone formation. In addition, bacterial enzyme breakdown of free fatty acids and subsequent precipitation of calcium palmitate has been shown to be an important aspect of brown pigment gallstone formation (Fig. 23.2). However, little is known about the factors which regulate these processes. Moreover, research in this area has been inhibited by the lack of commercially available bilirubin diglucuronide [5]. One or both of these avenues are likely to open, however, leading to significant advances in our knowledge and ability to prevent and/or treat pigment stones.

Indications for treatment

A primary goal of research in gallstone pathogenesis is prevention of gallstone formation. Reasons to consider prevention include:
1 the considerable cost of treatment;
2 significant morbidity in terms of pain and anxiety;
3 disease complications such as acute cholecystitis and gallstone pancreatitis;
4 treatment complications such as bile duct injury;
5 mortality [5].
Although efforts to prevent gallstones will certainly have their own cost, prevention should be less expensive than current therapeutic measures and should decrease morbidity and mortality. Prevention may take the form of a drug, lifestyle changes or genetic manipulations.

Approximately two-thirds of patients who have gallstones are asymptomatic. Natural history studies suggest that these patients become symptomatic at a rate of only 1–3% per year [6, 7]. Moreover, computerized cost-effectiveness analyses suggest that expectant management has a better outcome. Therefore, most experts have recommended that asymptomatic patients should not undergo cholecystectomy. Similarly,

Table 23.1 Gallstone risk factors

General factors		Specific factors		
Major	Motility	Cholesterol	Black pigment	Brown pigment
Age	Sphincter dysfunction	Multiparity	Hemolytic disorders	Parasites
Gender	Diabetes	Estrogens	Cirrhosis	Biliary strictures
Diet	Vagotomy	Obesity	Ileal disorders	Biliary cysts
Genetics	Chagas disease	Cholesterol drugs	Parenteral nutrition	Sclerosing cholangitis

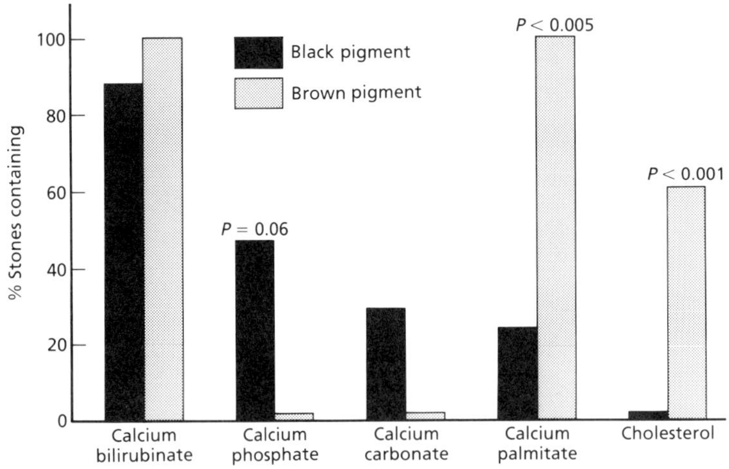

Fig. 23.2 Percentage of black (n = 17) and brown (n = 5) pigment stones containing individual calcium salts and cholesterol. Statistical analysis compares black and brown pigment stone groups. From Kaufman *et al.* [2].

non-operative options and laparoscopic cholecystectomy have not been recommended for asymptomatic patients. An argument can be made, however, for treating some particularly high-risk groups (Table 23.2). As newer treatments become more effective and less costly, these patients may be reasonable subjects for treatment even when stones are asymptomatic.

Most authorities agree that symptomatic patients should be treated. Natural history studies suggest that once symptoms have begun the chance of developing a complication is 6–8% per year [6–8]. As a result, most authorities recommend that symptomatic patients should be treated. However, the outcome of cholecystectomy is dependent upon the pre-operative symptoms. Patients with typical abdominal pain are more likely to be relieved of their symptoms by cholecystectomy than are those with non-specific symptoms such as dyspepsia, bloating, and belching [9, 10]. Even symptomatic patients may be subclassified into those with relatively mild symptoms with recent onset, as opposed to those with severe and/or long-standing symptoms. As treatment options become less invasive and more effective, a trend toward treatment of younger, healthier, less symptomatic patients will most likely be observed.

Table 23.2 High-risk gallstone patients

Native American women
Multiparous postpartum women
Obese—rapid weight loss
Diabetics with complications
Ileal disorders
Long-term parenteral nutrition

Non-operative treatment

During the 1980s, a wave of enthusiasm for non-operative therapies challenged open cholecystectomy which was celebrating its 100th anniversary. Many options, which have been detailed in this book, became available and were employed as alternatives to open cholecystectomy. In general, these alternatives can be put into three broad categories:

1 oral dissolution agents;
2 percutaneous contact techniques;
3 extracorporeal shock wave lithotripsy (ESWL).

Each of these options had one or more limitations, however, which inhibited its broad acceptance (Table 23.3). Moreover, with the introduction of laparoscopic cholecystectomy these shortcomings

Table 23.3 Limitations of non-operative treatments

Patient eligibility
Efficacy
Stone recurrence
Cost-effectiveness

became more pronounced when compared to the new less invasive surgical option.

Two oral bile acids, chenodeoxycholic acid (CDCA or cheno) and ursodeoxycholic acid (UDCA or urso), have been approved by the Food and Drug Administration in the USA. UDCA has supplanted CDCA because cheno has side-effects which include diarrhoea, abnormal liver chemistries and elevated low-density lipoprotein cholesterol levels. Ideal patients for urso treatment are thin women with small radiolucent gallstones in a gallbladder visualized by oral cholecystography (OCG). In addition, these stones float when observed by OCG or are of low density on computed tomography (CT) [11]. Unfortunately, these various criteria make only about 20% of the gallstone population eligible for oral dissolution agents [12]. Even with these restrictive criteria, only 60–70% of patients will have their gallstones dissolved in two years. In addition, up to 70% of patients whose stones have dissolved will develop recurrent stones over a 10-year period. Moreover, this non-operative therapy is expensive and, therefore, not very cost-effective.

Percutaneous contact techniques may approach the gallbladder transhepatically or transperitoneally. Gallstones may be dissolved with methyl tert-butyl ether (MTBE), disintegrated with a rotary lithotrite or extracted via the access tract with the aid of a scope or fluoroscopy. To be eligible for MTBE, gallstones should be composed largely of cholesterol and low density on CT scan. With these criteria, again, only about 20% of patients with gallstones are eligible for MTBE [11]. A large percentage of patients should be eligible for the other percutaneous techniques. However, the relative invasiveness, complications, residual debris, and high recurrence rates have limited the widespread acceptance of these percutaneous techniques [11]. Similarly, newer laparoscopic approaches which remove stones and leave the gallbladder will have problems with stone recurrence. In theory, subgroups of patients likely to have a low recurrence rate could be defined, but even in these patients cholecystectomy should be more cost-effective.

Extracorporeal shock wave lithotripsy (ESWL) was introduced as a treatment for gallstones in the mid-1980s. As with oral bile salts, only approximately 20% of gallstone patients are eligible for this therapy [12]. This group differs, however, in that ESWL has generally been applied to patients with one, two or three radiolucent stones from 5–30 mm in diameter in a functioning gallbladder. A National Biliary Lithotripsy study in the USA confirmed the need for oral bile salts to dissolve residual fragments, but stone clearance rates were lower than initially reported from Europe [13]. The reported stone recurrence rates have been somewhat lower for patients undergoing ESWL, perhaps because of a different patient population with fewer stones. As a result of problems with initial efficacy, the need for up to 2 years of oral bile acids, and stone recurrence, ESWL has not been shown to be cost-effective when compared with open cholecystectomy [14].

In addition to oral bile acids, percutaneous contact techniques and ESWL, a number of theoretical therapies may become available in the future (Table 23.4). These potential new treatments may be divided into four general categories:

1 gallbladder emptying;
2 lipid manipulations;

Table 23.4 Future therapies for cholelithiasis

Gallbladder emptying	Lipid manipulations	Protein manipulations	Calcium/bilirubin
Cholecystokinin	Oral bile acids	Aspirin	Calcium chelation
Motilin	Cholesterol lowering drugs	NSAIDS	Bilirubin alteration
Erythromycin	Fish oils	Mucolytic agents	Gallbladder absorption
Cisapride		Nonmucin glycoproteins	
		Immunoglobulins	

3 protein manipulations;
4 calcium/bilirubin alterations.
The fact that cholecystokinin (CCK), as a single daily injection, can prevent gallstone formation in animal models has been known since the early 1980s. In addition, CCK has been able to prevent biliary sludge in both prairie dogs and humans maintained on long-term total parenteral nutrition [15]. One of the problems to date with CCK is the need for parenteral administration. However, newer delivery systems including nasal, sublingual and/or transdermal are likely to become available in the not too distant future. Moreover, CCK-receptor agonists which can be given orally may be on the horizon.

In addition to CCK, motilin is another hormone which influences gallbladder and sphincter of Oddi motility [16]. Moreover, erythromycin, a motilin agonist, has been suggested as an upper gastrointestinal prokinetic agent that may improve gallbladder emptying. Although erythromycin is not as effective as CCK in emptying the gallbladder, ongoing research on other macrolide antibiotics as potential prokinetic agents may result in more effective oral gallbladder emptying agents. Cisapride is another prokinetic agent which is presently available and has been shown to prevent gallstone formation in an animal model [17]. This general strategy of preventing gallstone formation by regular gallbladder emptying may have application for:
1 postpartum women with asymptomatic stones or sludge;
2 obese patients undergoing rapid weight loss;
3 patients receiving parenteral nutrition.

While ursodeoxycholic acid is presently the most effective oral bile acid, newer designer bile acids may be developed as gallstone dissolution agents. Serum cholesterol lowering drugs have variable effects on biliary cholesterol. Ongoing development of these agents may result in drugs which inhibit biliary cholesterol secretion. Similarly, agents directed at HMG CoA reductase, the rate limiting enzyme for biliary cholesterol secretion, may be a fruitful avenue for research. In addition to bile salts, phospholipids help keep cholesterol in solution. Fish oil has been shown to prevent gallstone formation in animal models [18], and dietary manipulations of lipids, as has been recommended for atherosclerosis, may also prevent gallstone formation.

Another potentially fruitful avenue for future manipulations will be to influence the proteins in bile which affect the nucleation of cholesterol and, perhaps, calcium bilirubinate. Aspirin has been employed both experimentally and clinically because of its presumed effects on gallbladder mucus. Similarly, non-steroidal anti-inflammatory drugs (NSAIDs) have been shown to be effective in reducing intragallbladder pressure in patients with acute cholecystitis, and NSAIDs could play a role in preventing gallstone formation. In theory, mucolytic agents might be helpful for contact dissolution or, perhaps, as systemic drugs. In addition to mucin glycoproteins, nonmucin glycoproteins are thought to be potent pronucleators of cholesterol [19]. Once this puzzle has been solved and the source of these proteins has been identified, methods to eliminate or enhance these proteins may be possible. The fact that some pronucleating nonmucin glycoproteins are immunoglobulins may also mean that immunosuppressive agents may be helpful.

The fourth major area where ongoing research may lead to new methods for gallstone prevention and/or treatment is the precipitation of calcium and bilirubin. Calcium chelating agents have been used in combination with other drugs for contact dissolution. Oral calcium has also been shown to enhance pigment gallstone formation in the prairie dog model [20]. Thus, methods to influence calcium metabolism or dietary calcium may help prevent or treat gallstones. Efforts to impact on haem breakdown and, therefore, bilirubin excretion may also be undertaken. Whether light could be used to alter bilirubin is another interesting speculation. Finally, the gallbladder is very efficient at absorbing water and, therefore, at concentrating calcium and bilirubin. Thus, treatments directed at inhibition of gallbladder absorption may impact on pigment and cholesterol gallstone formation.

Operative therapy

For slightly more than 100 years, open cholecystectomy was the gold standard for the management of symptomatic cholelithiasis. As mentioned, during the 1980s, several non-operative treatments challenged this procedure, but the overall rate of cholecystectomy was relatively constant. With the introduction of laparoscopic cholecystectomy in the late 1980s dramatic changes have occurred. By 1992, two dramatic changes had occurred [21]. Firstly, within a few short years over 75% of the cholecystectomies were being performed laparoscopically (Fig. 23.3). Secondly, the overall rate of cholecystectomy had increased by approximately 25%. These trends are likely to continue in the near future. How long they will persist is a matter of considerable conjecture.

Presently, patients that are still undergoing open cholecystectomy include those with severe acute cholecystitis, significant bleeding disorders or bleeding problems during laparoscopy, prior major upper abdominal surgery, unusual anatomy, or other problems requiring open surgery. Even in patients with acute cholecystitis, the majority are now being performed with laparoscopic techniques [22]. As experience continues to be gained, the percentage of patients undergoing open cholecystectomy should continue to decrease to, perhaps, as low as 10% of the patients. Conversely, some of the problems with laparoscopic cholecystectomy such as bile duct, vascular and bowel injury should decrease, and the overall

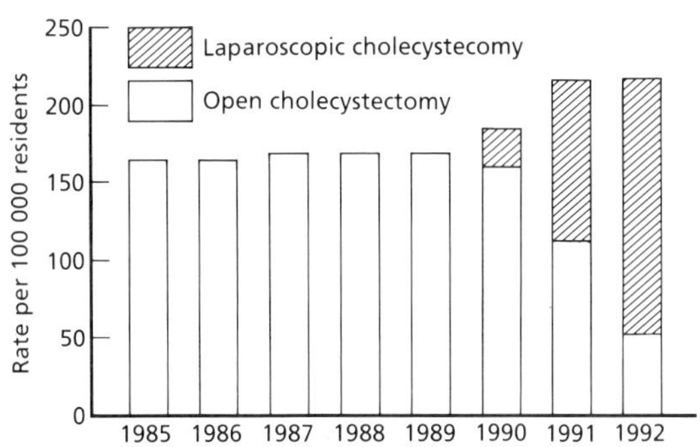

Fig. 23.3 Rates of open and laparoscopic cholecystectomy in the state of Maryland, USA, from 1985 through 1992. Increased overall rate of cholecystectomy in 1991 and 1992 is significant ($P < 0.01$). After Steiner *et al.* [21].

percentage of patients managed laparoscopically should increase to 90%.

A fascinating phenomenon that has accompanied the introduction of laparoscopic cholecystectomy has been an overall increase in the rate of cholecystectomy [21]. Patients undergoing the procedure laparoscopically have tended to be younger, healthier and to have less complicated gallstone disease. An initial cost-effective analysis, before this phenomenon was appreciated, suggested that laparoscopic cholecystectomy was likely to be less costly and more effective than open cholecystectomy [23]. Concerns have been raised, however, that overall costs will increase if more cholecystectomies are performed. On the other hand, the increased rate of cholecystectomy may be a transient phenomenon and/or may lower overall costs by reducing the severity of disease. For the near future, laparoscopic equipment and techniques should improve, and the popularity of this option should continue. Undoubtedly, newer therapies, some of which were outlined above, will ultimately challenge the predominance of laparoscopic cholecystectomy.

Bile duct stones

More than 85% of stones found in the bile ducts are secondary stones which formed in the gallbladder. The likelihood of finding stones in the bile ducts increases with age and varies from 5–20%. In the era of open cholecystectomy the incidence of associated choledocholithiasis was usually in the range of 10–15%. Interestingly, in recent years with the introduction of laparoscopic cholecystectomy common duct stones have been found in only 5–10% of patients [24]. This fact is another indication that patients are undergoing surgery earlier in the disease process. The minority of patients with choledocholithiasis have primary stones which form in the bile duct itself. In a small percentage of patients a gallbladder stone forms a nidus around which a larger primary brown pigment stone forms.

Pathogenesis

In Western countries brown pigment stones form

predominantly in the common bile duct. In East Asia brown pigment stones are found most often in the intrahepatic ducts. For these stones to form, two factors are required: bile stasis; and bacterial infection [1, 2]. In the West, sphincter of Oddi motility disorders including peri-Vaterian duodenal diverticula, which lower sphincter pressure and allow duodenal reflux, are the usual cause of stasis. In East Asia biliary parasites, including *Clonorchis sinensis* and *Ascaris lumbricoides*, or intrahepatic strictures may contribute to biliary stasis. Stasis facilitates bacterial infection and the accumulation of both mucin gel and bacterial cytoskeletins (Fig. 23.4). Bacterial hydrolases catalyze the hydrolysis of lipids that contain amide or ester linkages. Phospholipase A1 produces palmitic and stearic acid from phospholipids, glucuronidase produces unconjugated bilirubin from bilirubin glucuronides, and bile acid hydrolases produce free (unconjugated) from conjugated bile acids. These anions then precipitate with calcium.

Indications for treatment

As with stones in the gallbladder, the ultimate goal for choledocholithiasis is prevention. Because the vast majority of common duct stones start out in the gallbladder, new strategies that prevent gallbladder stone formation should also eliminate bile duct stones. With respect to prevention of primary brown pigment common duct stones, stasis and infection are known aetiological factors. Thus, biliary prokinetic agents and, perhaps, antibiotics might be considered in high-risk patients such as those with peri-Vaterian duodenal diverticula.

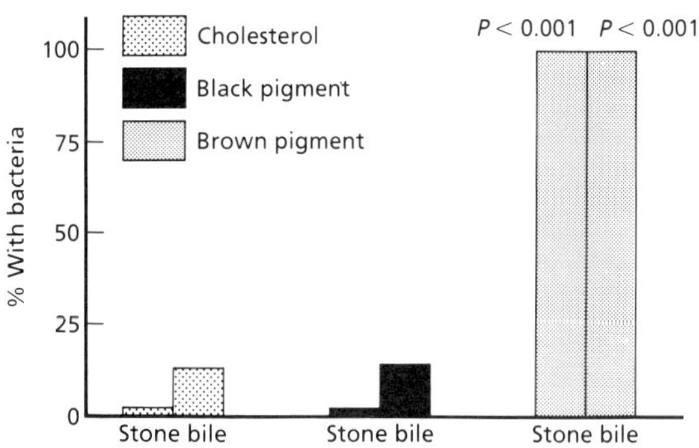

Fig. 23.4 Percentage of bacteria seen within stones by scanning electron microscopy or cultural from gallbladder or common duct bile. Statistical analysis compares brown pigment stones and bile with both cholesterol and black pigment stones and bile, respectively. From Kaufman *et al.* [2].

Most common duct stones cause symptoms and/or liver function test abnormalities. Biliary pain, jaundice, fever, and chills are the symptoms that occur when bile duct stones cause obstruction. However, some small common duct stones may be silent and are discovered only with routine operative cholangiography. When open cholecystectomy was being performed, most of these patients with silent common duct stones underwent open cholecystectomy and stone retrieval. Now that laparoscopic cholecystectomy is the norm, some authorities have questioned whether small, silent common duct stones should be removed endoscopically without a sphincterotomy or simply observed [25].

Common duct stones that are causing pain, jaundice, cholangitis or pancreatitis should all be treated. Debate continues about the type and timing of treatment, but endoscopists, radiologists and surgeons agree that symptomatic choledocholithiasis is an indication for therapeutic intervention. Pain and jaundice tend to be transient in these patients, and therapy can usually be undertaken between attacks. The spectrum of cholangitis is quite wide, and varies from mild, intermittent, low-grade fevers to life-threatening septic shock. Obviously, the urgency of treatment will vary with the severity of disease. Similarly, gallstone pancreatitis is usually mild but may be severe. Debate continues about the type and timing of intervention, but most experts agree that treatment should be completed during the initial hospitalization because the chance of recurrence within 6 weeks is very high [27, 28].

Non-operative treatment

Multiple options are presently available for the management of choledocholithiasis. Non-operative options include endoscopic, percutaneous, extracorporeal and pharmacological approaches.

Operative alternatives also include open choledochotomy, and open transduodenal exploration of the bile duct. In choosing from among these various options several factors should be considered (Table 23.5) [26]. Presently, the treatment of choice for patients with common duct stones who have previously undergone cholecystectomy is endoscopic sphincterotomy. Debate continues, however, about the proper management of patients with an intact gallbladder. Endoscopic sphincterotomy alone may be appropriate for very elderly patients with multiple medical problems. However, a strong argument can be made for removing the gallbladder in younger patients with both gallbladder and common duct stones.

Pre-operative endoscopic sphincterotomy followed by open cholecystectomy has not been shown to have any advantage over open cholecystectomy and common duct exploration [26]. Nevertheless, popular treatment algorithms now combine pre- or postoperative endoscopic sphincterotomy with laparoscopic cholecystectomy for patients with cholelithiasis and choledocholithiasis. In theory, however, the combination of the two less-invasive procedures might have a higher morbidity and mortality as well as cost when compared to open cholecystectomy and choledochotomy. Thus, future prospective, randomized trials should be designed to address this question. However, the design and conduct of such a study may be quite difficult because of physician and patient biases.

The second important question in deciding whether a non-operative or operative approach is appropriate is the severity of symptoms. This factor applies both to patients with cholangitis and to those with gallstone pancreatitis. A prospective randomized trial of endoscopic sphincterotomy versus open choledochotomy in patients with severe toxic cholangitis has favoured the non-operative approach [29]. Similarly, patients with severe gallstone pancreatitis may be helped by early endoscopic sphincterotomy [28, 30]. On the other hand, debate continues about the need for cholangiography in patients with mild gallstone pancreatitis whose episode has resolved in a few days. Most of these patients will be cured by laparoscopic cholecystectomy alone and will have passed their common duct stone within a few days after the attack. Even though good randomized trials have been performed on patients with gallstone pancreatitis, new studies are indicated now that laparoscopic cholecystectomy has become part of this equation.

Table 23.5 Questions to consider in managing choledocholithiasis

Is the gallbladder intact?
How severe are the symptoms?
What are the results of various options?
What is the local expertise?

Carefully selected patients with choledocholithiasis may also be candidates for percutaneous or extracorporeal management of bile duct stones. In patients with a retained stone after open choledochotomy who have a T-tube in place, percutaneous extraction is usually the treatment of choice. Similarly, in patients who have previously undergone a gastrectomy with a Billroth II reconstruction and a cholecystectomy, percutaneous transhepatic removal of common duct stones may be the best option. For patients with very large or inaccessible bile duct stones, ESWL may also be considered for adjuvant therapy. The overall success of ESWL in these difficult cases has been approximately 75% [31]. Electrohydraulic lithotripsy has also been used in conjunction with endoscopic and percutaneous approaches, and this technology should receive more widespread application in the future.

As with cholelithiasis, a long list of potential non-operative therapies for choledocholithiasis can be constructed (Table 23.6). Pharmacological methods to relax sphincter of Oddi baseline pressure should improve in the future. Presently, cholecystokinin and glucagon are available for parenteral administration. Motilin has been used experimentally, and the motilin agonist, erythromycin, which can be given orally, also affects sphincter of Oddi motility [32]. Again, research continues on more effective CCK and motilin agonists that can be administered orally. In the meantime both nifedipine and cisapride have been shown to affect sphincter of Oddi motility and are available as oral medications.

Table 23.6 Future therapies for choledocholithiasis

Sphincter emptying	Antibiotics	Lipid manipulations	Calcium/bilirubin
Cholecystokinin	Amoxicillin clavulanate	Oral bile acids	Calcium chelation
Motilin	Fluroquinolones	Cholesterol lowering drugs	Bilirubin alteration
Nifedipine	Trimethoprim/sulphamethoxazole	Fish oils	Cholerhesis
Cisapride		Ethyl proprionate	

Since brown pigment primary common duct stones contain 10–15% cholesterol by weight, newer oral bile acids and serum cholesterol lowering agents may be useful for patients who are at high-risk such as those with benign strictures or congenital cysts. In addition, alteration in dietary fats, such as an increase in fish oil and a decrease in butter fat, may be helpful for these patients. For contact dissolution, newer chemicals such as ethyl propionate may also be helpful in the future. The use of oral antibiotics whose spectrum covers the Gram-negative aerobes and anaerobes may be wise in selected high-risk patients. Among the antibiotics listed in Table 23.6, amoxicillin clavalanate may have the best spectrum for the organisms likely to play a role in brown pigment stone formation. Calcium chelating agents have already been used for contact dissolution. Effective methods to alter bilirubin production or composition would also impact on the prevention and treatment of common duct stones. Finally, effective choleretic agents should also help by diluting the calcium and bilirubin available for precipitation.

Operative therapy

Until the 1970s, open choledochotomy was essentially the only method for managing common duct stones. During the 1980s, endoscopic sphincterotomy was employed with increased frequency especially in patients who had previously undergone cholecystectomy. With the introduction of laparoscopic cholecystectomy even fewer patients have undergone open choledochotomy in the early 1990s. Early in the laparoscopic experience many groups employed pre-operative endoscopic cholangiography in patients suspected of having common duct stones and sphincterotomy when stones were found [24, 33]. Over a relatively few years, however, more patients are undergoing laparoscopic common bile duct exploration and more small stones are being allowed to pass spontaneously (Fig. 23.5).

Laparoscopic common duct exploration (LCDE) was developed in the early 1990s [34]. Laparoscopic cholangiography is an important first step in this process. In recent years laparoscopic ultrasound has also been employed by some groups to identify and localize common duct stones. In most reported series the majority of LCDEs have been performed via the cystic duct. Fogarty catheters, Dormia-type baskets and small, flexible choledochoscopes are used to identify and retrieve stones. Stones may also be flushed or

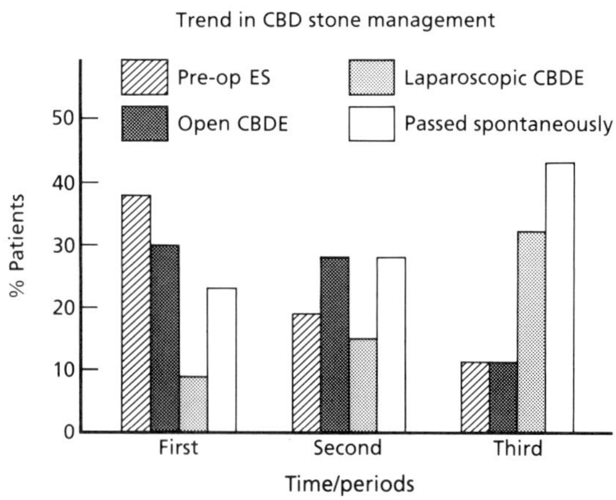

Fig. 23.5 Trend in common bile duct stone management over a 40 month period after the introduction of laparoscopic cholecystectomy. The first, second, and third time-periods are equal. ES = endoscopic sphincterotomy, CBDE, common bile duct exploration. After Voyles *et al.* [33].

pushed through the sphincter into the duodenum with the aid of glucagon to relax the sphincter. If the cystic duct cannot be sufficiently dilated to allow instrumentation, a small, longitudinal choledochotomy is made in a standard fashion. After the LCDE, a T-tube is inserted and sutured in place. In the reported series of LCDE, stones have been cleared in 85–95% of the cases. Undoubtedly, laparoscopic common duct exploration will become more popular in the years of come. Whether the majority of common duct stones encountered at laparoscopic cholecystectomy will eventually be managed laparoscopically remains a matter of debate. Moreover, more data are needed on the strategy of allowing small stones to pass spontaneously.

Conclusions

During the past 25 years, our knowledge of both gallstone pathogenesis and the clinical management of gallstone disease has advanced significantly. For cholesterol gallstones, cholesterol supersaturation of bile, gallbladder motility problems and nucleation of cholesterol crystals by biliary proteins are presently thought to be the key pathogenic mechanisms. For black pigment gallstones, the precipitation of calcium with bilirubin and other anions in bile is key, but the factors regulating this process are poorly understood. For brown pigment stones, biliary stasis and bacterial enzyme breakdown of free fatty acids are thought to be the important pathogenic elements. Clinical management of gallbladder stones has evolved dramatically from open cholecystectomy toward non-operative techniques to laparoscopic cholecystectomy. The treatment of choledocholithiasis is presently in a state of flux with trends away from open choledochotomy and pre-operative endoscopic sphincterotomy and toward laparoscopic common duct exploration and observation of small asymptomatic common duct stones.

During the next 25 years, the rapid pace of research advancements should continue, non-operative options will proliferate, and minimally invasive surgical techniques will improve. As a result, the pendulum is likely to continue to swing. Non-operative treatments presently on the horizon that will impact on gallbladder and/or sphincter of Oddi motility and manipulations of biliary lipids are likely to have moderate success. Manipulations of biliary proteins, calcium and bilirubin are farther in the future but may produce significant breakthroughs. High-risk populations with asymptomatic stones will be targets for these new non-operative therapies. Cost-effectiveness will continue to be an important issue for these new treatments. At the same time, endoscopy, interventional radiology and surgery will continue to evolve. New technologies may be costly, but these costs will be moderated by the overall pressures to reduce the cost of medical care.

Finally, the ultimate goal of primary prevention of gallstones will continue. Wellness issues related to prevention of obesity through diet, regular small meals and exercise that have been directed at atherosclerosis should also impact on the incidence of gallstones. The present initiative to define the human genome should also spill over to gallstone pathogenesis research. As a result, the genetic factors responsible for the disease should become clear, and larger subsets of high-risk populations should be defined. With this knowledge and the proliferation of gene therapy for other diseases, such as cancer, primary prevention should be an achievable goal in the 21st century.

References

1 Carey MC. Pathogenesis of gallstones. *Am J Surg* 1993;165:410–19.
2 Kaufman HS, Magnuson TH, Lillemoe KD, Frasca P, Pitt HA. The role of bacteria in gallbladder and common duct stone formation. *Ann Surg* 1989;209:584–92.
3 Doty JE, Pitt HA, Kuchenbecker SL, DenBesten L. Impaired gallbladder emptying prior to gallstone formation in the prairie dog. *Gastroenterology* 1983;85: 168–74.
4 Harvey PRC, Upadhya GA, Strasberg SM. Immunoglobulins as nucleating proteins in the gallbladder bile of patients with cholesterol gallstones. *J Biol Chem* 1991;266:13996–4003.
5 Hofmann AF. Primary and secondary prevention of gallstone disease: implications for patient management and research priorities. *Am J Surg* 1993;165:541–8.
6 Sama C, Labate AMM, Taroni F, Barbara L. Epidemiology and natural history of gallstone disease. *Semin Liver Dis* 1990;10:149–58.

7 Friedman GD. Natural history of asymptomatic and symptomatic gallstones. *Am J Surg* 1993;**165**:399–404.

8 Ransohoff DF, Gracie WA. Management of patients with symptomatic gallstones: a quantitative analysis. *Am J Med* 1990;**88**:154–60.

9 Gilliland TM, Traverso LW. Modern standards for comparison of cholecystectomy with alternative treatments for symptomatic cholelithiasis with emphasis on long term relief of symptoms. *Surg Gynecol Obstet* 1990;**170**:39–44.

10 Traverso LW. Clinical manifestations and impact of gallstone disease. *Am J Surg* 1993;**165**:405–9.

11 Schoenfield LJ, Marks JW. Oral and contact dissolution of gallstones. *Am J Surg* 1993;**165**:427–30.

12 Magnuson TH, Lillemoe KD, Pitt HA. How many Americans will be eligible for biliary lithotripsy? *Arch Surg* 1989;**124**:1195–1200.

13 Schoenfield LJ, Berci G, Carnovale RL *et al.* The effect of ursodiol on the efficacy and safety of extracorporeal shock wave lithotripsy of gallstones. The Dornier National Biliary Lithotripsy Study. *N Engl J Med* 1990;**323**:1239–45.

14 Bass EB, Steinberg EP, Pitt HA *et al.* Cost-effectiveness of extracorporeal shock wave lithotripsy vs. cholecystectomy for symptomatic gallstones. *Gastroenterology* 1991;**101**:1189–99.

15 Sitzmann JV, Pitt HA, Steinborn PA, Pasha ZR, Sanders RC. Cholecystokinin prevents parenteral nutrition-induced gallbladder sludge. *Surg Gynecol Obstet* 1990;**170**:25–31.

16 Muller EL, Grace PA, Conter RC, Roslyn JJ, Pitt HA. The influence of motilin and cholecystokinin on sphincter of Oddi and duodenal pressures in the prairie dog. *Am J Physiol* 1987;**253**:G679–83.

17 Xu Q, Shaffer EA. Cisapride improves gallbladder contractility and bile lipid composition in an animal model of gallstone disease. *Gastroenterology* 1993;**105**: 1184–91.

18 Magnuson TH, Lillemoe KD, High RC, Pitt HA. Fish oil prevents cholesterol crystal nucleation and gallstone formation. *Gastroenterology* 1989;**96**:625. (Abstract).

19 Lipsett PA, D'Souza MP, Kaufman HS *et al.* Differences in biliary nonmucin glycoproteins in patients with and without gallstones. *Gastroenterology* 1992;**102**:A319. (Abstract).

20 Magnuson TH, Lillemoe KD, Peoples GE, Pitt HA. Oral calcium promotes pigment gallstone formation. *J Surg Res* 1989;**46**:286–91.

21 Steiner C, Bass EB, Talamini MA, Pitt HA, Steinberg EP. Laparoscopic cholecystectomy in Maryland: trends in surgical rates and operative mortality. *N Engl J Med* 1994;**330**:403–8.

22 Zucker KA, Flowers JL, Bailey RW, Graham SM, Buell J, Imbembo AL. Laparoscopic management of acute cholecystitis. *Am J Surg* 1993;**165**:508–14.

23 Bass EB, Pitt HA, Lillemoe KD. Cost-effectiveness of laparoscopic cholecystectomy versus open cholecystectomy. *Am J Surg* 1993;**165**:466–73.

24 Lillemoe KD, Yeo CJ, Talamini MA, Wang BH, Pitt HA, Gadacz TR. Selective cholangiography: current role in laparoscopic cholecystectomy. *Ann Surg* 1992;**215**: 669–76.

25 Cotton PB. Endoscopic retrograde cholangiopancreatography and laparoscopic cholecystectomy. *Am J Surg* 1993;**165**:474–8.

26 Pitt HA. Role of open choledochotomy in the treatment of choledocholithiasis. *Am J Surg* 1993;**165**:483–6.

27 Pellegrini CA. Surgery for gallstone pancreatitis. *Am J Surg* 1993;**165**:515–18.

28 Carr-Locke DL. Role of endoscopy in gallstone pancreatitis. *Am J Surg* 1993;**165**:519–21.

29 Lai ES, Mok FPT, Tan ESY *et al.* Endoscopic biliary drainage for severe acute cholangitis. *N Engl J Med* 1993;**326**:1582–6.

30 Fan ST, Lai ECS, Mok FPT, Lo CM, Zheng SS, Wong J. Early treatment of acute biliary pancreatitis by endoscopic papillotomy. *N Engl J Med* 1993;**328**:228–32.

31 Moody FG. Lithotripsy in the treatment of biliary stones. *Am J Surg* 1993;**165**;479–82.

32 Kaufman HS, Ahrendt SA, Pitt HA, Lillemoe KD. The effect of erythromycin on motility of the duodenum, sphincter of Oddi gallbladder. *Surgery* 1993;**114**: 543–8.

33 Voyles CR, Sanders DS, Hogan RM. The evolution of common bile duct evaluation in laparoscopic cholecystectomy. *Ann Surg* 1994;**219**:744–52.

34 Petelin JB. Laparoscopic approach to common duct pathology. *Am J Surg* 1993;**165**:487–91.

Index

Page references to figures appear in *italic* type and those for tables appear in **bold** type.